T0181540

HANDBOOK OF DENTAL THERAPEUTICS

Dental practitioners require a comprehensive understanding of the drugs used in clinical practice in order to safely prescribe and manage medication use in and by their patients. *Handbook of Dental Therapeutics* provides practical education and advice regarding medications use in dentistry, with commentary tailored for dental students throughout their degree, and for dentists in professional practice.

This text draws together the latest recommendations for Australia and Aotearoa New Zealand, covering the common drugs that dental practitioners administer and prescribe, perioperative management considerations, oral adverse effects and drug safety. Dedicated chapters on how therapeutics affect children, pregnant and breastfeeding women, and elderly patients enable readers to safely prescribe and administer medications across the lifespan of their patients.

The text is concisely written and is a practical guide that includes dosage recommendations and tips for drug use in patient care. Diagrams, graphs and tables summarise complex information to ensure readers have readily accessible information on the drugs most commonly used in dentistry.

Handbook of Dental Therapeutics is an essential text that equips dental students and practitioners with succinct and clinically relevant information about all aspects of drugs in dentistry.

Leanne Teoh is a Senior Lecturer in Dental Therapeutics at The University of Melbourne, as well as a practising dentist and registered pharmacist.

Geraldine Moses AM is Consultant Pharmacist to the Australian Dental Association and Adjunct Associate Professor in the Schools of Pharmacy at The University of Queensland and Queensland University of Technology, and the Dental School at The University of Western Australia.

Michael McCullough is Professor in Oral Medicine at the Melbourne Dental School at The University of Melbourne.

Cambridge University Press acknowledges the Australian Aboriginal and Torres Strait Islander peoples of this nation. We acknowledge the traditional custodians of the lands on which our company is located and where we conduct our business. We pay our respects to ancestors and Elders, past and present. Cambridge University Press is committed to honouring Australian Aboriginal and Torres Strait Islander peoples' unique cultural and spiritual relationships to the land, waters and seas and their rich contribution to society.

Cambridge University Press acknowledges the Māori people as *tangata whenua* of Aotearoa New Zealand. We pay our respects to the First Nation Elders of New Zealand, past, present and emerging.

HANDBOOK OF DENTAL THERAPEUTICS

Leanne Teoh

Geraldine Moses

Michael McCullough

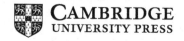

CAMBRIDGE
UNIVERSITY PRESS

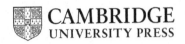

Shaftesbury Road, Cambridge CB2 8EA, United Kingdom

One Liberty Plaza, 20th Floor, New York, NY 10006, USA

477 Williamstown Road, Port Melbourne, VIC 3207, Australia

314–321, 3rd Floor, Plot 3, Splendor Forum, Jasola District Centre, New Delhi – 110025, India

103 Penang Road, #05–06/07, Visioncrest Commercial, Singapore 238467

Cambridge University Press is part of Cambridge University Press & Assessment,
a department of the University of Cambridge.

We share the University's mission to contribute to society through the pursuit of
education, learning and research at the highest international levels of excellence.

www.cambridge.org
Information on this title: www.cambridge.org/highereducation/isbn/9781009060059

© Cambridge University Press & Assessment 2024

This publication is copyright. Subject to statutory exception and to the provisions
of relevant collective licensing agreements, no reproduction of any part may take
place without the written permission of Cambridge University Press & Assessment.

First published 2024

Cover designed by Tanya De Silva
Typeset by Lumina Datamatics Ltd

A catalogue record for this publication is available from the British Library

A catalogue record for this book is available from the National Library of Australia

ISBN 978-1-009-06005-9 Paperback

Additional resources for this publication at www.cambridge.org/highereducation/
isbn/9781009060059/resources

Reproduction and communication for educational purposes
The Australian *Copyright Act 1968* (the Act) allows a maximum of one chapter or 10%
of the pages of this work, whichever is the greater, to be reproduced and/or communicated
by any educational institution for its educational purposes provided that the educational
institution (or the body that administers it) has given a remuneration notice to Copyright
Agency Limited (CAL) under the Act.

For details of the CAL licence for educational institutions contact:

Copyright Agency Limited
Level 12, 66 Goulburn Street
Sydney NSW 2000
Telephone: (02) 9394 7600
Facsimile: (02) 9394 7601
E-mail: memberservices@copyright.com.au

Cambridge University Press & Assessment has no responsibility for the persistence
or accuracy of URLs for external or third-party internet websites referred to in this
publication and does not guarantee that any content on such websites is, or will
remain, accurate or appropriate.

....

Every effort has been made in preparing this book to provide accurate and up-to-date
information which is in accord with accepted standards and practice at the time of publication.
Although case histories are drawn from actual cases, every effort has been made to disguise the
identities of the individuals involved. Nevertheless, the authors, editors and publishers can make
no warranties that the information contained herein is totally free from error, not least because
clinical standards are constantly changing through research and regulation. The authors, editors
and publishers therefore disclaim all liability for direct or consequential damages resulting from
the use of material contained in this book. Readers are strongly advised to pay careful attention
to information provided by the manufacturer of any drugs or equipment that they plan to use.

CONTENTS

ABOUT THE AUTHORS

Dr Leanne Teoh is both a practising dentist and registered pharmacist. At The University of Melbourne, she holds the position of Senior Lecturer in Dental Therapeutics at the Melbourne Dental School and coordinates the Dental Therapeutics program for the Doctor of Dental Surgery and Bachelor of Oral Health courses. She has published over 30 peer-reviewed articles on medicine use in dentistry, and her main research interest is dental prescribing, with a focus on antibiotic and opioid stewardship. She was a member of the Expert Group for the Australian *Therapeutic Guidelines Oral and Dental (Version 2)* and is on the Editorial Board for the journal *BMC Oral Health*. As an invited speaker, Dr Teoh has presented both locally and internationally in various forums, including the Australian Therapeutic Goods Administration, FDI World Dental Federation and the International Association for Dental Research. She continues to provide educational lectures, webinars and podcasts for various health professional groups around Australia. She also maintains clinical work in private practice dentistry.

Adjunct Associate Professor Geraldine Moses AM is a consultant clinical pharmacist with an extensive background in medicines information and education. Since 2013, Dr Moses has provided the drug information and advisory service called 'Pharma Advice' for the Australian Dental Association. She has published over 30 peer-reviewed journal articles and continues to write regular articles, and present webinars and podcasts for pharmacy and dental organisations throughout Australia and Aotearoa New Zealand. Dr Moses maintains her clinical expertise working part-time at the Mater Public Hospital in Brisbane. She also holds the position of Adjunct Associate Professor in the Schools of Pharmacy at The University of Queensland and Queensland University of Technology and in the Dental School at The University of Western Australia. She was a member of the Expert Group for the Australian *Therapeutic Guidelines Oral and Dental (Version 3)* and has been appointed to the writing group for Version 4. She also consults to various organisations such as the Department of Veterans Affairs, the New Zealand Dental Association and the Australian Commission for Safety and Quality in Healthcare. In 2019, Dr Moses was made a Member of the Order of Australia (AM) for her significant service to medicine and the community as a pharmacist.

Professor Michael McCullough is Professor in Oral Medicine at the Melbourne Dental School at The University of Melbourne and convenes the oral medicine program for the Doctor of Clinical Dentistry. Professor McCullough has published over 210 articles in peer-reviewed scientific journals and was on the Expert Panel for the first two editions of the *Therapeutic Guidelines Oral and Dental*. He was an editor on the comprehensive textbook *Contemporary Oral Medicine*, authoring several chapters. He is an Oral Medicine Clinical Consultant to the Royal Dental Hospital of Melbourne and the Royal Melbourne Hospital.

PREFACE

'Dental therapeutics' is the term used to describe the use of medicines and other pharmacologically active substances for the treatment of dental conditions. Although medicines are usually considered second-line to dental interventions, therapeutics remains a significant and sometimes critical part of managing dental patients. As a result, a comprehensive understanding of the drugs used in dentistry is required for safe and appropriate advising, prescribing, administering, and supplying medicines in dental practice.

While the fundamental principles of therapeutics have not changed much in recent decades, increasing availability of new drug classes, a greater focus on managing drugs in the perioperative setting, and with more patients taking a wider variety of medicines, drug knowledge in dentistry is more important and relevant than ever. Our intention is that the *Handbook of Dental Therapeutics* provides a concise and all-inclusive reference regarding all practical aspects of drugs encountered in dental practice today.

Our book starts with a discussion of the key therapeutic principles of pharmacology and toxicology, as these concepts form the basis of every aspect of appropriate and safe medication use in any health-related field. Chapter 2 outlines the steps that govern appropriate and rational prescribing, including prescribing competencies and the factors that contribute and prevent medication errors. This leads into a description of legislation governing prescribing practices in Australia and Aotearoa New Zealand, as well as how this relates to off-label prescribing.

Our book draws together information regarding the most common drugs that dentists administer and prescribe—including local anaesthetics, antimicrobials, drugs for pain management and anxiolytics—and focuses on the relevant use of drugs in dentistry. Prescribing and other considerations for particular patient groups, such as children, the elderly, pregnant and breastfeeding women, are also presented, including concise but detailed information on oral adverse effects and drug safety.

Key chapters target dental practice including drugs that contribute to bleeding risk and medication-associated osteonecrosis of the jaw, both of which are continually evolving issues. Perioperative management considerations are presented in its own chapter to assist dental practitioners with the management of patients taking medications for common conditions, such as diabetes, and those taking immunosuppressants or medicines for cancer therapy.

It is our hope that the *Handbook of Dental Therapeutics* will provide a succinct, practical and readily accessible source of drug information for both dental students and clinicians in professional practice. This comprehensive but concise handbook is the ultimate reference to carry a dental practitioner from their university course through to working life.

Dr Leanne Teoh
Adjunct Associate Professor Geraldine Moses
Professor Michael McCullough

ACKNOWLEDGEMENTS

This book is the fulfillment of our dream to create a comprehensive, succinct and practical guide to the use of drugs in dentistry for dental practitioners and students in their studies at university and chairside with patients. Our robust and fruitful collaboration, brilliantly led by Leanne, has culminated in what we believe to be a very worthwhile resource, ultimately aiding the safe treatment of dental patients.

We are very grateful for the support of Cambridge University Press and their belief in this book. We particularly thank Emily Baxter and Lucy Russell for their patience and guidance throughout the writing process.

Finally, we are indebted to each of our families for their love and support. We fully appreciate their understanding of our passion for this book and their patience over the two years that we have dedicated to its completion.

The authors and Cambridge University Press would like to thank the following for permission to reproduce material in this book.

Figures 1.3, **9.2** and **9.3**: These figures were published in Ritter J, Flower R, Henderson G, Loke YK, MacEwan D, Rang HP. *Rang and Dale's Pharmacology*. 9th edition. Elsevier; 2020. Copyright Elsevier 2020. Reproduced under STM licence.

Figure 1.4: This figure was published in Rang HP, Dale MM, Ritter J, Flower RJ, Henderson G. *Rang and Dale's Pharmacology*. 7th edition. Elsevier; 2012. Copyright Elsevier 2012. Reproduced under STM licence.

Figure 1.5: This figure was published in Brenner GM, Stevens CW. *Pharmacology*. 4th edition. Elsevier; 2018. Copyright Elsevier 2018. Reproduced under STM licence.

Figure 1.6: From Dolton MJ, Roufogalis BD, McLachlan AJ. Fruit juices as perpetrators of drug interactions: the role of organic anion-transporting polypeptides. *Clinical Pharmacology & Therapeutics*. 2012;92(5):622–630. doi:10.1038/clpt.2012.159. © 2012 John Wiley & Sons Ltd. Reproduced with permission from Wiley.

Figure 2.1: From Gazarian M, Kelly M, McPhee JR et al. Off-label use of medicines: consensus recommendations for evaluating appropriateness. *Medical Journal Australia*. 2006;185(10):544–548. © 2006 AMPCo Pty Ltd. Reproduced with permission from Wiley.

Figure 5.1: This figure was published in Brenner GM, Stevens CW. *Pharmacology*. 5th edition. Elsevier; 2018. Copyright Elsevier 2018. Reproduced under STM licence.

Figure 5.3: Nephron diagram © Getty Images/Stocktrek Images.

Figure 9.1: From Fortier K, Shroff D, Reebye UN. Review: An overview and analysis of novel oral anticoagulants and their dental implications. *Gerodontology*. 2018;35(2):78–86. © 2018 John Wiley & Sons A/S and The Gerodontology Association. Reproduced with permission from Wiley.

Figure 10.1: Reprinted from Baron R, Ferrari S, Russell RG. Denosumab and bisphosphonates: Different mechanisms of action and effects. *Bone*. 2011;48(4):677–692, copyright 2011, with permission from Elsevier.

Figure 11.1: © Australian and New Zealand College of Anaesthetists 2021. Reproduced with permission from the Australian and New Zealand College of Anaesthetists (ANZCA).

ANZCA is the organisation leading a collaboration of medical colleges and societies in the development of a Diploma in Perioperative Medicine.

Figure 12.1: From McAlinden J, Masson C. Keep within sight and reach: teaching paediatric prescribing. *Prescriber*. 2021 Oct;32(10):28–33. doi/10.1002/psb.1948. © 2021 John Wiley & Sons Ltd. Reproduced with permission from Wiley.

Table 3.2: Reproduced under Creative Commons Attribution-NonCommercial 4.0 International (CC BY-NC 4.0), https://creativecommons.org/licenses/by-nc/4.0/.

Table 4.1: From Teoh L, Stewart K, Marino R, McCullough M. Antibiotic resistance and relevance to general dental practice in Australia. *Aust Dent J*. 2018;63(4):414–421. © 2018 Australian Dental Association. Reproduced with permission from Wiley.

Table 5.8: This table was published in Ritter J, Flower R, Henderson G, Loke YK, MacEwan D, Rang HP. *Rang and Dale's Pharmacology*. 9th edition. Elsevier; 2020. Copyright Elsevier 2020. Reproduced under STM licence.

Tables 9.4 and **9.5**: From Teoh L, Moses G, McCullough MJ. A review of drugs that contribute to bleeding risk in general dental practice. *Aust Dent J*. 2020;65(2):118–130. © 2020 Australian Dental Association. Reproduced with permission from Wiley.

Table 10.3: Reprinted from Nicolatou-Galitis O, Schiodt M, Mendes RA et al. Medication-related osteonecrosis of the jaw: Definition and best practice for prevention, diagnosis, and treatment. *Oral Surg Oral Med Oral Pathol Oral Radiol*. 2019;127(2):117–135, copyright 2019, with permission from Elsevier.

Table 11.3: From Scottish Dental Clinical Effectiveness Programme. *Management of Dental Patients Taking Anticoagulants or Antiplatelet Drugs*. 2nd edition. 2022. https://www.sdcep.org.uk/published-guidance/anticoagulants-and-antiplatelets/. © Scottish Dental Clinical Effectiveness Programme (SDCEP), NHS Education for Scotland.

Table 11.8: Adapted with permission from Corticosteroids: considerations for oral and dental procedures. In Oral and Dental Expert Group. *Therapeutic Guidelines Oral and Dental (Version 3)*. Therapeutic Guidelines Pty Ltd; 2019. Accessed June 23, 2023. https://www.tg.org.au.

Table 12.2: © 2019 Australian Medicines Handbook Pty Ltd. This content was originally published in the *Australian Medicines Handbook* (AMH).

Table 14.1: From Therapeutic Goods Administration. *Prescribing medicines in pregnancy database*. 2022. https://www.tga.gov.au/products/medicines/find-information-about-medicine/prescribing-medicines-pregnancy-database, used by permission of the Australian Government. Copyright notice: © Commonwealth of Australia. This work is copyright. You may download, display, print and reproduce the whole or part of this work in unaltered form for your own personal use or, if you are part of an organisation, for internal use within your organisation, but only if you or your organisation do not use the reproduction for any commercial purpose and retain this copyright notice and all disclaimer notices as part of that reproduction. Apart from rights to use as permitted under the *Copyright Act 1968* or allowed by this copyright notice, all other rights are reserved and you are not allowed to reproduce the whole or any part of this work in any way (electronic or otherwise) without first being given specific written permission from the Commonwealth to do so. Requests and inquiries concerning reproduction and rights are to be sent to the TGA Copyright Officer, Therapeutic Goods Administration,

PO Box 100, Woden ACT 2606 or emailed to tga.copyright@tga.gov.au. Disclaimer: The Australian categorisation system and database for prescribing medicines in pregnancy have been developed by medical and scientific experts based on available evidence of risks associated with taking particular medicines while pregnant. This information is presented for the use of health professionals prescribing medicines to pregnant women, rather than for the general public to use. It is general in nature and is not presented as medical advice to health professionals or the public. It is not intended to be used as a substitute for a health professional's advice.

Tables 15.1–15.8: From Teoh L, Moses G, McCullough MJ. A review and guide to drug-associated oral adverse effects—Dental, salivary and neurosensory reactions. Part 1. *J Oral Pathol Med.* 2019;48(7):626–636. © 2019 John Wiley & Sons A/S. Reproduced with permission from Wiley.

Tables 15.9–15.15: From Teoh L, Moses G, McCullough MJ. A review and guide to drug-associated oral adverse effects—Oral mucosal and lichenoid reactions. Part 2. *J Oral Pathol Med.* 2019;48(7):637–646. © 2019 John Wiley & Sons A/S. Reproduced with permission from Wiley.

Extracts from *The Poisons Standard* February 2022 and *Therapeutic Goods (Poisons Standard—February 2023) Instrument 2023*: Sourced from the Federal Register of Legislation and reproduced under Creative Commons Attribution 4.0 International (CC BY 4.0). For the latest information on Australian Government law please go to https://www.legislation.gov.au.

Every effort has been made to trace and acknowledge copyright. The publisher apologises for any accidental infringement and welcomes information that would redress this situation.

BASIC CONCEPTS IN PHARMACOLOGY AND THERAPEUTICS

1

KEY POINTS

- Drugs and pharmacology are relevant to dentistry, not only in what is prescribed but also in how the patients' medicines impact on oral health, dental diagnosis and procedures.
- Fundamental concepts of pharmacology are important for understanding appropriate management of drugs in dentistry.
- Drug interactions are increasingly relevant in dentistry as they are an important yet often-ignored source of adverse drug events.

1.1 Introduction

Drugs are a part of everyday life and may be defined as 'any pharmacologically active substance intended for use in the diagnosis, cure, mitigation, treatment, or prevention of disease' (1). Whether a drug is a conventional medicine, a herbal remedy, or the caffeine in your coffee, drugs are an integral part of human existence and have been since ancient times. Drugs may be synthetic in origin or naturally derived from plants, animals, or biotechnology. A 'medicine' is a pharmaceutical product containing one or more pharmacologically active substances in a formulation administered for a therapeutic purpose.

1.2 Role of drugs in dentistry

In clinical practice, dentists interact with drugs and medicines in four main ways. These interactions are with the patient's own medicines, with the medicines used during a procedure, the medicines used in the practice for medical emergencies, and the medicines prescribed for patients for use after a consultation or procedure. Although dental practitioners do not prescribe medicines very often, with tertiary level education about drugs and broad prescribing privileges, dentists are expected to have a comprehensive understanding of the science of drugs and how their use can impact on dental conditions and procedures. As drugs may be administered by dentists during dental procedures or in the event of a medical emergency in the dental practice, dentists have a responsibility to understand how to use them safely and effectively, their side effects, drug interactions, place in therapy, and their impact on patient care.

1.2.1 What is pharmacology?

The term 'pharmacology' is derived from the Greek word *pharmakon* ('drug, poison' and -λογία, -logia 'study of', 'knowledge of') and refers to the study of drugs. In pharmacology, the chemical structures of pharmacologically active substances are elucidated, their mechanisms of action and target sites examined, and their route around the body mapped to eventually become the drug's pharmacodynamics and pharmacokinetics.

1.2.2 What is the study of therapeutics?

Therapeutics is the science of treatment and care of a patient for the purpose of preventing and combating disease or injury (1). Medical Britannica states that 'the term "therapeutics" comes from the Greek *therapeutikos*, which means "inclined to serve"' (1). In the area of pharmacology, therapeutics involves the application of drug knowledge to patient care through the judicious, safe, appropriate, economic, and effective use of medicines. This area is also referred to as 'pharmacotherapeutics'.

1.2.3 How is pharmacology different from therapeutics?

Pharmacology and therapeutics are similar disciplines in that both require an understanding of the properties and actions of pharmacologically active substances. However, pharmacology places more emphasis on the mechanisms of action, chemical structures, and movement of the drug around the body, while therapeutics focuses on the practical aspects of safe and effective medicines use in clinical practice.

1.2.4 How is pharmacy different from pharmacology?

Pharmacy is the study of medicines, from their design and development to their regulation and distribution in the community and finally to their safe use by prescribers and consumers. Pharmacy training covers all aspects of drug usage including pharmacology, manufacture, acquisition, storage, dispensing, administration, and disposal of medicines—as well as patient aspects such as management of adverse effects, drug interactions, prevention and management of medication error, medication review and deprescribing. Those who study pharmacy typically become pharmacists who prepare and dispense medication and collaborate with other healthcare providers to optimise medication use in patient care (4). Many pharmacists work in non-dispensing roles as well: in hospitals, community pharmacies, general medical practice, residential aged care, government, regulatory authorities, academia, the armed forces and the pharmaceutical industry. Those who study pharmacology, however, are qualified as scientists and generally work in research settings or incorporate their qualification into another health-based degrees. For example, clinical pharmacologists are medical practitioners who have specialised in pharmacology and usually work in hospitals.

1.2.5 What is toxicology?

Toxicology is the study of the harmful effects of chemicals, drugs and poisons on living organisms. Toxicologists are medical experts in poisons and poisoning and are consulted to analyse and advise on the treatment of ingestions, bites, and stings from acute or chronic drug or toxin exposure (3). Poisons information centres are operated by toxicologists and pharmacists trained in toxicology.

1.2.6 The importance of patient-centred care

One of the key themes of pharmacotherapeutics in the 21st century is patient-centred care. This type of care moves away from the prescriber being the focus of treatment choices towards the patient being at the centre of decision-making. Treatments are tailored to individual patient characteristics with patients' treatment goals and health-related beliefs respected. Some of the move towards patient-centred care has been driven by medico-legal considerations in healthcare, but also a greater understanding that respect for patient rights and responsibilities, preferences and consent leads to better health outcomes. This is further encouraged with greater understanding that medications work differently in different people and are used more safely if prescribed in a way that is considerate of each patient's medical history, pharmacogenetic profile, co-morbidities, and concomitant medications.

1.3 The fundamentals of drug response

Many factors contribute to inter-individual differences in drug response. These are broadly divided into three principal areas:

1. Pharmacodynamics = the actions of drugs (what the drug does to the body).
2. Pharmacokinetics = the movement of drugs (what the body does to the drug).
3. Pharmacogenetics = the influence of genes and their protein products on drug dynamics and kinetics.

1.3.1 What is pharmacodynamics?

Marino, Jamal and Zito describe pharmacodynamics as 'the study of a drug's molecular, biochemical, and physiologic actions' (4). The term is derived from the Greek words *pharmakon* which means 'drug' and *dynamikos* meaning 'power.' (4) The pharmacodynamics of a drug are its pharmacological actions and effects, often described as 'what the drug does to the body'.

Drugs work by binding to a variety of targets including external receptors on target tissues, active sites on enzymes, cell surface signalling proteins, and molecules circulating in the blood stream. The pharmacological aim is that, subsequent to the drug-target interaction, downstream dynamic effects occur which can be measured by biochemical or clinical means such as decrease in pain, killing of infectious organisms, reduction of blood pressure or lowering of blood-glucose levels (4).

1.3.2 What is pharmacokinetics?

The pharmacokinetics of a drug are its movements around the body, which are described in terms of four steps: absorption, distribution, metabolism and excretion (5). It is also described as 'what the body does to the drug'. The term 'pharmacokinetics' is derived from the Greek words *pharmakon* meaning 'drug' and *kinisi* meaning 'movement' (4).

1.3.2.1 Key pharmacokinetic parameters

Key parameters of every drug's pharmacokinetics are its bioavailability, maximum serum concentration reached (Cmax), time to maximum concentration (Tmax), volume of distribution and half-life (see Section 1.3.2.3).

These parameters are used to describe how a drug's disposition changes over time, or in certain disease and physiological states. For example, drug use in renal and liver impairment is guided by the changes in a drug's pharmacokinetics depending on the degree of organ impairment.

The pharmacokinetics of paracetamol, for example, can be described as follows: Orally administered paracetamol is rapidly and almost completely absorbed, attaining peak blood levels (Tmax) at 1–3hrs, with negligible binding to plasma proteins. It is widely and almost uniformly distributed in the body (volume of distribution ~ 1L/kg); extensively metabolised in the liver and the metabolites are excreted renally.

Pharmacokinetics also guide drug use in pregnancy and breastfeeding as it helps to measure to what extent a drug distributes across the placenta or into breastmilk, and when drug concentrations peak in the breastmilk in order to plan the timing of breastfeeding.

1.3.2.2 Bioavailability

Bioavailability describes how much of the originally administered drug reaches the systemic circulation and is expressed as a fraction or percentage. It depends largely on the physicochemical properties of the substance such as its lipophilicity, route of administration and whether the drug is passively or actively transported across the gut wall. Other factors that affect bioavailability include drug formulation, the presence or absence of food, pharmacogenomic variations in metabolic enzymes and drug transporters, gastric motility, and mesenteric blood flow.

For example, drugs administered intravenously have 100% bioavailability as they are delivered directly into the blood stream, with all the administered drug entering the systemic circulation. Drugs administered orally must navigate the gastrointestinal (GI) tract, survive gastric acid and digestive enzymes, achieve drug transport across the gut wall and survive first pass metabolism in the gut and liver. As a result, only a small amount of orally administered drugs may reach the systemic circulation.

1.3.2.3 Cmax and Tmax

As shown in Figure 1.2, Cmax describes the maximum serum concentration reached after a single dose of the drug and Tmax describes the time taken to reach peak concentration (Cmax) after a single dose of the drug (6). Cmax will be reached more quickly for intravenously administered drugs than for those administered orally. So, drugs administered intravenously have a shorter Tmax than the oral drugs, but both could have the same Cmax (see Figure 1.1).

Figure 1.1 Graphical representation of Cmax, Tmax and AUC and half-life as they vary with time and drug concentration.

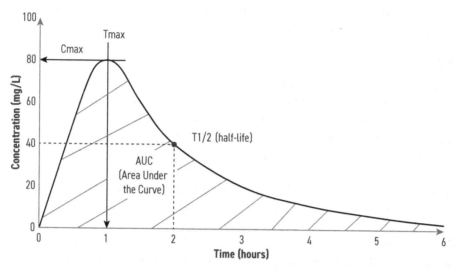

Figure 1.2 Graphical differences between Tmax and Cmax for the same drug administered via IV and oral routes.

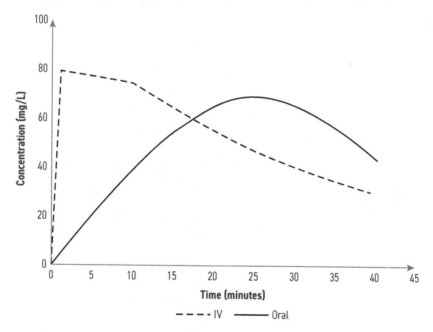

1.3.2.4 Area under the Curve (AUC)

AUC represents the total amount of drug absorbed into the systemic circulation from a single dose. AUC is determined by mapping plasma concentrations of the drug over the entire dosage interval, then measuring the area under the plasma concentration time curve (see Figure 1.1). AUC can be a useful tool for comparing different formulations of the same drug and dose; for example, a capsule versus a tablet. Plasma concentration time curves show how drug concentrations from each formulation vary over time, and how the AUCs from the two different products compare.

1.3.2.5 Half-life

The half-life (T1/2) of a drug is the time it takes for the drug's serum concentrations to decrease to half its Cmax. Although this is a mathematical parameter, it forms the basis for calculating how long each drug dose persists in the body, for determining drug dosing interval, and to calculate when a drug is completely eliminated. The convention for the latter is to multiply the half-life by 5, as this is when the drug is 98.5% eliminated (i.e. close enough to 100%). Drugs that linger in specific compartments in the body (e.g. bone or fat) will have a different half-life for each one of those compartments.

1.3.2.6 Steady state

When a drug is administered repeatedly, it eventually reaches a plateau, which is called 'steady state'. This is where an equilibrium is reached between the amount of drug entering the body and the amount excreted with each dose. Steady state is usually achieved after approximately five half-lives (see Figure 1.3). Knowing a drug's half-life and steady state allows clinicians to predict when a drug's effects will stabilise and, if the drug is ceased, when its effects wear off.

Figure 1.3 Drug concentrations with repeated administration. Adapted from (6).

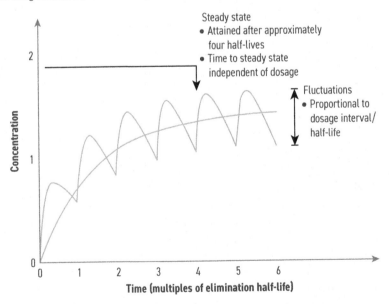

1.4 Administration and absorption of drugs

Drugs can be administered by many different routes, after which they are absorbed into the blood for delivery to their site of action. Common routes of administration include oral (swallowed), sublingual (under the tongue), oromucosal/buccal (via the inside of the cheek), rectal, transdermal, parenteral (intravenous, intramuscular, subcutaneous, intrathecal), or via inhalation (see Figure 1.4).

Figure 1.4 Drug absorption, distribution and elimination sites (32).

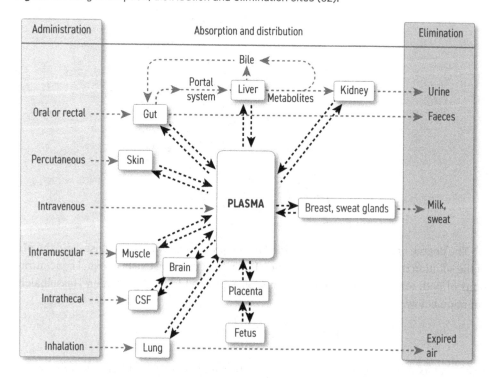

1.4.1 Oral drug absorption

The term 'absorption' describes the transfer of a drug from its site of administration into the blood stream. For drugs administered directly into the blood stream, there is no absorption phase. Absorption of drugs administered via the skin or muscle will have an absorption phase dependent on the administration site. Most drugs used in dentistry are prescribed for oral administration, so their absorption will involve transit through the GI tract.

After swallowing, these formulations transit into the stomach where they might be absorbed or transit further down in the small intestine. Factors that affect oral drug absorption include the drug's degree of ionisation, availability of active and passive transporters in the intestinal wall, GI motility, the presence or absence of food, mesenteric blood flow, formulation, and physicochemical properties of the drug (6).

1.4.2 Absorption of weak acids and bases

Many drugs are weak acids or weak bases; for example, local anaesthetics are all weak bases. Weak acids and bases exist in both ionised and unionised forms and their absorption through barriers such as the gut wall, skin or nerve fibres, depends on their lipophilicity and degree of ionisation. Figure 1.5 shows how ionisation influences the absorption of weak acids and weak bases. The more lipophilic a drug and the less it is ionised, the greater its ability to penetrate through a lipid bilayer such as a nerve fibre (6).

Figure 1.5 Oral absorption of weak acids and bases (20).

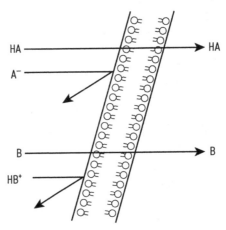

The degree of ionisation is determined by the pK_a of weak acids and bases and the pH of the solution they are in. Each pK_a is the pH at which the drug exists in equal concentrations of both ionised and unionised forms, as expressed in the Henderson-Hasselbalch equation below:

$$\log\frac{[\text{ionised form}]}{[\text{unionised form}]} = pK_a - pH$$

The Henderson-Hasselbalch equation is used to calculate the pH of buffer solutions:

$$pH = pK_a + \log\frac{[\text{base}]}{[\text{acid}]}$$

Acidic drugs will have a pK_a <7, and basic drugs will have a pK_a >7.

For example, local anaesthetics, which are weak bases, are better absorbed in basic conditions as this pH promotes conversion to the unionised state. At their site of action, the presence of infection such as an abscess can change the local tissue pH to acidic conditions, which is thought to be one reason why a local anaesthetic injected into an abscess is less effective and less well absorbed (see Section 7.3).

1.4.3 Absorption via drug transporters

The movement of drugs and endogenous molecules across cell membranes in almost every part of the body is dependent on transporters. Transporters are membrane-bound proteins that play a key role in the absorption, distribution, and excretion of drugs. Some transporters pump drugs into a cell (uptake) and others pump them out (efflux).

Drug transporters not only play an important role in individual drug pharmacokinetics, but also in their vulnerability to drug–drug interactions. This is because certain drugs can inhibit and/or induce the action of drug transporters, interrupting the absorption of the victim drug (see Section 1.14).

1.4.4 Other factors influencing GI absorption

A range of other factors influence drug absorption in the gut, including GI motility, the presence or absence of food, mesenteric blood flow, drug formulation, physiochemical properties of the drug and competitive drug interactions (6).

Increased GI motility speeds up GI transit time, decreases drug-villus contact time and decreases drug absorption. Conversely, slowed GI motility prolongs gastric transit time, increases drug-villus contact time and increases overall drug absorption. Excessively rapid movement of the GI tract (e.g. diarrhoea) can reduce drug absorption completely.

Co-administration of many drugs with food slows down their oral absorption and reduces their Cmax. For example, when non-steroidal anti-inflammatory drugs (NSAIDs) and paracetamol are administered in the presence of food, their Cmax is reduced by about 30% and their Tmax delayed by about one hour (7). Therefore, in acute pain, it is preferable to administer these drugs on an empty stomach, as this promotes a faster onset of action and higher Cmax which confers faster and more effective pain relief. There is also little evidence that administration with food improves safety.

Conversely, some drugs are absorbed better in the presence of food. For example, the antifungal itraconazole requires a low pH for maximal absorption so it is recommended to be orally administered immediately after a meal (8). For the antifungal griseofulvin, less than 50% of the oral dose is usually absorbed, but ingestion with a fatty meal increases the rate and extent of its absorption substantially (9).

Mesenteric or 'splanchnic' blood flow (i.e. the blood supply to abdominal organs including the stomach, liver, spleen, pancreas, small intestine, and large intestine) affects the passage, absorption and removal of drugs from the body. In some conditions where there is a reduction in blood flow to the gut (e.g. hypovolaemia), a reduction in drug absorption is seen. Splanchnic blood flow tends to increase after a meal, which may increase drug absorption (10).

Certain formulations can influence the rate of release and absorption of drugs such as transdermal patches or sustained release tablets. Prolonged release preparations usually present drugs via coated tablets, multi-layered preparations or embedded in a waxy matrix which release the drug slowly over a prolonged period. Drugs formulated with an 'enteric' coating are designed to stay intact while they traverse the acidic pH of the stomach (enteric) but dissolve once they pass into the more alkaline pH of the small intestine.

Drugs of a relatively smaller particle size and/or increased lipophilicity are more likely to cross the lipid bilayer of the intestine by diffusion. Prior disintegration of drug formulations is often required for drugs to be optimally absorbed, so liquid formulations that are already disintegrated can provide better drug absorption than tablets that require disintegration to take place with prior chewing or in the stomach.

Drug interactions can increase or decrease drug absorption in the gut. This can be used to an advantage; for example, the absorption of drugs taken in overdose onto activated charcoal to prevent the drug from being absorbed. Drug interactions occurring via competition, inhibition or induction of drug transporters can alter drug absorption. Pharmacogenomic variability in drug transporters and transport mechanisms can also affect the oral absorption of drugs.

1.5 First pass metabolism

'First pass metabolism' is a broad term given to the overall effect of drug destruction and elimination by transporters and metabolic enzymes in the gut wall and the liver that prevent a drug from reaching the systemic circulation (see Figure 1.6).

Figure 1.6 Overview of first pass transport and metabolism (11).

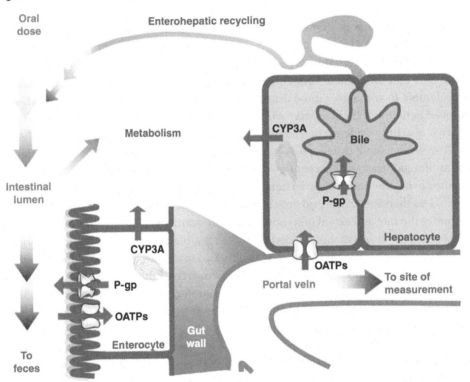

After a drug is administered orally it is taken up into enterocytes in the gut wall, either by passive diffusion or by drug transporters. Within the enterocyte, the drug may pass through unchanged but may also be metabolised to active or inactive metabolites. If it survives this process, the drug is transported out of the enterocyte into the portal circulation and carried via the portal artery to the liver, where it is transported into hepatocytes and can be further metabolised (11). If the drug survives all this, it can be transported out of the hepatocyte into the general circulation. The fraction that survives is considered 'bioavailable' and, when expressed as a percentage, describes the drug's oral bioavailability. Drug interactions can occur at any step in a drug's 'first pass' and are further described in Section 1.14.

1.6 Oromucosal drug administration and absorption

Sublingual administration involves drug delivery under the tongue, where there are numerous blood vessels and very thin mucosa. Physiological characteristics of this area permit highly effective drug absorption directly into the blood stream, bypassing the GI tract and first pass metabolism. Only a few drugs can be administered via this route. They are often used when a drug is needed to act rapidly; for example, glyceryl trinitrate sublingual spray in the management of acute angina.

Drugs can be applied topically to the oral mucosa (e.g. local anaesthetic) to produce a local effect; however, systemic absorption from this site must be considered. Corticosteroids in the form of topical ointments and creams (the same products used on external skin) are a well-tolerated and efficacious treatment of aphthous ulcers and oral lichen planus with negligible systemic absorption due to infrequent administration. Local anaesthetics can be applied topically to oral mucosa before injectable local anaesthetics are administered. However, it should be noted that absorption still occurs from topical administration, and some may also be swallowed. For example, topical local anaesthetic has oral bioavailability of about 30–35% so, if swallowed, about one-third of the dose applied topically will reach the systemic circulation (12). This may be negligible in adults, but in teething babies or infants the dose absorbed could confer serious adverse effects.

1.7 Parenteral drug administration

Parenteral means 'away from the intestines'. Drugs administered parenterally are given via routes other than the GI tract, which is generally by injection, infusion, or injectable implant. Drugs given directly into a blood vessel have no absorption phase as they bypass the barriers of the gut and liver. Therefore, these drugs have 100% bioavailability and produce an immediate effect. Drugs given into muscle (intramuscular), under the skin (subcutaneous) or as an implant, however, must first diffuse through the muscle and layers of the skin in order to reach and enter the local blood flow, which slows their rate of absorption and delays the onset of their effect.

1.8 Pro-drugs

A pro-drug is one that does not exert its main pharmacological effect until it has been converted, usually by enzymatic action, to its active form. There are broadly two kinds of pro-drugs: those that are converted to their active form *inside* cells, such as antiviral medicines converted inside a virus or inside human liver cells (30). Then there are pro-drugs whose conversion occurs extracellularly; for example, in digestive fluids or in the systemic circulation. Many drugs in clinical use are pro-drugs, including codeine, tramadol and clopidogrel (13).

Codeine, an opioid commonly used in dentistry for pain management, is a pro-drug. Also known as 3-methyl-morphine, codeine has no analgesic effect until it is converted to its active metabolite, which is morphine. After oral absorption, codeine is transported to the liver where its demethylation to morphine occurs via CYP2D6 enzymes.

1.9 Drug distribution

After drugs are absorbed into the blood stream, they are then distributed around the body either bound or unbound to plasma proteins. When they arrive at different organs and body compartments, they are transported in and out of these compartments via active or passive drug transport. Both transport via the blood and the passage of drugs in and out of different compartments accounts for drug distribution.

1.9.1 Volume of distribution (V_D)

V_D is a pharmacokinetic parameter used to describe and quantify the extent of drug distribution between plasma and other tissues. It is defined as 'the volume that would contain the total body content of the drug (Q), at a concentration (C) equal to that present in the plasma' (6).

1.9.2 Plasma protein binding

Many drugs are transported around the systemic circulation bound to plasma proteins. However, only the unbound fraction of a drug can diffuse into interstitial fluid and thereby exert pharmacodynamic effects. The concentration of free drug, the affinity of the drug for protein-binding sites, and the concentration of plasma proteins all influence the ratio of bound to unbound drug in the circulation (6).

The most abundant plasma protein is albumin. Being alkaline, albumin tends to bind acidic drugs such as warfarin, penicillin, and diazepam (14). Other plasma proteins that bind drugs include alpha-1 acid glycoprotein and beta globulin (6). Alpha-1 acid glycoprotein is an acute phase reactant, produced in times of illness and inflammation. Being acidic, it tends to bind basic and neutral drugs/substances such as iron and propranolol. As such, the free fraction of these drugs can decrease during times of illness and inflammation so measurement of their serum levels (which can only measure the free fraction) might be transiently and falsely low (15).

Plasma protein binding of drugs becomes clinically important in situations when the amount of plasma protein available greatly increases or decreases. In these situations, the degree of protein binding of a drug can affect its clinical performance as well as potential toxicity (16).

1.9.3 Drug transporters

Drug transporters are important contributors to pharmacokinetics. Transporters are proteins found in membranes of various compartments and organs around the body whose primary function is to facilitate the movement of molecules in and out of cells. Key transporters discussed in drug literature include P-glycoprotein (P-gp); breast cancer resistance protein (BCRP); organic anion transporters (OAT1 and OAT3); organic cation transporter (OCT2); and organic anion transporting polypeptides (OATP1B1 and OATP1B3).

Because transporters are involved in drug absorption, distribution and excretion, it is important to know which transporters are responsible at each step to understand the drug's movement and disposition and its vulnerability to drug interactions—all of which may account for inter-individual differences in drug responses.

1.9.4 The blood–brain barrier

The blood–brain barrier (BBB) is a term used to describe the layers of neural tissue, blood vessels, drug transporters and metabolic enzymes that collectively prevent the transition of drugs and other substances in and out of the central nervous system (CNS) (17).

Small lipid soluble drugs such as inhalational anaesthetics (e.g. methoxyflurane or nitrous oxide) can cross the BBB by simple diffusion due to small particle size and very high lipid solubility. Larger molecules, such as antibiotics, require active transport into the CNS but may be actively transported out again, thus achieving little or no detectable CNS concentrations.

1.10 Drug metabolism and excretion

Drug elimination is defined as the irreversible loss of the drug from the body, which is comprised of two processes: metabolism and excretion (6). Metabolism is the conversion of the drug into another chemical entity by the action of enzymes (6). In the liver, these are described as Phase 1 and Phase 2 reactions. As mentioned previously, after a drug is orally administered, it can be metabolised in the gut wall or liver, which constitutes its first pass metabolism. Drugs can be metabolised at other sites in the body, such as in the blood itself by serum proteases, which is how many local anaesthetics and antibody-based medicines are metabolised.

1.10.1 Phase 1 reactions

Phase 1 metabolic reactions are broadly grouped into three categories: oxidation, reduction, and hydrolysis. Most small molecule drugs are lipophilic in nature. Metabolic enzymes, mostly in the gut and the liver, convert these drugs into more water-soluble compounds that can be more readily excreted. Oxidation is the most common Phase 1 reaction and the cytochrome P450 enzymes (CYP) are the most thoroughly studied of these (6). Individual enzymes within the CYP system are identified via the nomenclature involving a number, a letter and a number (e.g. CYP2D6).

1.10.2 Phase 2 reactions

Phase 2 reactions occur in the liver and involve conjugation of a drug with an endogenous substrate (e.g. glucuronyl, sulphate or acetyl) to further increase the hydrophilicity of the drug, making it more readily excreted (6). While some drugs are substrates for both Phase 1 and 2 reactions, some will not be substrates for Phase 1 metabolism but only Phase 2, and vice versa.

1.11 Drug excretion

Drug excretion can occur via the skin, hepatobiliary system, and lungs, but is primarily achieved through the kidneys in the urine. Renal clearance of drugs is defined as the 'volume of plasma containing the amount of substance that is removed from the body by the kidneys in unit time' (6). As many drugs are renally cleared, their excretion is dependent on the patient's kidney function.

Drugs can be filtered passively through the glomerulus into the filtrate to be excreted. Large molecules and protein-bound drugs (e.g. warfarin, which is 99% protein bound) will not be filtered. These unfiltered drugs will pass on to the proximal tubule of the nephron, where non-selective active transporters can actively pump acidic and basic drugs into the filtrate (6). This active tubular secretion is the predominant method of drug elimination as drugs are secreted against their concentration gradient (6).

As the filtrate forms in the nephron and the drug is excreted, water and various small substances such as sodium and glucose are also reabsorbed. Drugs that are permeable to the tubule lumen can be reabsorbed passively (e.g. more lipophilic drugs) down their concentration gradient, while more hydrophilic drugs tend to stay in the urine (6).

1.12 Pharmacodynamics

As mentioned earlier, the term 'pharmacodynamics' describes the physiological actions and effects of drugs, which are often expressed in terms of drug-receptor relationships. A drug or a substrate interacts with a receptor in order to produce a physiological effect. Receptors are target molecules that combines with the drug or substrate. The fit is specific, like two pieces of a puzzle, and on binding a conformational change is produced. Receptors are usually membrane-bound protein molecules that interact with endogenous substrates or drug targets (6).

1.12.1 Receptor affinity, drug potency and clinical response

When a drug or substrate interacts with the target receptor, it can either cause activation of the receptor to elicit a physiological response or it can block the receptor to prevent a tissue response.

The strength with which drugs interact with their target receptor can be expressed using two parameters: affinity and potency.

'Affinity' describes how well a drug can bind to the receptor, or a measure of the strength of the binding of the drug to the receptor (20). A drug with a higher affinity will be more extensively bound to the receptor compared with a drug with a lower affinity, where less will be bound (see Figure 1.7).

'Potency' indicates the affinity that a drug has for the receptors and the ability to elicit a physiological response (6). It is measured by the concentration of the drug that produces 50% of the maximal response known as the half maximal effective concentration (EC50). This is a laboratory method of measuring potencies in order to compare drugs and relative potencies *in vitro* (20). It is a measure of how much drug is required to produce a particular response; the lower the dose required to produce the response, the more potent the drug.

1.12.2 Interactions with the receptor

Drugs interact with receptors in four different ways:

- **Agonist:** is a drug/substrate that will initiate a physiological response when combined with a receptor and has affinity for the receptor.
- **Antagonist:** is a drug/substrate that has affinity for the receptor but blocks the effect of an agonist for that receptor.

Figure 1.7 Low versus high receptor affinity.

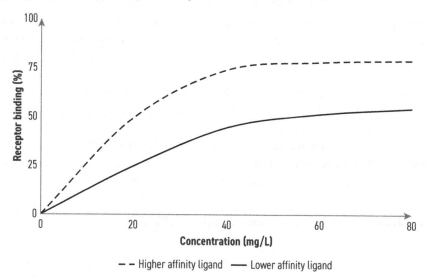

— — Higher affinity ligand   —— Lower affinity ligand

- **Inverse agonist (or negative antagonist):** is a drug/substrate that has affinity, so binds with the receptor but produces the opposite effect of that as expected for that receptor. An example is flumazenil which is an inverse agonist of the GABA benzodiazepine receptor. Flumazenil is used to reverse the sedation induced by benzodiazepines during general anaesthesia or after benzodiazepine overdose.
- **Partial agonists:** is a drug/substrate that has affinity for the receptor, but sub-maximal efficacy. It also blocks the action of the full agonist, thereby producing a submaximal effect (20). Buprenorphine is an example of a partial opioid receptor agonist, which is used for pain management and to treat opioid dependence. The latter is possible as buprenorphine activates opioid receptors with submaximal effect which confers less abuse potential (21).

1.12.3 Therapeutic index

A drug's therapeutic index (TI) is the ratio of the dose that is lethal in animal studies for 50% of a population compared with dose that is effective for 50% of the population. The equation used is LD_{50}/ED_{50}.

Unfortunately, this strict definition of a drug's TI is not very helpful in daily thera-peutics as it is largely based on animal studies and therefore not relevant to humans. However, it can be useful for comparing drugs generally by describing them as a having a 'narrow' or 'wide' TI. A drug with a narrow TI is one for which there is only a small difference between the minimum effective blood concentration and the minimum toxic concentration. With such drugs, a small increase in dose or blood concentration can lead to toxic effects. Examples of drugs with a narrow TI include digoxin, warfarin, clozapine, apixaban, rivaroxaban, dabigatran, lithium, carbamazepine, gentamicin and many more. A drug with a wide TI has a large difference between the minimum effective and the mini-mum toxic blood concentrations. Drugs like this include amoxicillin and omeprazole for which there is a big difference between their therapeutic and toxic doses.

1.13 What are pharmacogenetics and pharmacogenomics?

Pharmacogenetics is the study of how drug responses are affected by single gene variations in a person's DNA. Pharmacogenomics is a broader term that relates to the effects of multiple genes or the entire genome on drug response (2). A relevant example in dentistry is the pharmacogenetics of codeine, as this drug is converted to its active form of morphine by the enzyme CYP2D6, which is subject to significant genetic variations among different populations. People who do not carry the genetic alleles that code for CYP2D6—known as 'slow metabolisers'—cannot convert codeine to morphine and will therefore find it ineffective for pain. Those with multiple copies of the alleles coding for CYP2D6 gene—known as 'ultrafast metabolisers'—convert codeine quickly to morphine and will likely to find it effective for pain relief but experience more side effects.

1.14 Drug interactions and drug response

Drug interactions are common because taking more than one drug at a time is a frequent event. It can be as easy as taking a medicine with a cup of tea, as the medicine may interact with the caffeine, tannins, catechins or heat in the tea! What matters is that health professionals, including dentists, are aware of drug interactions and how they arise, how to assess them, when and how to intervene and, most of all, how to prevent them.

'A drug interaction is said to occur when the effects of one drug are changed by the presence of another drug, herbal medicine, food, drink, nutrient, medical condition, pharmaceutical or environmental agent' (22). Interactions have also been defined as 'the clinical result of a drug combination which is different from either agent alone' (23).

The high prevalence of polypharmacy in modern healthcare increases the chance of drug interactions. However, the contribution of self-medication with non-prescription drugs and complementary medicines (~60% population) is increasingly making drug interactions more difficult to predict. Greater understanding of pharmacogenetics (i.e. the role our genes play in individual response to drugs) adds another layer of complexity to predicting drug response.

It's not so much the drug interaction that matters, but the outcome to the patient, which can be harmful or beneficial depending on the context. Although most drug interactions do not result in serious impact, occasionally they do, so health professionals should try to prevent drug interactions since their outcomes can be very serious, including:

- adverse drug effects such as sudden death, seizures, arrhythmias, serotonin syndrome, respiratory depression, neuroleptic malignant syndrome, and delirium
- exaggeration of drug side effects such as dry mouth, cognitive impairment, sedation
- impaired drug efficacy
- misdiagnosis of symptoms as disease-related rather than drug-induced
- withdrawal symptoms due to declining serum drug concentrations.

1.14.1 Kinetic versus dynamic mechanisms

There are two main mechanisms of drug interactions: pharmacokinetic and pharmacodynamic. These are not mutually exclusive mechanisms. Either or both can occur with a particular drug combination.

1.14.1.1 Kinetic interactions

Kinetic interactions are those that occur due to altered movement of the drugs around the body, resulting in increased or decreased drug concentrations. Drug interactions can occur at each of the four steps of pharmacokinetics: absorption, distribution, metabolism, and excretion. Interactions occurring at any of those steps interfere with the 'victim' drug's ability to progress to its next kinetic step.

Drug interactions are neither good nor bad per se. What matters is the clinical outcome of the interactions for the patient. Elevated drug concentrations can cause increased drug side effects and toxicity but may also boost the drug's efficacy and cost-effectiveness per dose. Reduced drug concentrations may, on the other hand, decrease a drug's efficacy but may also reduce side effects and make it more tolerable.

For example, the cholesterol-lowering drug simvastatin is a substrate for CYP3A4, and the antibiotic erythromycin is a potent inhibitor of this enzyme. If simvastatin and erythromycin are used at the same time, erythromycin can increase the levels and toxicity of simvastatin by inhibiting its CYP3A4-mediated metabolism. A study in healthy volunteers found that erythromycin increased simvastatin AUC and Cmax approximately by 6.2- and 3.4-fold, respectively (18). In addition, several cases of rhabdomyolysis have been reported with the concurrent use of simvastatin and erythromycin and one case consequently developed renal failure (19). Concomitant use is not recommended and if erythromycin is needed as a short antibacterial course, simvastatin therapy should be suspended. Some examples of pharmacokinetic interactions are outlined in Table 1.1.

Table 1.1 Common pharmacokinetic drug interactions.

Interaction	Mechanism	Outcome to the patient	Resolution
Flucloxacillin + food	Food increases gastric acid which decreases flucloxacillin absorption and efficacy	Impaired treatment of infection	Take flucloxacillin an hour before or 2 hours after food
Oral bisphosphonates + calcium/magnesium/ iron/zinc (cationic minerals)	Cationic minerals chelate with oral bisphosphonates and significantly reduce their absorption	Impaired treatment of osteoporosis	Separate administration of cationic minerals from oral bisphosphate by at least 2 hours
Codeine + paroxetine	Paroxetine inhibits CYP2D6, which prevents codeine conversion to morphine	Inadequate analgesia	If an opioid is required, use oxycodone instead of codeine

A significant example of a pharmacokinetic interaction relevant to dentistry is the interaction between miconazole oral gel and warfarin. Miconazole is well absorbed through oral mucosa when applied on gums and lips. Like all azole antifungals, miconazole inhibits several CYP enzymes in the liver, and warfarin is dependent on these enzymes for its metabolism. In the presence of miconazole, warfarin concentrations can rise, increasing bleeding risk. Deaths from this interaction have been reported (31).

1.14.1.2 Dynamic interactions

Dynamic drug interactions occur due to the overlapping actions of combined drugs, resulting in increased or decreased effects. The results of combining two drugs together can be conceptualised as follows:

1. Additive (1 + 1 = 2) = when effects of two drugs add together.
2. Antagonistic (1 + 1 <2) = when effects of drugs oppose each other.
3. Synergistic (1 + 1 >2) = when the combined effect of two drugs is greater than just adding them together.

Additive dynamic drug interactions result in increased actions or effects of the combined drugs, which can be experienced as increased efficacy and/or exaggerated side effects. A common example of this would be multiple antihypertensive drugs used in the one patient to enhance their efficacy to lower blood pressure and, as a result, be able to prescribe lower than usual doses of each drug.

Antagonistic interactions occur when the actions of the drugs oppose each other, which usually result in both drugs being less effective. A common example of this is the concomitant use of stimulants and sedatives, often seen in people who have a cup of caffeinated tea just before taking their sleeping tablet at night. No wonder the sleeping tablet does not work!

Synergistic dynamic interactions are those that result in drug effects much greater than that expected from simply adding the effects of the two drugs together. Well-known examples of drug combinations that confer synergistic effects include amoxicillin and clavulanic acid, trimethoprim and sulfamethoxazole, and levodopa and carbidopa.

Dynamic interactions are always dose-related, so management of these interactions is often simply a matter of adjusting the dose of one or both the drugs, depending on the clinical situation. Ceasing one of the drugs may also be a more appropriate intervention as well.

1.14.2 How often do drug interactions occur?

Most drug–drug interaction (DDI) studies have been conducted in institutional settings such as hospitals or nursing homes. In those settings, it is known that approximately 1% of all hospital admissions and 2–5% of hospitalisations of elderly patients are caused by DDIs. Once in hospital, up to 90% of elderly patients experience a DDI during their hospital stay (25).

In the nursing home setting, van Dijk et al. found that 32% of residents were exposed to one or more combinations of drugs that could lead to clinically adverse outcomes (26). More recently, Dolton et al. found potentially harmful DDIs for 6.1% of 3876 residents of Australian residential aged care facilities (27).

Regarding DDIs in the community, a recent Polish study examined potential drug–drug interactions (pDDIs) with analgesics (28). The study found 23.3 million prescriptions for analgesics were dispensed on the Polish national scheme in 2018. Of these, approximately 2.5 million (6.47%) involved pDDIs. The most prevalent pDDI are caused by NSAIDs + antihypertensives (4.12%), followed by NSAIDs + NSAIDs (1.40%) and NSAIDs + glucocorticoids (0.56%). On average, 76.63% of pDDIs were ordered by the very same prescribers, indicating the drug interactions were being ignored.

1.14.3 Polypharmacy and culprit drugs

Overall, the two main risk factors for DDIs are polypharmacy and the use of drugs more prone to interactions. The latter are sometimes called 'culprit' drugs (CDs). Although it seems obvious that the risk of DDIs increases with polypharmacy, a handy rule of thumb comes from an often-quoted study by Cadieux et al., which stated that once a person is taking eight drugs or more, there is a 100% of a drug interaction (29).

There are three types of CDs:

1. Those prone to dynamic interactions.
2. Those prone to kinetic interactions.
3. Those with a narrow therapeutic index.

CDs that contribute to dynamic drug interactions are those with very broad and pronounced pharmacological effects, such that they easily interfere with or override other drugs. A common example would be corticosteroids such as prednisone/olone or dexamethasone. These drugs do their own potent anti-inflammatory and immunosuppressant actions extremely well. However, they also confer a range of other effects including immunosuppression and increased risk of infection, impaired wound healing, hyperglycaemia, increased blood pressure, mood instability and insomnia. So, they can counteract the effects of many other drugs that might be taken by the patient at the same time.

Examples of additive interactions:

- benzodiazepines + opioids → increased sedation, CNS and respiratory depression
- aspirin + turmeric + fish oil → increased risk of bleeding
- amitriptyline + oxybutynin → increased risk of dry mouth
- angiotensin converting enzyme inhibitors (ACEIs) + thiazide diuretic → added BP lowering effects
- SSRI + tramadol → increased risk of serotonin excess

Examples of antagonistic interactions:

- antihypertensives + NSAIDS → NSAIDs increases BP and makes antihypertensives less effective
- sedatives + caffeine → both less effective
- warfarin + vitamin K → vitamin K is the antidote to warfarin
- corticosteroids + hypoglycaemics → corticosteroids increase blood sugar levels and make drugs for diabetes less effective

In practice, CDs tend to cause more significant kinetic than dynamic drug interactions. This occurs by the CDs interfering with the one or more of the four steps of kinetics, as follows:

1. **Absorption:** via chelation, binding, competition and altered gastric pH to other drugs
2. **Distribution:** by blocking or stimulating drug transport through the gut wall or other body compartments such as the liver, brain, kidneys, or by altering serum protein binding

3. **Metabolism:** by blocking or stimulating metabolic enzymes in the gut wall, liver, or both
4. **Excretion:** by blocking or stimulating passive and active transport in the liver, bile or kidney, or by altering urine pH to manipulate excretion rate

Table 1.2 Examples of drugs prone to kinetic interactions: culprits and victims.

Drug family	Culprit or victim	Drugs significantly involved	Mechanism
Anticonvulsants	Culprit	Carbamazepine, phenobarbital, phenytoin	Induction of liver metabolism
Antiarrhythmics	Culprit	Amiodarone, flecainide	Inhibition of drug transport and metabolism
Azole antifungals	Culprit	Miconazole, ketoconazole, itraconazole, fluconazole	Inhibition of liver metabolism
Macrolide antibiotics	Culprit	Erythromycin, clarithromycin	Inhibition of drug transport and liver metabolism
Opioid analgesics	Victim	Codeine	Subject to CYP2D6 metabolism
Anticoagulants	Victim	Warfarin, apixaban, rivaroxaban, dabigatran	Subject to drug transport and liver metabolism
Corticosteroids	Culprit and victim	Dexamethasone, prednisone/olone	Induction and substrate of liver metabolism

The third type of CD is one with a narrow TI. This is a drug for which there is only a small difference between the minimum effective concentration and the minimum toxic concentrations in the blood. With such drugs, just a small increase in dose or in blood concentration can lead to toxic effects. Examples include digoxin, warfarin, clozapine, apixaban, rivaroxaban, dabigatran, lithium, carbamazepine, gentamicin and many more.

Well-known CDs, which all inhibit metabolic enzymes, include the following:

- anticonvulsants: carbamazepine, phenobarbital, phenytoin
- antiarrhythmics: amiodarone
- immunosuppressants: cyclosporine, tacrolimus
- HIV: ritonavir
- azole antifungals: ketoconazole, itraconazole, fluconazole, miconazole
- macrolide antibiotics: clarithromycin, erythromycin, azithromycin
- oral contraceptives
- quinolones: ciprofloxacin, norfloxacin
- rifampicin
- St John's wort, turmeric, quercetin, green tea
- warfarin, rivaroxaban, apixaban, dabigatran

1.14.4 When to suspect a drug interaction and when to intervene

There are two main scenarios when drug interactions should be suspected. First, whenever a new drug is added to a patient's drug regimen, the prescriber and the dispenser should check for drug interactions. This is usually done by manually scanning for culprit drugs and listing all the drugs into a drug interaction database or calculator to check for interactions.

The second scenario is when the patient is experiencing unexpected symptoms of an adverse event, so drug interactions should be included in the differential diagnosis. Since drug interactions are frequent but only occasionally significant, the key issue is knowing when to make a fuss. The following scenarios would be situations when a suspected DDI should be acted upon:

- when the patient is symptomatic of the interaction's predicted outcome
- if the predicted outcome of the interaction is serious
- if the medicines involved in the interaction have a narrow TI
- if the patient is currently frail, unstable or currently unwell, or
- if the patient is very young or very old, and thus less able to maintain homeostasis

1.14.5 Applying this to patient care: what is the process?

Step 1: Establish why you are investigating potential drug interactions

- Is the patient unwell? Do they have worrying symptoms?
- Is there diagnostic uncertainty?
- Do the drugs look suspicious?
- Are you just curious?

Step 2: Take a comprehensive medication history

You can only assess drug interactions accurately by looking at all the drugs the patient is on. The assessment relies on taking a comprehensive, accurate and up-to-date medication history. The medications must include all prescription and non-prescription drugs such as those bought in a pharmacy, supermarket or online, as well as vitamins, herbal remedies and nutritional supplements. Make sure that not just oral products are documented, but also any other medicines used systemically, such as medicated inhalers, eyedrops, drug-eluting implants and injections.

In addition to the name of each medication (preferably the active ingredient, followed by brand name), the history should also record the dose taken, how long the drug has been used and what they are taking it for. Smoking, alcohol, caffeine and recreational drug consumption can also be documented in a medication history.

Step 3: Identify the drugs frequently prone to interactions (culprit/victim)

Culprit drugs are those prone to drugs interactions (potent inhibitors/inducers of metabolic enzymes/transporters) or those with a narrow TI. Victim drugs are those that have a narrow TI and thus could easily cause toxicity or share potential dynamic or kinetic interactions with the culprit drug.

Step 4: Manually identify any potential dynamic or kinetic interactions
Based on first principles, examine the list for potential interactions that could be expected from these combinations. For any interactions identified, determine if action is warranted based on the current clinical situation.

Step 5: Confirm potential interactions using drug interaction calculators
Based on your manual investigation, confirm this assessment by running the medication list through drug interaction calculators (DICs). Although many excellent DICs are available online or embedded into drug information resources, none are completely up to date or comprehensive. Therefore, in order to confirm their results, use at least two calculators to determine whether the information derived from these tools agrees.

Step 6: Tease out confirmed drug interactions to their outcome and management
Once an interaction has been identified, it is important to tease it out to its outcome, significance and evidence base and what, if anything, should be done to manage it. One of the authors of this book, Geraldine Moses, has developed a mnemonic to help tease out drug interactions into their separate issues. This assists in the clinicians thinking slowly and deliberately about each issue, leading to the final step of how the interaction should be managed.

For each individual interaction, tease it out using the mnemonic DMOSES:

- **Drugs**: what are the drugs involved?
- **Mechanism**: what is the mechanism of the interaction?
- **Outcome**: what is the outcome of the interaction to the patient?
- **Significance**: what is the significance of this outcome?
- **Evidence**: how strong is the evidence that claims this interaction occurs?
- **Strategy**: what solution will you provide to manage this interaction?

Examples of worked through interactions are given below.

D = Tramadol + sertraline

- M = increased serotonin in synaptic cleft
- O = agitation, flushing, sweating, seizures
- S = occurs on spectrum from negligible to serious
- E = well-documented from evidence in case series and primary research
- S = cease unnecessary drugs or reduce the dose

D = NSAIDs + ACEIs + diuretic

- M = constriction of afferent arteriole, dilatation of efferent arteriole, reduce glomerular filtration
- O = reduced blood flow through glomerulus causing kidney damage and systemic hypertension
- S = very significant interactions: can cause acute renal failure
- E = well-documented from evidence in case series and primary research
- S = avoid combination. If necessary, monitor renal function frequently

FURTHER READING

Dawoud B, Roberts A, Yates J. Drug interactions in general dental practice—considerations for the dental practitioner. *British Dental Journal*. 2014;216:15–23. doi:10.1038/sj.bdj.2013.1237

Tannenbaum C, Sheehan NL. Understanding and preventing drug–drug and drug–gene interactions. *Expert Review of Clinical Pharmacology*. 2014;7(4):533–544. doi:10.1586/17512433.2014.910111

REFERENCES

1. Rakel RE. *Therapeutics—Medicine Britannica*. Accessed August 24, 2021. https://www.britannica.com.science/therapeutics
2. NHMRC. *Medical Genetic Testing—Information for health professionals*. 2010. Accessed August 24, 2021. http://nhmrc.gov.au?file/download
3. National Institutes of Environmental Health Sciences. *Toxicology*. 2019. Accessed August 25, 2021. https://www.niehs.nih.gov/health/topics/science/toxicology/index.cfm
4. Marino M, Jamal Z, Zito PM. *Pharmacodynamics*. 2021. Accessed August 25, 2021. https://www.ncbi.nlm.nih.gov/books/NBK507791/
5. Grogan S, Preuss CV. *Pharmacokinetics*. 2021. Accessed August 25, 2021. https://www.ncbi.nlm.nih.gov/books/NBK557744/
6. Ritter J, Flower R, Henderson G, Loke YK, MacEwan D, Rang H. *Rang and Dale's Pharmacology*. 9th edition. Elsevier; 2020.
7. Moore RA, Derry S, Wiffen PJ, Straube S. Effects of food on pharmacokinetics of immediate release oral formulations of aspirin, dipyrone, paracetamol and NSAIDs—a systematic review. *Br J Clin Pharmacol*. 2015;80(3):381–388. doi:10.1111/bcp.12628
8. Sporanox® Capsules. *Registered product information*. https://www.ebs.tga.gov.au/ebs/picmi/picmirepository.nsf/pdf?OpenAgent=&id=CP-2010-PI-01501-3&d=20230805172310101
9. Grisovin® Tablets. *Registered product information*. https://www.ebs.tga.gov.au/ebs/picmi/picmirepository.nsf/pdf?OpenAgent=&id=CP-2022-PI-02452-1
10. Crouthamel W, Doluisio JT, Johnson RE, Diamond L. Effect of mesenteric blood flow on intestinal drug absorption. *J Pharm Sci*. 1970;59(6):878–879. doi:10.1002/jps.2600590642
11. Dolton MJ, Roufogalis BD, McLachlan AJ. Fruit juices as perpetrators of drug interactions: the role of organic anion-transporting polypeptides. *Clin Pharmacol Ther*. 2012;92(5):622–630. doi:10.1038/clpt.2012.159
12. Curtis LA, Dolan TS, Seibert HE. Are one or two dangerous? Lidocaine and topical anaesthetic exposures in children. *J Emerg Med*. 2009;37:32–9. doi:10.1016/j.jemermed.2007.11.005
13. Grond S, Sablotzki A. Clinical pharmacology of tramadol. *Clin Pharmacokinet*. 2004;43(13):879–923. doi:10.2165/00003088-200443130-00004
14. Larsen MT, Kuhlmann M, Hvam ML, Howard KA. Albumin-based drug delivery: harnessing nature to cure disease. *Mol*. 2016;4:3. doi:10.1186/s40591-016-0048-8
15. Smith SA, Waters NJ. Pharmacokinetic and Pharmacodynamic Considerations for Drugs Binding to Alpha-1-Acid Glycoprotein. *Pharm Res*. 2018;36(2):30. doi:10.1007/s11095-018-2551-x
16. Coumadin® tablets. *Registered product information*. https://www.ebs.tga.gov.au/ebs/picmi/picmirepository.nsf/pdf?OpenAgent&id=CP-2010-PI-02588-3
17. Daneman R, Prat A. The blood-brain barrier. *Cold Spring Harb Perspect Biol*. 2015;7(1):a020412. doi:10.1101/cshperspect.a020412

18. Kantola T, Kivisto KT, Neuvonen PJ. Erythromycin and verapamil considerably increase serum simvastatin and simvastatin acid concentrations. *Clinical Pharmacology and Therapeutics*. 1998;64:177–182. doi:10.1016/S0009-9236(98)90151-5

19. MHRA. *Drug Safety Update*. Simvastatin: updated advice on drug interactions. 2014. Accessed August 28, 2021. https://www.gov.uk/drug-safety-update/ statinsinteractions-and-updated-advice-for-atorvastatin

20. Brenner GM, Stevens CW. *Pharmacology*. 4th edition. Elsevier; 2018.

21. Rossi S (ed). *Australian Medicines Handbook*. Australian Medicines Handbook Pty Ltd; 2021.

22. Preston CL (ed). *Stockley's Drug Interactions*. 12th edition. Pharmaceutical Press; 2021.

23. Zwart-van Rijkom JE, Uijtendaal EV, ten Berg MJ, van Solinge WW, Egberts AC. Frequency and nature of drug–drug interactions in a Dutch university hospital. *Br J Clin Pharmacol*. 2009;68(2):187–193. doi:10.1111/j.1365-2125.2009.03443.x

24. Bailey E, Worthington HV, van Wijk A, Yates JM, Coulthard P, Afzal Z. Ibuprofen and/or paracetamol (acetaminophen) for pain relief after surgical removal of lower wisdom teeth. *Cochrane Database Syst Rev*. 2013;12(12):CD004624. doi:10.1002/14651858.CD004624.pub2

25. de Oliveira LM, Diel JDAC, Nunes A, da Silva Dal Pizzol T. Prevalence of drug interactions in hospitalised elderly patients: a systematic review. *Eur J Hosp Pharm*. 2021;28(1):4–9. doi:10.1136/ejhpharm-2019-002111

26. van Dijk KN, de Vries CS, van den Berg PB, Brouwers JRBJ, Jong De Van den Berg LTW. Occurrence of potential drug-drug interactions in nursing home residents, *International Journal of Pharmacy Practice*. 2001;9(1):45–52.

27. Dolton MJ, Pont L, Stevens G et al. Prevalence of Potentially Harmful Drug Interactions in Older People in Australian Aged-Care Facilities. *J Pharm Pract Res*. 2015;April. doi:10.1002/j.2055-2335.2012.tb00128.x

28. Kardas P, Urbański F, Lichwierowicz A et al. The Prevalence of Selected Potential Drug-Drug Interactions of Analgesic Drugs and Possible Methods of Preventing Them: Lessons Learned From the Analysis of the Real-World National Database of 38 Million Citizens of Poland. *Front Pharmacol*. 2021;18(11):607852. doi:10.3389/fphar.2020.607852

29. Cadieux RJ. Drug interactions in the elderly: how multiple drug use increases risk exponentially. *Postgrad Med*. 1989;86:179–186.

30. Wu KM. A New Classification of Prodrugs: Regulatory Perspectives. *Pharmaceuticals (Basel)*. 2009;2(3):77–81. doi:10.3390/ph2030077

31. Pemberton M. Morbidity and mortality associated with the interaction of miconazole oral gel and warfarin. *Br Dent J*. 2018;225:129–132. doi:10.1038/sj.bdj.2018.534

32 Rang HP, Dale MM, Ritter J, Flower RJ, Henderson G. *Rang and Dale's Pharmacology*. 7th edition. Elsevier; 2012.

PRESCRIBING ESSENTIALS

2

KEY POINTS

- Prescribing is a complex process that requires consideration of the specific patient's medical condition and other medications, the clinical scenario, communication with the patient, review of the patient and satisfaction of legal requirements.
- Medication errors can lead to inappropriate medication use or patient harm; they can occur at any part of the medication usage and prescribing pathway; they are the most common cause of preventable patient harm.
- While there is national registration of dental practitioners in Australia, legislation governing the prescribing, supply, use, possession and administration of drugs is different in each state and territory.
- Medicines in Australia are classified into Schedules that are detailed in *The Poisons Standard* and subsidised through the Pharmaceutical Benefits Scheme.
- Prescribing in Aotearoa New Zealand is regulated by the *Medicines Act 1981*, *Medicines Regulations 1984* and *Medicines (Standing Order) Regulations 2002*; subsidisation of medicines occurs through PHARMAC and is then listed in the *Pharmaceutical Schedule*.

2.1 Introduction

Dentists are permitted to obtain, supply, possess, administer, and prescribe medicines for the management of their patients' oral health. In Australia, dental prescribing and provision of medicines are regulated by individual state and territory drug legislation, as well as through national rules and regulation through the Dental Board of Australia, the Pharmaceutical Benefits Scheme (PBS) and the Therapeutic Goods Administration (TGA).

In Aotearoa New Zealand, subsidisation of medicines is determined through the Pharmaceutical Management Agency (PHARMAC) and categorisation of medicines and legalities around their availability is determined by the *Medicines Act 1981*, with listing of approved medicines in the *Pharmaceutical Schedule*.

2.2 What is prescribing?

By definition, 'prescribing is an iterative process involving the steps of information gathering, clinical decision making, communication and evaluation which results in the initiation, continuation or cessation of a medicine' (1, 2).

A prescription may include recommendation for medicines that are available without a prescription, or other treatments such as exercise or wound care, but the process of prescribing necessitates an understanding of the decision-making process of choosing and recommending a treatment for a health condition (3).

2.2.1 Appropriate, effective and rational prescribing

Appropriate and effective prescribing is guided by following 'the six rights': the right drug, for the right patient, at the right time, at the right dose, for the right duration, in the right way (3). It is a complex process that requires consideration of the specific patient, their medical condition and other current medications, the clinical scenario, the communication with the patient, and the review and consideration of legal requirements (4).

2.2.2 Framework for prescribing and core competencies

Prescribing is a high-risk intervention that requires cognitive and decision-making processes. In dentistry, drugs are adjunctive, and the role of drugs come after diagnosis, determination of the therapeutic objective, and dental treatment (5).

Rather than being an isolated event or an afterthought at the end of an appointment, prescribing is a continuous process that involves four stages, as described by Coombes et al. (Section 2.2.2.1), where each stage affects the subsequent stage (6).

2.2.2.1 Stages of prescribing

1. Information-gathering
   - Obtain relevant patient information to make a safe prescribing decision, such as medical history, current and past medications, allergies, adverse drug reactions, and information on the presenting complaint
2. Decision-making
   - Determine the clinical need for drugs
   - Use knowledge of clinical pharmacology to select the appropriate medication. Tailor this decision to the patient and involve the patient in the decision
   - Consider the ideal treatment (pharmacological and non-pharmacological), taking into account contraindications/concerns: drug–patient, drug–disease, drug–drug, and allergy interactions
   - Select the drug and treatment regimen
3. Communicating the decision
   - Communicate the prescribing decision to the patient and/or carer, so they have a clear understanding of the rationale for treatment, how to take the medication, any potential adverse effects and where to seek help if adverse effects arise
   - Ensure that the prescription to the pharmacist is accurate and legible
4. Monitoring and reviewing
   - Review the patient within an appropriate time frame for outcomes, adherence to the instructions, reviewing the diagnoses, dose adjustments or change of therapy (6, 7)

2.2.2.2 Prescribing competencies

The *Prescribing Competencies Framework* (2) describes the skillset, knowledge and tasks needed to perform safe and effective prescribing while ensuring quality use of medicines. The *Framework* focuses on the person receiving the prescription (i.e. the patient), the relationship between the prescriber and patient, and other health professionals involved in the prescribing process. The four stages of prescribing as described by Coombes et al. are incorporated into the *Framework*, which includes information-gathering, clinical decision-making, communicating the decision, and monitoring and reviewing (6). Seven competency areas are also included. These describe the expectations for prescribers to prescribe safely and competently, to adapt as required for the specific individual, and to consider any legal and professional considerations (2).

Competency Areas 1–5 detail the requirements needed to prescribe at the level of the prescriber, including understanding the patient and their needs, management options, the shared-decision process to prescribe, communicating the decision and reviewing treatment outcomes (2). Competency Areas 6 and 7 detail the practice environment and overarching support that allows the prescriber to prescribe safely and effectively (2). All dentists are recommended to prescribe according to this *Framework* (see Further Reading).

2.2.3 Inappropriate prescribing

Inappropriate prescribing can lead to unsuccessful treatment, adverse effects, hospitalisation, opportunities for overdose, and, in the worst-case scenario, even death (3, 8).

Examples of inappropriate prescribing include using medicines:

- in combination, or instead of dental treatment, when dental procedures alone would be more appropriate
- of unclear or limited clinical benefit
- whose risks outweigh their benefit
- in inappropriate doses, duration or frequency
- that are inappropriate for the clinical scenario
- that interact negatively with the patient's other medications or medical conditions (3)

Prescribing decisions are complex and are influenced by both clinical and non-clinical factors. For example, prescribing of antibiotics is fraught with considerations of necessity, tolerability, interactions, and antimicrobial resistance. Nevertheless, overprescribing of antibiotics, which is the unnecessary or inappropriate use of antimicrobial medicines, is common. In Australia, it has been shown that around 55% of antibiotics are overprescribed by dentists (9). This is mostly due to the prescribing of antibiotics for localised infections when dental treatment alone would suffice (9). Similar overprescribing has been seen in other countries; for example, in the UK up to 79% of therapeutic prescribing was unnecessary (10), and 80% of dental prophylactic antibiotics were overprescribed in the US (11). Non-clinical factors also influence inappropriate prescribing by dentists such as clinical time pressure, fear of losing patients, and patient expectations and demands.

2.3 Medication errors and safety

Medication errors are defined by the World Health Organization (WHO) (adopted from the United States National Coordinating Council for Medication Error Reporting and Prevention) as:

> any preventable event that may cause or lead to inappropriate medication use or patient harm while the medication is in the control of the health care professional, patient, or consumer. Such events may be related to professional practice, health care products, procedures, and systems, including prescribing, order communication, product labelling, packaging, and nomenclature, compounding, dispensing, distribution, administration, education, monitoring, and use (12).

Medication errors are the most preventable cause of patient harm (13). Medication errors can occur anywhere in the medication usage pathway from the point of manufacture to their use by patients. They can occur just as much in hospitals as in community settings. In Australia, medication-related problems account for 250,000 hospital admissions annually, costing $1.4 billion, with 50% of these issues identified as preventable and therefore avoidable (14).

In 2017, the WHO announced its third WHO Global Patient Safety Challenge, 'Medication Without Harm', with the objective to reduce 'severe, avoidable, medication-related harm by 50%' over the prospective five years worldwide (4, 15). Australia is involved in this initiative, aiming to improve all areas of the medication use process (which also affects dentistry), including prescribing, dispensing, administering, monitoring and reviewing (15).

2.3.1 Reasons for error

Medication errors are rarely caused deliberately. They are known to be caused by two main problems: human factors and system failures (16).

Three types of human errors are most common: slips, lapses, or mistakes. Slips and lapses are skills-based errors that occur due to erroneous performance of a task (slips) or inadequate attention (lapses) (17). Examples of slip error include prescribing one drug while thinking of another, accidently adding a zero to the strength of a dose (e.g. 50mg instead of 5mg), and prescribing an incorrect dose due to an erroneous calculation. A lapse may occur due to incorrectly writing a dose or forgetting to administer a medication. Mistakes are errors that are knowledge-based (wrong or inadequate knowledge) or rule-based (using an inappropriate rule or misapplying an appropriate rule). For example, not following a guideline due to lack of awareness or following an outdated treatment guideline (18).

Many errors due to system failures are generated by sequential weaknesses within a process that cascade into errors and result in patient harm (16). A flawed working environment can predispose the practitioner to error—such as excessive workload, frequent interruptions, and unclear handwriting—and then result in mistakes at the expense of the patient. In the event of a medication error, the system (rather than the individual) should be blamed and analysed to determine where the weaknesses lie, how the weaknesses predisposed to error, and how the system can be strengthened to prevent the error from happening again (18). Table 2.1 highlights areas of medication use that are the most frequently cited sources of medication error (19).

Table 2.1 Elements of medication use that can be a source of error. Adapted from (19).

Element of medication use		Example of error
Source of medication error	Preventative action	
1. Inadequate patient information	Obtaining a thorough medical and drug history from the patient prior to prescribing reduces preventable adverse drug events	A dentist may not be informed about a patient's full list of medications and prescribes a drug which adversely interacts with one that was omitted
2. Insufficient drug information	Accurate, up-to-date and readily accessible sources of drug information are necessary for all prescribers	A dentist prescribes 'Tooth Mousse', without knowing it contains milk proteins, to a child with a confirmed allergy to milk proteins, and the child has an anaphylactic allergic reaction (20)
3. Poor communication of drug information	Ensuring accurate communication between prescribers, pharmacists and patients to reduce medication error	Illegibility of handwritten orders leading to the wrong drug being dispensed and administered Placement of decimal points without a leading zero is a common source of error: '.5g' can be mistaken for '5g', resulting in an overdose
4. Similar drug labelling, packaging and nomenclature	Being aware that medication names that look alike and sound alike or have similar packaging are often confused and are a source of error	A prescription for 'clindamycin' can be mistaken for 'clarithromycin'
5. Drug device acquisition, use and monitoring	Drug delivery devices (e.g. inhalers, infusion pumps, injections) should be checked and standardised to minimise errors	Pre-filled syringes of similar-looking substances, such as sodium hypochlorite and saline, may be unlabelled and then incorrectly selected and the wrong product used
6. Environmental factors that predispose to error	Being aware that distractions, interruptions, fatigue, and an excessive workload can contribute to errors	Frequent disruptions and distractions, as well as being hungry, angry, late or tired, can lead to errors, such as giving the wrong dose of a drug, mishearing the patient, writing a prescription for the wrong patient, or making notes in the wrong patient's file

Table 2.1 (cont.)

Element of medication use		Example of error
Source of medication error	Preventative action	
7. Professional competency and education	Continuing professional education for prescribers is necessary to ensure knowledge about medications, as well as medication safety, errors, and current protocols for medication use	A dentist being unaware of new medications that increase risk of MRONJ, then performing a dentoalveolar surgical procedure and increasing MRONJ risk
8. Appropriate patient education and consent	Patients should receive advice and education about their medicines from their prescribers and their pharmacist to ensure they understand treatment, are happy to take the medication, and can administer their medicines appropriately	Patients not understanding instructions on how to take their medication, resulting in inappropriate drug administration or dose of an antibiotic or pain relief medicine. Insufficient education may lead to non-adherence
9. Quality processes and risk management	Systems and processes should be designed to eliminate errors, instead of blaming the error on the individual	A new staff member is asked to sterilise equipment through the autoclave. This is a complex task but there is no checklist. Being unfamiliar with the process, he/she accidentally skips a step, sterilisation is not completed appropriately, and the equipment needs to be autoclaved again

Note: MRONJ: medication-related osteonecrosis of the jaw.

2.4 Drugs and poisons legislation in Australia

Despite the union of all Australian states into one federation in 1901, the eight separate states and territories each have their own legislation for regulation of medicines and poisons (5, 21). Each state has a Health Act that enacts the drugs and poisons regulations, which govern drug manufacture, wholesaling, distribution, ordering, prescribing, supply, dispensing, and administration. While there are many similarities between each state's acts and regulations, there are also important differences between the various jurisdictions, which become relevant when professionals practice in different states. Dentists who work in different states and territories need to be aware of the requirements dictated by drug and poisons legislation in the relevant states and territories (22, 23). The current state or territory Acts and Regulations are shown in Table 2.2.

Table 2.2 Current legislation for each Australian state or territory.

State or territory	Current legislation
Australian Capital Territory	*Drugs of Dependence Act 1989* *Drugs of Dependence Regulation 2009* *Medicines, Poisons and Therapeutic Goods Act 2008* *Medicines, Poisons and Therapeutic Goods Regulations 2008*
New South Wales	*Poisons and Therapeutic Goods Act 1966* *Poisons and Therapeutic Goods Regulation 2008*
Northern Territory	*Medicines, Poisons and Therapeutic Goods Act 2012* *Medicines, Poisons and Therapeutic Goods Regulations 2014*
Queensland	*Medicines and Poisons Act 2019* *Medicines and Poisons (Medicines) Regulation 2021*
South Australia	*Controlled Substances Act 1984* *Controlled Substances Regulations 2011*
Tasmania	*Poisons Act 1971* *Poisons Regulations 2008*
Victoria	*Drugs, Poisons and Controlled Substances Act 1981* *Drugs, Poisons and Controlled Substances Regulations 2017*
Western Australia	*Medicines and Poisons Act 2014* *Medicines and Poisons Regulations 2016*

2.4.1 *The Poisons Standard*

In Australia, medicines are classified into Schedules, as set out in the *System for Uniform Scheduling of Medicines and Poisons* (SUSMP) (also known as *The Poisons Standard*), that was originally published in 1986. This national classification system is managed by the Therapeutic Goods Administration (TGA) and regulates availability and advertising of medicines and other chemicals in the interests of public health and safety (24).

The Poisons Standard reflects decisions made by the TGA's Advisory Committee on Medicines Scheduling and the Advisory Committee on Poisons Scheduling regarding the classification of drugs and poisons into Schedules. *The Poisons Standard* also details labelling and packaging requirements for each Schedule, and various degrees of control on advertising, use, supply and possession (24).

There are currently 10 Schedules in *The Poisons Standard* that may carry over to variations in each state. For example, New South Wales has a Schedule 4D and Victoria has Schedule 11 in their respective Acts that the other states do not. It should be noted that scheduling of drugs and poisons is dependent on the products they are presented in, so individual substances can be in more than one Schedule depending on their dose, concentration and pack size.

Substances in Schedules 2, 3, 4 and 8 tend to be human medicines, while those in Schedules 5, 6 and 7 tend to be industrial chemicals and substances in agriculture or veterinary medicine.

Definitions of each Schedule and examples of drugs included are shown in Table 2.3 (41).

Table 2.3 Description of Schedules and examples of drugs included. Adapted from (41).

Poisons Schedule	Label statement	Description of Schedule	Examples
Schedule 1	This schedule is intentionally blank		
Schedule 2	Pharmacy medicines	'Substances, the safe use of which may require advice from a pharmacist and which should be available from a pharmacy or, where a pharmacy service is not available, from a licensed person' These substances may also be sold by a registered dentist or doctor	Large packs of paracetamol, lidocaine/prilocaine ('Emla') cream, xylometazoline nasal spray
Schedule 3	Pharmacist only medicines	'Substances, the safe use of which requires professional advice but which should be available to the public from a pharmacist without a prescription' These substances may also be sold by a registered dentist or doctor	Salbutamol inhaler ('Ventolin'), high strength fluoride toothpaste (5000 ppm), miconazole oral gel
Schedule 4	Prescription only medicines, or prescription animal remedies	'Substances, the use or supply of which should be by or on the order of persons permitted by State or Territory legislation to prescribe and should be available from a pharmacist on prescription' These substances may also be supplied by a registered dentist or doctor	Antibiotics, codeine-based combination analgesics
Schedule 5	Caution	'Substances with a low potential for causing harm, the extent of which can be reduced through the use of appropriate packaging with simple warnings and safety directions on the label'	Acetone, sodium hypochlorite and hydrochloric acid in various specific concentrations
Schedule 6	Poisons	'Substances with a moderate potential for causing harm, the extent of which can be reduced through the use of distinctive packaging with strong warnings and safety directions on the label'	4-amino-m-cresol in hair dyes and eyebrow/ eyelash colouring preparations, cleaning products such as benzalkonium chloride in specific concentrations

Table 2.3 (cont.)

Poisons Schedule	Label statement	Description of Schedule	Examples
Schedule 7	Dangerous poisons	'Substances with a high potential for causing harm at low exposure and which require special precautions during manufacture, handling or use. These poisons should be available only to specialised or authorised users who have the skills necessary to handle them safely. Special regulations restricting their availability, possession, storage or use may apply'	Some concentrations and forms of arsenic, cyanides
Schedule 8	Controlled drugs	'Substances which should be available for use but require restriction of manufacture, supply, distribution, possession and use to reduce abuse, misuse and physical or psychological dependence'	Opioids (e.g. oxycodone, methadone)
Schedule 9	Prohibited substances	'Substances which may be abused or misused, the manufacture, possession, sale or use of which should be prohibited by law except when required for medical or scientific research, or for analytical, teaching or training purposes with approval of Commonwealth and/or State or Territory Health Authorities'	Heroin, desomorphine, cannabis in specific forms and concentrations
Schedule 10	Substances of such danger to health as to warrant prohibition of sale, supply and use	'Substances which are prohibited for the purpose or purposes listed for each poison'	Formaldehyde in specific forms, uses and concentrations, silicones for injection/ implantation except when in Schedule 4

The Schedules relevant to dentistry are as follows.

Schedule 2: Pharmacy medicines. Medicines in Schedule 2 can only be sold in a pharmacy, by a pharmacist or a person under the direction of a pharmacist, but do not require a prescription. They can also be sold by a medical or dental practitioner. These include small packs of simple analgesics in specific concentrations per dosage form and pack sizes, such as ibuprofen and paracetamol.

Schedule 3: Pharmacist only medicines. This Schedule includes medicines and other products that can only be sold in a pharmacy under the direction of a pharmacist and the products are located behind the counter. Schedule 3 medicines can also be sold by a medical or dental practitioner. These substances require professional advice to be provided to the patient but do not require a prescription. These include simple analgesics in specific concentrations per dosage form and pack sizes, such as diclofenac, ibuprofen in combination with paracetamol, and also includes high concentration fluoride toothpaste (5000ppm).

When supplying a Schedule 3 medicine, the health professional is required to (24):

- provide adequate instructions for use, either written or verbal at the time of supply or sale
- label the container from which it was sold or supplied either with the business name and address or in some states (e.g. Qld and ACT) a full dispensing label, as per Appendix D of *The Poisons Standard*. If required by regulation, make a record of the transaction in a prescription book or other approved recording system
- ensure no advertising of the product is undertaken, unless the product is specifically exempted, as per Appendix H of *The Poisons Standard*

Schedule 4: Prescription only medicines. These medicines are only available to the public by prescription from an authorised health professional, such as a doctor, nurse practitioner or dentist. A pharmacist dispenses these medicines in response to a prescription. Many regulations and requirements regarding labelling, storage and availability apply to medicines in this Schedule. Medicines in this category in dentistry will relate mostly to antibiotics and some pain relief. Dentists may 'supply' Schedule 4 medicines directly to the patient; however, the patient must be provided with all the labelling and advice expected from a pharmacist.

Schedule 8: Controlled drugs. Schedule 8 drugs have many restrictions on their manufacture, supply, distribution, possession and use to reduce abuse, misuse and physical or psychological dependence (24). Examples of Schedule 8 drugs include codeine as a single ingredient, oxycodone, hydromorphone and tapentadol.

Schedule 10: Substances of such danger to health as to warrant prohibition of sale, supply and use. Each poison is prohibited for the purpose as listed in this Schedule. *The Poisons Standard* states that this includes:

> hydrogen peroxide (excluding its salts and derivatives) in teeth whitening preparations containing more than 6 per cent of hydrogen peroxide **except** in preparations manufactured for, and supplied solely by, registered dental practitioners as part of their dental practice (41).

2.4.2 The Pharmaceutical Benefits Scheme

The Australian Pharmaceutical Benefits Scheme (PBS) began in 1948 as a post-war effort to help subsidise the cost of medicines for consumers, especially veterans. This system was modelled on the British National Health Service (NHS) and the Australian scheme provided a small list of 'life-saving and disease preventing' drugs at no charge to the patient at the time (29). Today, the PBS subsidises around 75% of medicines and is a fundamental part of Australia's National Medicines Policy framework that aims to ensure the National Strategy for Quality Use of Medicines while maintaining a viable medicines industry (25, 26). The aim of the PBS is to provide all Australians with timely, affordable and necessary medicines (27), and is administered by the Australian Government Department of Health.

Not all drugs on the Australian market are subsidised by the PBS and not all drugs on the PBS are subsidised for prescribing by dentists. The PBS has a sub-schedule, titled the Dental Schedule, that is a list of medicines in specific doses, dose forms and quantities that, when prescribed by dentists, can be subsidised for patients through the PBS. It is of note that the current list of medicines for dental prescribers has not been updated for many years and is therefore somewhat out of step with current dental practice guidelines and should not be used to indicate appropriateness of medication choice or regimen (5, 28, 29).

2.4.3 The prescription

A prescription is a communication tool from a prescriber to a pharmacist detailing what is to be dispensed to the patient and how the medication is to be used (5). Prescriptions can be either handwritten or computer-generated through approved prescribing software—the latter of which can either be printed or sent as a e-token to the patient's phone or email, but there are the same requirements for both.

The requirements for dental prescriptions vary slightly depending on the different laws for each state or territory in Australia but, in general, the requirements are (5, 30):

- name and address of the patient (as registered on their Medicare card)
- name, clinic address and PBS prescriber number of the dentist
- medication details: drug name, strength, frequency, dose form (e.g. tablets/liquid) and quantity
- instructions on the medication regimen, in English (not abbreviated Latin terms)
- handwritten signature of the prescriber
- date of the prescription (prescriptions cannot be forward or back dated)
- for dental prescriptions, the words 'For Dental Treatment Only'
- for drugs of dependence, the patient's date of birth

Under the PBS all Australian dentists are not permitted to write repeat prescriptions (23, 27). Most states also specify in legislation that a legitimate therapeutic need for a medicine should be established prior to prescribing (23).

Medicines written on the prescription can only be for the person named in the prescription. If more than one family member needs the same medication, another prescription for the other member should be written. Recent changes require antibiotic prescriptions to be detailed with the exact duration of therapy, not simply stating 'until the pack is all finished'.

In order to improve communication regarding medicines, active ingredient prescribing (AIP) was introduced in Australia on 1 February 2021 as a requirement of all PBS prescriptions. AIP occurs when the drugs prescribed are referred to by their active ingredient or generic name rather than their brand name. Handwritten prescriptions have been exempted from AIP, but it is recommended that prescribers prescribe by active ingredient regardless.

2.4.4 Record-keeping

As dentists often use scheduled medicines as part of their practice (e.g. local anaesthetic), there are requirements for record-keeping of the administration of these medicines that vary by state and territory. In general, requirements include:

- the date of the administration
- name, form, strength and quantity of the medicine
- name and address or location of the patient who received the administered drug

Records need to be completed soon after the administration of the drug. Legislation varies between states and territories on the storage requirements of scheduled medicines in the dental clinic. Individual legislation should be consulted for these requirements on both storage and record-keeping.

2.4.5 Prescriptions for drugs of dependence

Various legislative requirements exist in the different states and territories for the writing of prescriptions for drugs of dependence. Some requirements for prescriptions of drugs of dependence in each state and territory are outlined below in Table 2.4.

Real-time prescription monitoring (RTPM) is now active in all Australian states and territories, although dentists are currently not actively involved in Victoria or Tasmania. These databases are referred to as Safescript (in NSW, Victoria and Tasmania), QScript (Queensland), ScriptCheckWA (Western Australia), Script Check SA (South Australia), and NTscript (Northern Territory). RTPM provides data regarding the monitored medicines dispensed to patients in real time. This data is provided as a tool to support clinical decision-making and does not tell the prescriber what to do. In most Australian states, it is required that these programs are accessed prior to prescribing, supply, or administration of a treatment dose of monitored medicines or drugs of dependence.

Dentists should also be aware that several states have restrictions on prescribing drugs of dependence to patients with a history of high-risk drug or drugs of dependence use. Individual relevant legislation should be consulted when practising in each state. Under the PBS, dentists are not permitted to self-prescribe controlled drugs (27).

2.4.6 Off-label prescribing

Off-label or 'off-licence' prescribing (OLP) is the term used to describe prescription of medicines outside their legally approved product information (PI) (31). Examples include using a medicine for a different purpose, in a different dose, for a different patient group, or administering via a different route of administration from that which has been legally approved by the regulatory authority in that country. 'Labelling' refers to 'any written material that may accompany a medical product such as prescribing information, a package insert[s], and professional product instructions' (40).

Table 2.4 Terminology differences and some requirements of prescriptions for drugs of dependence. Adapted from (23).

State/Territory	Terminology	Points of note
Australian Capital Territory	Controlled medicine	• Prescriptions are restricted to 'not more than the quantity approved'
New South Wales	Drug of addiction	• Quantity and/or strength of drug is written in both numerals and words • Drugs of addiction that can be prescribed by dentists are those listed on the PBS, with the exception being if the patient is in hospital • The prescribed drug of addiction must be listed on its own prescription
Northern Territory	Unrestricted or restricted Schedule 8 substance	• Quantity and/or strength of drug is written in both numerals and words • Patient's date of birth is required on the prescription • The prescribed Schedule 8 substance must be listed on its own prescription
Queensland	Controlled or restricted drugs or poisons	• Patient's date of birth is required on the prescription • The prescribed controlled drug must be listed on its own prescription
South Australia	Controlled drug or drug of dependence	• Quantity and/or strength of drug is written in both numerals and words • Patient's date of birth is required on the prescription
Tasmania	Drug of dependence or narcotic	• Patient's date of birth is required on the prescription • The prescribed drug of dependence must be listed on its own prescription
Victoria	Drug of dependence	• Quantity of drug is written in both numerals and words • Can only prescribe to a patient under the dentist's care • Dentist to establish that a therapeutic need exists • Patient's date of birth is required on the prescription
Western Australia	Drug of addiction or Schedule 8 or Schedule 4 reportable poison	• Patient's date of birth is required on the prescription • The prescribed drug of addiction must be listed on its own prescription

OLP is common in dentistry as few drugs other than those specifically packaged for dental use have registered dental indications. Common examples are antibiotics and analgesics that have registered medical uses, but not dental uses.

Examples of OLP in dentistry (which may or may not be substantiated by reasonable evidence) include:

- oral administration of midazolam injection fluid where it is only legally registered for IV administration
- use of methoxyflurane as an anti-anxiety agent where it is only registered for management of acute pain associated with emergencies or surgical procedures
- use of tranexamic acid tablets as a mouth rinse where tablets are only registered for systemic administration to treat heavy menstrual bleeding, bleeding in the eye or in patients with established coagulopathies undergoing surgery
- use of dexamethasone tablets to pre- or postoperatively reduce post-extraction pain and swelling

2.4.7 Appropriate and inappropriate off-label prescribing

Poorly substantiated OLP can raise significant professional, ethical and therapeutic issues.

Three broad categories of appropriate OLP are as follows:

- that which is justified by high-quality evidence of efficacy and safety
- that which is within the context of a formal research proposal
- exceptional prescribing justified by individual clinical circumstances (32)

Gazarian et al. (32) state that in all three categories of OLP, an informed consent process should be employed to support the patient and their carer/s in their understanding and agreement to the process. Informed consent provides an opportunity for the prescriber not only to explain the situation but also for the patient and carer/s to:

- agree, or not, with the unapproved use
- accept, or not, the potential risks accompanying drug use outside its registered limits
- understand the justification for OLP, and
- be empowered to deal with the circumstances if the off-label use is questioned

For longer-term off-label medication use, the prescriber should remain aware of their responsibility to monitor the medication's tolerability, safety and efficacy and 'report any significant adverse events to the TGA to help develop a comprehensive profile of the medication prescribed in the off-label' setting (33).

2.4.8 Location of a drug's registered indications

Legally registered indications are those approved by the TGA that are then listed in each drug's TGA-approved product information (PI). The PI also contains age group restrictions, special patient population indications, approved doses and routes of administration. Registered product information is readily available online, via the TGA website in Australia, via websites such as NPS MedicineWise, as well as in drug compendia. It is important to note that PI varies between countries, so approved indications and uses may also vary.

2.4.9 Process for OLP

The suggested process for OLP is as follows:

1. Determine whether your prescribing is off-label or not. This can be done by following the flow chart in Figure 2.1.

Figure 2.1 Assessing appropriateness for OLP (32).

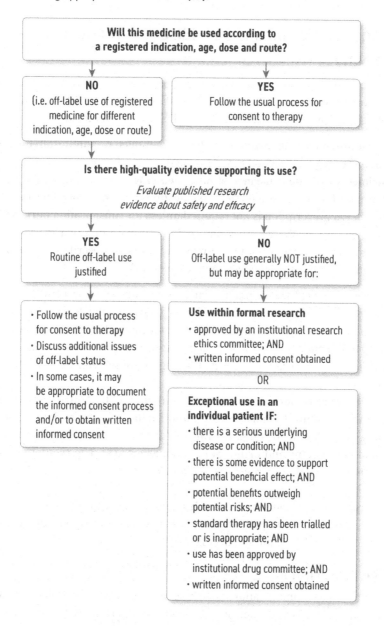

2. Ensure that your prescribing is supported by substantial evidence. Gazarian et al. state that 'as a general rule, the less serious the clinical need, the higher the level of evidence needed to support off-label use' (23).

3. If the prescriber thinks OLP is required, ensure that the potential benefit outweighs the potential harm by checking the PI and other prescribing resources for warnings, precautions, adverse effects and drug interactions.
4. Inform the patient/carer when you are prescribing off-label: explain the rationale for this, the evidence supporting this practice, and how the benefit outweighs the risk. If the patient has reservations, reconsider prescribing. If the patient consents, ensure this is adequately documented.

2.5 Drugs legislation and subsidisation in Aotearoa New Zealand

Drugs are regulated in Aotearoa New Zealand by the *Medicines Act 1981, Medicines Regulations 1984* and *Medicines (Standing Order) Regulations 2002* (34). The *Medicines Act 1981* details the classification categories for medicines, which includes:

- **Prescription medicine**: medicine only sold, supplied or administered from a prescription from an authorised prescriber (34).
- **Restricted medicine (pharmacist-only medicine)**: medicine sold or supplied by a pharmacist or in a hospital. These medications can be supplied by an authorised prescriber; a prescription is not required unless for subsidisation purposes (34).
- **Pharmacy-only medicine**: medicine sold or supplied in a pharmacy or hospital. These medications can be supplied by an authorised prescriber; a prescription is not required unless for subsidisation purposes (34).

While prescription drugs are the main medicines subsidised under PHARMAC, patients can also receive a subsidy for non-prescription pharmaceuticals, therapeutic devices and other health-related products. PHARMAC determines the subsidisation depending on the listing of the medicine on the *Pharmaceutical Schedule*. If the medicine is not listed on the *Pharmaceutical Schedule*, there is no funding for these items even if a prescription is written (34).

Oral health practitioners are registered and regulated by Aotearoa New Zealand's Dental Council Te Kaunihera Tiaki Niho, and include 'dentists, dental specialists, dental therapists, dental hygienists, oral health therapists, clinical dental technicians, dental technicians and orthodontic auxiliaries' (35). The regulation of dental professionals is carried out under the *Health Practitioner Competence Assurance Act 2003* (36).

In Aotearoa New Zealand, dentists are legally permitted to sell, supply or administer prescription medicines to patients, but need to comply with the storage, labelling, recording and advertising requirements (34, 37).

2.5.1 The prescription

The prescription is a communication tool between a prescriber and a pharmacist, detailing instructions for the exact dispensing of a medication. From the *Medicines Regulations 1984* (37), the requirements on a prescription in Aotearoa New Zealand are:

- name and address of the patient
- for a child older than 13 years of age, their date of birth
- name, street address and telephone number of the prescriber, or postal address of the prescriber if there is no work address listed
- medication details: drug name, strength/dose, frequency and quantity, or total period of supply
- the method of administration: e.g. injection, swallowing, external use
- instructions on the medication regimen
- handwritten signature of the prescriber
- date of the prescription

A dentist can write a prescription for the treatment of a patient under their care (37). If a dentist needs a patient to obtain medicines *urgently*, they can communicate the prescription details by telephone or in person with a pharmacist to whom the dentist is known. The dentist is required to supply a corresponding physical pre-scription to the pharmacist within 1 week to confirm the oral communication of the prescription (37).

2.5.2 Controlled drugs in Aotearoa New Zealand

Dentists are permitted to prescribe a controlled drug for a 'maximum period of supply (is) no greater than a quantity sufficient for use for a period of 7 days' (38, 39). Controlled drugs are classified into Class A, B and C drugs, and include opioids and benzodiazepines. The differences between the classes are determined by the degree of risk of harm they inherently possess to individuals or society by their misuse (38). The list of controlled drugs is available from the *Misuse of Drugs Act 1975*.

In addition to the above, prescriptions for controlled drugs also require the following:

- for children under 12 years of age, their age must be written in years and months.
- dispensing of prescriptions for Class A and Class B controlled drugs (e.g. oxyco-done) must take place within 7 days of the original prescription date.
- dispensing of prescriptions for Class C controlled drugs (e.g. temazepam) must take place within 6 months of the original prescription date.
- prescriptions must be handwritten on a specific form (currently triplicate con-trolled drugs prescription form H572) or on an electronically-generated form with an approved system that has a data connection to Medicines Control and Sector Operations within the Ministry of Health (39).

The relevant drug legislation in Aotearoa New Zealand is:

- *Medicines Act 1981*
- *Medicines Regulations 1984*
- *Medicines (Standing Order) Regulations 2002*
- *Misuse of Drugs Act 1975*

FURTHER READING

Johnstone M, Teoh L, Holden A. Prescribing drugs of dependence in dentistry: a review of legal and regulatory considerations. *Aust Dent J.* 2021;66(4):371–376. doi:10.1111/adj.12862

NPS MedicineWise. *Prescribing Competencies Framework: embedding quality use of medicines into practice.* 2nd edition. NPS MedicineWise; 2021.

Poisons Standard February 2022 (Cth).

REFERENCES

1. Health Workforce Australia. *Health Professionals Prescribing Pathway (HPPP) Project.* 2013. Final Report.
2. NPS MedicineWise. *Prescribing Competencies Framework: embedding quality use of medicines into practice.* 2nd edition. NPS MedicineWise; 2021.
3. Walker R, Whittlesea C. *Clinical Pharmacy and Therapeutics.* 4th edition. Churchill Livingstone; 2007.
4. Harrison C, Hilmer S. The Prescribing Skills Assessment: a step towards safer prescribing. *Aust Prescr.* 2019;42(5):148–150.
5. Oral and Dental Expert Group. *Therapeutic Guidelines Oral and Dental (Version 3).* Therapeutic Guidelines Pty Ltd; 2019.
6. Coombes ID, Reid C, McDougall D, Stowasser D, Duiguid M, Mitchell C. Pilot of a National Inpatient Medication Chart in Australia: improving prescribing safety and enabling prescribing training. *Br J Clin Pharmacol.* 2011;72(2):338–349.
7. Lum EMC, Coombes I. The competent prescriber: 12 core competencies for safe prescribing. *Aust Prescr.* 2013;36(1):13–16.
8. Editorial Advisory Committee. *Australian Medicines Handbook.* Australian Medicines Handbook Pty Ltd; 2021.
9. Teoh L, Marino RJ, Stewart K, McCullough MJ. A survey of prescribing practices by general dentists in Australia. *BMC Oral Health.* 2019;19(1):193.
10. Cope AL, Francis NA, Wood F, Chestnutt IG. Antibiotic prescribing in UK general dental practice: a cross-sectional study. *Community Dent Oral Epidemiol.* 2016;44(2):145–153.
11. Suda KJ, Calip GS, Zhou J et al. Assessment of the Appropriateness of Antibiotic Prescriptions for Infection Prophylaxis Before Dental Procedures, 2011 to 2015. *JAMA Netw Open.* 2019;2(5):e193909.
12. World Health Organization. *Medication Errors: Technical Series on Safer Primary Care.* 2016 Report.
13. Williams, DJP. Medication errors. *R Coll Physicians Edinb.* 2007;37:343–346.
14. Pharmaceutical Society of Australia. *Medication Safety: Take Care.* Pharmaceutical Society of Australia Ltd; 2019.
15. Australian Commission of Safety and Quality in Health Care. *Medication without harm— WHO Global Patient Safety Challenge.* 2019. Discussion paper for public consultation.
16. Velo GP, Minuz P. Medication errors: prescribing faults and prescription errors. *Br J Clin Pharmacol.* 2009;67(6):624–628.
17. Aronson JK. Medication errors: what they are, how they happen, and how to avoid them. *QJM.* 2009;102(8):513-521. doi:10.1093/qjmed/hcp052
18. Nichols P, Copeland TS, Craib IA, Hopkins P, Bruce DG. Learning from error: identifying contributory causes of medication errors in an Australian hospital. *Med J Aust.* 2008;188(5):276–279. doi:10.5694/j.1326-5377.2008.tb01619.x

19. Institute for Safe Medication Practices. *Key Elements of Medication Use 2021*. 2021. https://www.ismp.org/key-elements-medication-use

20. Australian Dental Association. *Allergy: A dental cautionary tale*. Australian Dental Association Inc; 2019.

21. Tooms A. Opinion: Why We Need A National Poisons Law. *Australian Journal of Pharmacy*. 31 October 2017.

22. Bernaitis NL, King MA, Hope DL. Interstate dispensing: a case for uniform, intuitive legislation. *J Law Med*. 2014;22(1):174–178.

23. Johnstone M, Teoh L, Holden A. Prescribing drugs of dependence in dentistry: a review of legal and regulatory considerations. *Aust Dent J*. 2021;66(4):371–376. doi:10.1111/adj.12862

24. Australian Government Therapeutic Goods Administration. *The Poisons Standard (the SUSMP)*. 2021. https://www.tga.gov.au/publication/poisons-standard-susmp

25. Australian Government, Department of Health and Aged Care. *National Medicines Policy*. 2022. https://www.health.gov.au/sites/default/files/2022-12/national-medicines-policy.pdf

26. Australian Commission for Safety and Quality in Healthcare. *Quality Use of Medicines: Overview, publications, guiding principles, national Indicators*. 2023. https://www.safetyandquality.gov.au/our-work/medication-safety/quality-use-medicines.

27. Australian Government Department of Health. *The Pharmaceutical Benefits Scheme: About the PBS*. 2021. https://www.pbs.gov.au/info/about-the-pbs

28. Teoh L, Stewart K, Marino RJ, McCullough MJ. Part 1. Current prescribing trends of antibiotics by dentists in Australia from 2013 to 2016. *Aust Dent J*. 2018. doi:10.1111/adj.12622

29. Teoh L, Stewart K, Marino RJ, McCullough MJ. Part 2. Current prescribing trends of dental non-antibacterial medicines in Australia from 2013 to 2016. *Aust Dent J*. 2018. doi:10.1111/adj.12613

30. Australian Government Department of Health. *Prescribing Medicines—Information for PBS Prescribers*. 2021. https://www.pbs.gov.au/info/healthpro/explanatory-notes/section1/Section_1_2_Explanatory_Notes

31. Seale JP. Off-label prescribing. *Med J Aust*. 2014;200(2):65.

32. Gazarian M, Kelly M, McPhee JR et al. Off-label use of medicines: consensus recommendations for evaluating appropriateness. *Med J Aust*. 2006;185(10):544–548.

33. Day R. Off-label prescribing. *Aust Prescr*. 2013;36:5–7.

34. New Zealand Ministry of Health. *Prescribing statement—legal requirements and subsidization*. 2021. https://www.health.govt.nz/our-work/regulation-health-and-disability-system/medicines-act-1981/prescribing-statement-legal-requirements-and-subsidisation

35. Dental Council. *Welcome*. 2021. https://www.dcnz.org.nz/

36. *Health Practitioners Competence Assurance Act 2018* (New Zealand).

37. *Medicines Regulations 1984* (New Zealand).

38. *Misuse of Drugs Act 1975* (New Zealand).

39. New Zealand Ministry of Health. *Controlled drugs*. 2019. https://www.health.govt.nz/our-work/regulation-health-and-disability-system/medicines-control/controlled-drugs

40. Academy of General Dentistry. *AGD Policies*. 2020. https://www.agd.org/advocacy/agd-priorities/agd-policies

41. Commonwealth of Australia. *Therapeutic Goods (Poisons Standard—February 2023)*. 2023. https://www.legislation.gov.au/Details/F2023L00067.

3 DRUG ALLERGY VERSUS ADVERSE REACTIONS

KEY POINTS

- Adverse events from medicines are frequent but are not always due to adverse drug reactions, as they may also be due to human and system errors in medication use.
- Adverse drug effects continue to be discovered after a drug is approved for use and as it becomes more widely used in diverse settings.
- Hypersensitivity is a disproportionate or aberrant immune response and a variety of different allergic reactions to drugs can occur. Hypersensitivity reactions are most commonly either a drug-IgE complex reaction or a cell-mediated response.
- Penicillin allergy is commonly reported, but seriously over-estimated and the overwhelming majority of adults who report a penicillin allergy can actually safely receive systemic penicillin treatment.
- Allergic reactions to local anaesthetics are extremely rare and often not true allergic reactions. However, when they legitimately occur, referral for preservative-free local anaesthetic allergy testing is recommended.

3.1 Introduction

It has been estimated that 2–3% of all hospital admissions in Australia are medication-related and 50% of these are preventable (1, 2). A recent review of data from 44 general medical practices in New Zealand demonstrated that 10.8% of patients experienced medication-related harms over a 3-year period. Most were deemed minor; however, one in five were moderate or severe events and three patients died due to medication harm (3). The almost two million Australians that suffer an adverse event from medicines each year (4) are not all due to adverse drug reactions (ADRs), but are also caused by human and system-related errors (see Table 3.1).

Patients claiming a history of drug allergy are a daily occurrence in dental practice, so this chapter includes a description of allergy physiology and various adverse drug reactions, with detail regarding immune-mediated allergic reactions, focussing on Type 1 and 4 reactions. Further, as many claimed allergic reactions are false, how to correctly diagnose and manage actual drug allergies will also be discussed.

Table 3.1 Adverse drug events. Adapted from (6).

Adverse drug events	Subtypes
Adverse drug reactions—no error involved	**Predictable** (Type A): approx 90% of ADRs; largely dose- and time-related
	Unpredictable (Type B): approx 10% of all ADRs; not dose- and time-related; tend to be immunologically (allergy) or neurologically mediated
Medication errors—human/system error	**Human error:** knowledge gaps, process slips, memory lapses, excess self-reliance, distractions, poor handwriting, etc
	System error: process too complex; look-alike sound-alike drug names; error opportunities within multiple systems; local, state, country, and global differences

3.2 Definition of adverse drug reactions

The World Health Organization (WHO) defines an ADR as 'a response to a medicine that is noxious and unintended and occurs at doses normally used or tested in humans' (5). A more extensive definition is as 'an appreciably harmful or unpleasant reaction resulting from use of a medicinal product; adverse effects usually predict hazard from future administration and warrant prevention, or specific treatment, or alteration of the dosage regimen, or withdrawal of the product' (49). All medications have the potential to cause ADRs (7). The key is to recognise that most ADRs are spontaneous and occur as an extension of the drug's pharmacology, not because anyone has made a mistake. However, as most ADRs are predictable and therefore preventable, every effort should be made to prevent them.

Patients attending a dental practice will usually be taking medications. It has been reported that 87.1% of Australians older than 50 years take one or more medicines, with polypharmacy escalating with increasing age (8, 45). As many drugs have adverse reactions that affect the oral cavity (9, 10), and dentists prescribe medications that can cause ADRs, dentists need to be aware of the medications' side effects so these reactions can be promptly identified, prevented where possible, and reported if necessary (11). A systematic review and meta-analysis has shown that ADRs affect nearly 16% of patients during hospitalisation (12) with substantial impact on public health (45).

The vast majority of ADRs (approximately 90%) occur as an extension of the drug's known pharmacology, and these can affect any body system and tend to be dose- and time-related (46). These predictable ADRs (Type A) are related to the specific drug's pharmacology and pharmacokinetics while it is present in the body, mostly occurring on initiation or with dose increase (13).

Unpredictable (Type B) reactions are unrelated to the expected pharmacologic actions of the drug and tend to be immunologically or neurologically mediated. They can occur at any dose and may occur at any time during or after drug exposure, even after the drug has ceased (14, 46). Drug idiosyncrasy—often due to pharmacogenetic reactions where a patient has idiosyncratic drug metabolism, excretion, or bioavailability—also results in unexpected effects.

3.3 Discovery of adverse drug effects and pharmacovigilance

All drugs have the potential for adverse effects because they are not 'magic bullets' and always have the chance to affect unintended physiological sites in unintended ways. The risk of adverse reactions from a drug can be reduced by avoiding its use in at-risk patients, giving it via more localised administration, and using drugs with greater specificity of action, such as monoclonal antibodies. Unfortunately, most drugs in current clinical practice are used in a wide range of patients, administered systemically, and have broad mechanisms of action that give them a high probability of causing adverse effects. So how do we ever know the side effects of a drug?

Previously, when drugs were discovered serendipitously from the natural world, adverse effects were only discovered when they occurred. Due to the restricted use of early medicines by 'learned men' only, it took centuries for the associations to be made between ancient medicines—such as opium, arsenic, and belladonna—and their side effects. Indeed, the adverse effects of ancient drugs on pregnancy and the developing foetus were only taken seriously in the early 20th century.

Fortunately, drugs today are developed through the process of clinical trials and the protocols designed so that subjects are encouraged to report unusual or untoward symptoms as potential side effects of the tested drug. Due to the limitations of clinical trials—such as the homogenous study populations, short time frames and the exclusion of other disease states and other drugs—pre-marketing clinical trials tend to only capture common and predictable (Type A) adverse effects. Less common or rare adverse effects with a frequency of 1 in 1,000 or less are unlikely to be identified. Long-term adverse effects (often termed 'Type C') are never identified, since clinical trials are usually conducted over weeks or months, not years. The true extent and severity of adverse effects are also not found in clinical trials, as more vulnerable subjects are usually excluded, such as the elderly or those with co-morbidities.

Therefore, it is vital for health professionals to be aware that adverse effects and their predisposing risk factors continue to be elucidated after a drug is approved, made available on the open market, and used by a wide variety of people in combination with different diseases and other drugs.

By the time a drug is granted marketing approval, on average only about 1,500 patients have taken it and clinical trials will have detected only the most common side effects (15). Therefore, there is a need to continue monitoring and collecting drug safety evidence after a drug is marketed in order to discover the less frequent and unpredictable (Type B) side effects. This process is called post-marketing surveillance or 'pharmacovigilance'.

The WHO defines pharmacovigilance as 'the science and activities relating to the detection, assessment, understanding and prevention of adverse effects or any other medicine/vaccine related problem' (5). Pharmacovigilance encompasses the many drug safety monitoring activities conducted in the post-marketing period, from publication of case reports and case series in the literature, structured surveillance programs, to analysis of hospital and medical practice records to reporting of adverse drug reactions to national regulatory agencies. These data are collated by the WHO and fed back to countries for incorporation into the drug product information as post-marketing drug safety data.

The most frequently used source for information on drug adverse effects is the registered product information (PI) from the drug's manufacturer. In consulting this source, it is important to recognise some of its limitations. The PI is written to meet the legal requirements of registering the drug for marketing approval. As such, they are a legal document not a clinical guide. The adverse effect data are obtained from the manufacturer's pre-marketing clinical trials. Therefore, they tend to include only the common and largely predictable side effects and do not represent proven adverse effects of the drug. It only represents what was reported by the subjects in those clinical trials and best understood as potential adverse effects.

The reported effects of adverse reactions are usually categorised into body systems, but these are not all inclusive, nor are they reported consistently across drug monographs. Typically, there is no category for oral and dental side effects, although they may be found under categories such as gastrointestinal, dermatological or musculoskeletal.

Adverse effects identified by post-marketing pharmacovigilance are often included in a separate section in the PI entitled 'Post-marketing experience'. This section must be consulted separately from the general section on adverse effects. Adverse drug reactions from clinical trials are listed according to the MedDRA organ class system. The corresponding frequency category for each adverse drug reaction is based on the following convention:

- very common (≥1/10)
- common (≥1/100 to <1/10)
- uncommon (≥1/1,000 to <1/100)
- rare (≥1/10,000 to <1/1,000)
- very rare (<1/10,000) (16)

It is important to note that many practitioners and consumers interpret the words 'common' and 'rare' as occurring much more frequently than the manufacturers.

It is difficult to access information about specific populations, such as the very young and very old, as the PI will usually give little advice on the use of a drug in more vulnerable populations until it has been on the market for many years. Clinicians therefore should consult the medical literature or pharmacovigilance agencies for this specific type of safety advice.

3.4 Immunological mechanisms for drug allergies

Allergies, also referred to as allergic diseases, are a number of conditions which result from hypersensitivity of the immune system to typically harmless substances in the environment (16). Reactions include both true allergic and other non-allergic reactions, and they can range in severity from mild to life threatening. Hypersensitivity is a reflection of disproportionate or aberrant immune responses (17).

Several types of allergic reactions to drugs are described in the medical literature, but the Gell and Coombs classification remains the most frequently used (18). It classifies hypersensitivity reactions into four categories of which allergic drug reactions tend to either be Types 1 or 4 (see Table 3.2).

Table 3.2 The Gell and Coombs classification system for drug hypersensitivity. Adapted from (43).

Classification	Mechanism	Clinical symptoms/Examples	Timing
Type I (Immediate)	Drug-IgE complex attachment to mast cells; mast cell degranulation occurs on re-exposure to the antigen releasing histamine and other inflammatory mediators	Urticaria, angioedema, bronchospasm, wheezing, pruritus, vomiting, diarrhoea, anaphylaxis Hay fever, asthma, eczema, bee stings, food allergies	minutes to hours
Type II (Cytotoxic)	IgG or IgM antibodies are directed to drug-hapten coated cells; drug-hapten complexes can bind to RBCs and platelets and become targets for IgG antibodies and lysis by components of the immune system (e.g. macrophages, resulting in RBC lysis)	Haemolytic anaemia, neutropenia, thrombocytopenia. Rh factor incompatibility	variable
Type III (Immune complex)	Antigen and antibody complexes deposit in blood; subsequent localised inflammatory response	Serum sickness, fever, rash, arthralgias, lymphadenopathy, urticaria, glomerulonephritis, vasculitis	1–3 weeks
Type IVa	Activation and recruitment of monocytes, predominately a T helper 1 response	Erythema and dermatitis Contact dermatitis, poison ivy/oak, latex allergy	2–7 days
Type IVb	Activation and recruitment of eosinophils, mediated by T helper 2 cells	Maculopapular rash (MPR) often with peripheral blood eosinophilia DRESS: drug rash with eosinophilia and systemic symptoms	MPR: 1–several days DRESS: 2–6 weeks
Type IVc	Activation and recruitment of CD4+ or CD8+ T cells	FDE: fixed drug reaction, erythematous plaques at the same site after each exposure SJS/TEN: Stevens Johnson syndrome/toxic epidermal necrolysis	FDE: 1–2 days SJS/TEN: 4–28 days
Type IVd	Activation and recruitment of neutrophils	AGEP	Usually 1–2 days (but can be longer)

Notes: RBC: red blood cell; DRESS: drug rash with eosinophilia and systemic symptoms; SJS/TEN: Stevens Johnson syndrome/toxic epidermal necrolysis; Ig: immunoglobulin; Rh: rhesus; AGEP: acute generalised exanthematous pustulosis (19–21).

3.4.1 Type I immediate hypersensitivity reactions

Type I hypersensitivity reactions are mediated by drug-specific antibodies and occur within minutes to hours after the administration of the medicine. These results from the cross-linking of the antigen, or drug, with the IgE on mast cells and basophils resulting in their degranulation (22). Initial exposure to the antigen results in B lymphocyte activation and the production of IgE-releasing plasma cells. Subsequent exposure to the same antigen results in enhanced activation of previously sensitised mast cells. The release of vasoactive ammines, histamine, lipid mediators and cytokines from mast cells causes blood vessel dilation, enhanced permeability to vessels and smooth muscle contraction (22). Type I hypersensitivity reactions range from allergic rhinitis, allergic dermatitis, food allergy, allergic conjunctivitis, and anaphylactic shock, and can be related to drug use.

Anaphylaxis is a medical emergency that can lead to acute life-threatening respiratory failure. This Type I hypersensitivity reaction is the most severe form of an IgE-mediated acute allergic reaction that causes mast cells to release an enormous amount of histamine causing intense bronchospasm, oedema of the larynx, angioedema, rash, hives, flushing, hypotension and shock. These rapid reactions (minutes–hours) can be initiated by anything; however, in the dental setting, the most common triggers include antibiotics, analgesics and latex (23).

3.4.2 Type II cytotoxic reactions

Type II cytotoxic reactions are an antibody-dependent process where specific antibodies bind to antigens on cell surfaces leading to cell lysis, tissue damage, and subsequent functional loss (24). The drug-hapten components attach to circulating blood components, including RBCs and platelets. These circulating complexes trigger complement activation, as well as antibody-dependent cell cytotoxicity (24). Following exposure to the agent inciting this response, autoantibodies such as IgG and IgM are produced (sensitisation phase) that ultimately culminate in disease (effector phase) (25). Medications, such as penicillin, cephalosporins, thiazides, and methyldopa, bind to the cell surface and direct the immune system to recognise these modified antigens as foreign (26).

In drug-induced lupus erythematosus, anti-red blood cell or anti-dsDNA antibodies are produced after the drug attaches to red blood cells. This can be a mild to moderately severe lupus-like syndrome that is directly related to the temporal exposure to the medication and resolves upon the cessation of the trigger drug.

3.4.3 Type III immune complex reactions

Immune complexes formed from antigen–antibody aggregates cause Type III hypersensitivity reactions. These complexes precipitate in tissues, such as skin, joints and vessels, and trigger complement activation provoking an inflammatory response with the chemo-attraction of leukocytes and, ultimately, tissue damage (27). If subsequently there is inadequate clearance of these complexes, an accumulation within small blood vessels and joints can result and progress to immune complex diseases. The distinguishing feature of Type III reactions is that the antigen–antibody complexes are preformed in the circulation prior to deposition into tissue where the resultant damage occurs.

Medications implicated in Type III hypersensitivity reactions include penicillins, cephalosporins, tetracycline, lincomycin, streptomycin, metronidazole, allopurinol, barbiturates, captopril, and carbamazepine (27, 28).

3.4.4 Type IV hypersensitivity

Type IV hypersensitivity (also known as delayed hypersensitivity) is a cell-mediated immune reaction; that is, 'it does not involve the participation of antibodies but is due primarily to the interaction of T cells with antigens' (29). T-helper cells are activated by antigen presenting cells with a major histocompatibility complex (MHC) class II protein (29). Recognition of this antigen results in further activation of T-helper cells which in turn activate macrophages and cytotoxic T cells to form an inflammatory response that may include the formation of multinucleated giant cells. In general, T-cell reactions are delayed and can manifest days to weeks after the drug exposure and are less severe compared to Type I reactions. However, there are some severe delayed T-cell reactions, such as Stevens-Johnson syndrome (SJS) and toxic epidermal necrolysis (TEN), which are extremely severe, and patients should avoid the drug if these reactions occur.

3.5 Penicillin allergy

Type I hypersensitivity to penicillin, the most 'common of the serious drug reactions, may be safely and effectively evaluated in appropriate patients' (2, 30, 31, 34).

Penicillin allergy is the most recorded drug-class allergy, reported by approximately 10% of patients (32, 33). The use of a drug provocation challenge for those patients who are considered low risk of a serious drug reaction, either because of the history of their reaction with or without a negative penicillin skin test, is considered the gold standard to ensure that the patient does not have a penicillin allergy (31). It has been clearly demonstrated in a recent meta-analysis that 94% of 5,056 people undertaking such a drug provocation challenge were able to tolerate systemic penicillin, and so the overwhelming majority of adults who report a penicillin allergy can actually safely receive systemic penicillin treatment (34).

Thus, many people unnecessarily avoid penicillin antibiotics and use alternative antibiotics. These alternative antibiotics often have a broader spectrum of action, are likely to be less effective, are more toxic, have the potential to contribute to microbial antibiotic resistance, and have a higher incidence of severe adverse effects, such as clindamycin or fluoroquinolones (30, 33, 35). Penicillin is the drug of choice for many infections, being highly effective, extremely well-tolerated, and much cheaper. Penicillin-allergy referral and testing is considered an important component of antibiotic stewardship programs (33).

True IgE-mediated penicillin allergy is rare however, with only 1% of the general population reacting positively to skin testing; a further 4–5% are likely to be Type IV reactions (33). Most penicillin allergies are diagnosed from an experience in childhood and this history can persist in a patient's medical record for many years without verification. However, studies have shown that approximately 90% of penicillin allergy labels on medical records are, for many reasons, incorrect, and at most 1% of the population have a true penicillin allergy (33, 36).

The most common reason for an incorrect allergy claim is that the person wasn't allergic in the first place, with many often describing any nasty medication experience as an 'allergy'. Rashes occurring as part of viral illness can often be mistaken for a drug reaction as opposed to being part of the disease itself. This is of course compounded as penicillin in the past was frequently incorrectly given to children suffering viral illnesses. Similarly, penicillin given during an Epstein Barr infection (glandular fever) carries a high risk of triggering a rash, which is considered a drug–disease interaction, not an allergy.

Health professionals can contribute to inadequate documentation of drug reactions by only asking about drug allergies in their medical/dental history-taking but no other types of adverse drug reactions.

Another way in which a penicillin allergy label may be incorrect is that the allergy may have worn off. In fact, few allergies are lifelong; it has been shown that approximately 50% of patients with IgE-mediated penicillin allergy lose their sensitivity after 5 years and approximately 80% lose it after 10 years (2). In fact, 'individuals who have lost skin test reactivity to penicillins are at negligible risk of becoming re-sensitised when exposed again to penicillin or other β-lactam antibiotics' (36, 37).

According to Trubiano et al. (36), 'most allergy and immunology specialists can provide skin testing and challenge procedures for individuals with a history of penicillin allergy' to confirm current allergy status.

3.5.1 Managing patients who claim a penicillin allergy

Writing the term 'allergy–penicillin' should now be avoided since this terse phrase provides insufficient information to make clinical decisions. All health professionals should review patients' drug allergy claims to ensure accuracy, since true allergies require long-term abstinence, whereas ADRs can often be managed simply by reducing the dose. Three details should be documented for each adverse reaction: a) the name of the drug the patient reacted to (brand name preferred); b) the nature of the reaction; and c) how long ago the reaction occurred.

Evaluation of a drug allergy involves a risk–benefit analysis based on history, allergy test results (where available) and, if indicated, a direct challenge under medical supervision. Dentists are not expected to perform allergy testing, but they are expected to explore a patient's drug allergy history, which should reveal enough information to be able to rate it as a low-, medium- or high-risk category (Table 3.3).

True penicillin allergy has the potential for cross-reactivity with other β-lactam antibiotics, such as cefalosporins, carbapenems and monobactams. Historically, it was thought that cross-reactivity of the penicillin antibiotics with cephalosporin antibiotics occurred at a rate of 10% due to the common β-lactam ring central to the structure of both antibiotic groups. However, research over the past 10 years has shown that it is the similarity of the R1 side chains attached to the β-lactam ring that largely determines which antibiotics exhibit cross-reactivity. It has now been shown that previously reported cross-reactivity between penicillins and cephalosporins may have been due to the fact that prior to 1980 many cephalosporins were contaminated with trace amounts of penicillin, thus overestimating the cross-reactivity (38).

Table 3.3 Risk stratification for penicillin allergy evaluation and treatment. Adapted from (48).

	Low risk [#]	Medium risk [##]	High risk [###]
History	Isolated adverse effects unlikely to be allergic, such as GI upset, headache, sedation, dizziness, itch without rash Reactions more than 10 years old with no features of IgE* Family history alone History of safe use of penicillin, despite claiming allergy	Urticaria or other itchy rashes Reactions with features of IgE, but not anaphylaxis	Anaphylactic symptoms Positive skin testing Recurrent reactions Reactions to multiple β-lactam antibiotics
Action	Prescribe unrelated cephalosporin or clindamycin Refer patients for review of penicillin allergy claim and testing if appropriate, depending on their reported reaction	Prescribe unrelated cephalosporin or clindamycin Recommend referral to allergy/infectious disease/immunology specialist for testing if allergic	Do not prescribe penicillin or cephalosporin Prescribe clindamycin or other indicated antibiotic Consider allergy/immunology referral for desensitisation

Notes:

* IgE features classically include cutaneous symptoms, such as itching, flushing, urticaria and angioedema, but also concomitant respiratory symptoms (rhinitis, wheezing, shortness of breath, bronchospasm), cardiovascular symptoms (arrhythmia, syncope, chest tightness), and severe GI symptoms (abdominal pain, nausea, vomiting, diarrhoea).

[#] Low risk: Low-risk histories are those citing non-allergic symptoms (e.g. GI symptoms), pruritus without rash, a family history of penicillin allergy, or remote (>10 years) unknown reactions without features suggestive of an IgE-mediated reaction. Patients with a low-risk history can generally be assured they are not allergic and can be prescribed penicillin or an unrelated cephalosporin.

[##] Medium risk: Medium-risk histories are those where urticaria (hives), other itchy rashes or reactions with features of IgE-mediated reactions (e.g. swelling, but not anaphylaxis) are reported. These patients can most likely be re-exposed to penicillin but only after testing has been conducted and the absence of penicillin allergy confirmed medically.

[###] High risk: These reactions are those where patients have experienced immediate or rapid onset of severe reactions, either through treatment or testing, for whom life-long avoidance of penicillin is preferred. Desensitisation to the specific drug can be conducted if penicillin treatment is necessary.

Prescribers previously considered that up to 20% of people would be allergic to both classes of antibiotics; it is now known that cross-reactivity between penicillins and cefalosporins occurs in 0.5–2% of patients and this is thought to be almost exclusively with cefalosporins that have similar R1 groups. In dentistry, the commonly prescribed penicillin antibiotics, amoxicillin and ampicillin, and the cephalosporins, cephalexin and cefaclor, have similar R1 side chains and exhibit cross-reactivity. For patients in a high-risk allergy group, both should be avoided (Table 3.4).

Table 3.4 Grouping penicillins and cefalosporins with similar R1 side chains: cross-reactions between agents in each group is possible.

Group 1	Group 2	Group 3	Group 4
Benzylpenicillin Cefalothin Cefoxitin	Amoxicillin Ampicillin Cefaclor Cefalexin	Cefepime Ceftizoxime Cefpirome Cefotaxime Cefpodoxime	Cefazolin

Therefore, if a patient gives a history of a previous non-severe, non-IgE-mediated penicillin reaction, cefalosporins and carbapenems with dissimilar side chains can be prescribed. Patients who have had a delayed severe penicillin or cephalosporin hypersensitivity reaction (e.g. DRESS, SJS, or TEN) should avoid all penicillins and cephalosporins.

3.6 Allergy to local anaesthetics

True IgE-mediated allergic reactions to local anaesthetics (LAs) are extremely rare (39). Nevertheless, many dental patients are labelled allergic and subsequently not provided these critical drugs. Mostly this is due to a previous non-allergic adverse reaction such as vasovagal responses, adrenaline reactions caused by inadvertent intravenous injection, or simply the anxiety associated with both the actual injection and the planned post-anaesthetic procedure (40).

There is some cross-reactivity among ester-type LAs, but none between amide LAs and there is no cross-reactivity between esters and amides (38). If the reaction history is consistent with a possible Type I reaction, skin testing followed by graded rechallenge testings should be performed with the same (adrenaline-free) LA intended for use (38). While there may be differences between the reported graded challenge procedures, a rapid and convenient protocol may consist of: a) an initial skin prick testing with the undiluted anaesthetic (then wait for 20 minutes to check reaction); b) if negative then administer an intradermal injection 0.04mL of 1:100 dilution of LA (then wait 20 minutes); c) if negative then administer a 1.0mL subcutaneous injection of saline as a placebo (then wait 20 minutes); d) if negative then administer 1.0mL of LA and observe the patient for 20 minutes (38, 41). There are reports that false-positive intra-cutaneous results can occur (42). Further, in very rare instances, individuals can have a positive skin test response to the methylparabens present in LAs, and some of these can be false-positive (41). It has been recommended to use a preservative-free LA for the skin testing/graded challenge for these patients. This type of testing should only be conducted by an appropriately trained medical specialist.

3.7 When to report ADRs

Dentists should report any suspected ADRs they encounter to the relevant national body to aid greater awareness and better understanding of drug tolerability. In Australia, reports can easily be submitted online at: tga.gov.au/reporting-adverse-events, and in New Zealand at: medsafe.govt.nz/regulatory/devicesnew/9adverseevent.asp. See Section 15.18 for more detail on reporting ADRs.

Post-marketing surveillance of drug safety relies on voluntary reporting of adverse effects by the public and health professionals to detect and quantify side effects after a drug is marketed. For example, MRONJ, associated with drugs such as bisphosphonates and denosumab, was only identified through post-marketing reporting. It is not necessary to be certain or prove an adverse event is drug-induced before reporting it. If the practitioner is suspicious that an adverse event has occurred as a result of a drug, then that is sufficient for it to be reported.

FURTHER READING

Devchand M, Trubiano JA. Penicillin allergy: a practical approach to assessment and prescribing. *Aust Prescr*. 2019;42(6):192–199.
Rose L, Hamm EMJ. Drug Allergy: Delayed Cutaneous Hypersensitivity Reactions to Drugs. *Allergy Immunol*. 2016;1(1):92–101.

REFERENCES

1. Roughead EE, Semple SJ. Medication safety in acute care in Australia: where are we now? Part 1: a review of the extent and causes of medication problems 2002–2008. *Aust New Zealand Health Policy*. 2009;6:18.
2. Lim R, Semple S, Ellett LK, Roughead L. *Medicine Safety: Take Care*. Pharmaceutical Society of Australia Ltd; 2019.
3. Leitch S, Dovey SM, Cunningham WK et al. Medication-related harm in New Zealand general practice: a retrospective records review. *Br J Gen Pract*. 2021;71(709):e626–e633.
4. Roughead EE, Lexchin J. Adverse drug events: counting is not enough, action is needed. *Med J Aust*. 2006;184:315–316.
5. World Health Organization. *Safety of Medicines: A Guide to Detecting and Reporting Adverse Drug Reactions—Why Health Professional Need to Take Action*. 2018. http://apps.who.int/medicinedocs/en/d/Jh2992e/
6. Coleman JJ, Pontefract SK. Adverse drug reactions. *Clin Med (Lond)*. 2016;16(5):481–485.
7. Editorial Advisory Committee. *Australian Medicines Handbook*. Australian Medicines Handbook Pty Ltd; 2022.
8. Morgan TK, Williamson M, Pirotta M, Stewart K, Myers SP, Barnes J. A national census of medicines use: a 24-hour snapshot of Australians aged 50 years and older. *Med J Aust*. 2012;196(1):50–53.
9. Teoh L, Moses G, McCullough MJ. A review and guide to drug-associated oral adverse effects—Dental, salivary and neurosensory reactions. Part 1. *J Oral Pathol Med*. 2019;48(7):626–636.
10. Teoh L, Moses G, McCullough MJ. A review and guide to drug-associated oral adverse effects—Oral mucosal and lichenoid reactions. Part 2. *J Oral Pathol Med*. 2019;48(7):637–646.
11. Teoh L, Stewart K, Marino R, McCullough M. Antibiotic resistance and relevance to general dental practice in Australia. *Aust Dent J*. 2018;63(4):414–421.

12. Miguel A, Azevedo LF, Araujo M, Pereira AC. Frequency of adverse drug reactions in hospitalized patients: a systematic review and meta-analysis. *Pharmacoepidemiol Drug Saf.* 2012;21(11):1139–1154.

13. Smith A, Al-Mahdi R, Malcolm W, Palmer N, Dahlen G, Al-Haroni M. Comparison of antimicrobial prescribing for dental and oral infections in England and Scotland with Norway and Sweden and their relative contribution to national consumption 2010–2016. *BMC Oral Health.* 2020;20(1):172.

14. Macy E, Blumenthal KG. Are Cephalosporins Safe for Use in Penicillin Allergy without Prior Allergy Evaluation? *J Allergy Clin Immunol Pract.* 2018;6(1):82–89.

15. Stricker BH, Psaty BM. Detection, verification, and quantification of adverse drug reactions. *BMJ.* 2004;329(7456):44–47.

16. MIMS. *Data Version.* August 2021. https://www.mims.com.au

17. Samuelsson B. Leukotrienes: mediators of immediate hypersensitivity reactions and inflammation. *Science.* 1983;220(4597):568–575.

18. Gell PGH. *Clinical Aspects of Immunology.* Blackwell; 1963.

19. Solensky RK, Khan D, Bernstein L et al. Drug allergy: An updated practice parameter. *Annals of Allergy, Asthma, and Immunology.* 2010;105(4):259–273.

20. Riedl MA, Casillas AM. Adverse drug reactions: types and treatment options. *Am Fam Physician.* 2003;68(9):1781–1790.

21. Hamm RL. Drug-hypersensitivity syndrome: diagnosis and treatment. *J Am Coll Clin Wound Spec.* 2011;3(4):77–81.

22. Ishizaka K, Ishizaka T. Immune mechanisms of reversed type reaginic hypersensitivity. *The Journal of Immunology.* 1969;103(3):588–595.

23. Tarlo SM, Sussman GL, Holness DL. Latex sensitivity in dental students and staff: a cross-sectional study. *Journal of Allergy and Clinical Immunology.* 1997;99(3):396–400.

24. Bajwa SF, Mohammed RHA. *Type II Hypersensitivity Reaction.* StatPearls Publishing; 2021.

25. Tomasiak-Łozowska MM, Klimek M, Lis A, Moniuszko M, Bodzenta-Łukaszyk A. Markers of anaphylaxis—a systematic review. *Adv Med Sci.* 2018;63(2):265–277.

26. Viel S, Pescarmona R, Belot A et al. A Case of Type 2 Hypersensitivity to Rasburicase Diagnosed with a Natural Killer Cell Activation Assay. *Front Immunol.* 2018;9:110.

27. Usman N, Annamaraju P. *Type III Hypersensitivity Reaction.* StatPearls Publishing; 2021.

28. Patterson-Fortin J, Harris CM, Niranjan-Azadi A, Melia M. Serum sickness-like reaction after the treatment of cellulitis with amoxicillin/clavulanate. *BMJ Case Rep.* 2016. doi:10.1136/bcr-2016-217608

29. Sommer S, Wilkinson S, Beck M, English J, Gawkrodger D, Green C. Type IV hypersensitivity reactions to natural rubber latex: results of a multicentre study. *British Journal of Dermatology.* 2002;146(1):114–117.

30. Sogn DD, Evans R 3rd, Shepherd GM et al. Results of the National Institute of Allergy and Infectious Diseases Collaborative Clinical Trial to test the predictive value of skin testing with major and minor penicillin derivatives in hospitalized adults. *Arch Intern Med.* 1992;152(5):1025–1032.

31. Torres MJ, Adkinson NF Jr, Caubet JC et al. Controversies in Drug Allergy: Beta-Lactam Hypersensitivity Testing. *J Allergy Clin Immunol Pract.* 2019;7(1):40–45.

32. Bourke J, Pavlos R, James I, Phillips E. Improving the Effectiveness of Penicillin Allergy De-labeling. *J Allergy Clin Immunol Pract.* 2015;3(3):365–334.e1. doi:10.1016j .jaip.2014.11002

33. Devchand M, Trubiano JA. Penicillin allergy: a practical approach to assessment and prescribing. *Aust Prescr.* 2019;42(6):192–199.

34. DesBiens M, Scalia P, Ravikumar S et al. A Closer Look at Penicillin Allergy History: Systematic Review and Meta-Analysis of Tolerance to Drug Challenge. *Am J Med.* 2020;133(4):452–462.

35. Macy E, Contreras R. Health care use and serious infection prevalence associated with penicillin 'allergy' in hospitalized patients: A cohort study. *J Allergy Clin Immunol.* 2014;133(3):790–796.

36. Trubiano JA, Adkinson NF, Phillips EJ. Penicillin Allergy Is Not Necessarily Forever. *JAMA.* 2017;318(1):82–83.

37. Solensky R, Earl HS, Gruchalla RS. Lack of penicillin resensitization in patients with a history of penicillin allergy after receiving repeated penicillin courses. *Arch Intern Med.* 2002;162(7):822–826.

38. Khan DA, Solensky R. Drug allergy. *J Allergy Clin Immunol.* 2010;125(2 Suppl 2):S126– S137. doi:10.1016/j.jaci.2009.10.028

39. Venemalm L, Degerbeck F, Smith W. IgE-mediated reaction to mepivacaine. *J Allergy Clin Immunol.* 2008;121:1058–1059.

40. Berkun Y, Ben-Zvi A, Levy Y, Galili D, Shalit M. Evaluation of adverse reactions to local anesthetics: experience with 236 patients. *Ann Allergy Asthma Immunol.* 2003;91(4):342–345.

41. Macy E, Schatz M, Zeiger R. Immediate hypersensitivity to methylparaben causing false-positive results of local anesthetic skin testing or provocative dose testing. *Permanente J.* 2002;6:17–21.

42. Incaudo G, Schatz M, Patterson R, Rosenberg M, Yamamoto F, Hamburger RN. Administration of local anesthetics to patients with a history of prior adverse reaction. *J Allergy Clin Immunol.* 1978;61(5):339–345.

43. Hamm RL. Drug Allergy: Delayed Cutaneous Hypersensitivity Reactions to Drugs. *EMJ Allergy Immunol.* 2016;1(1):92–101.

44. Theraputic Guidelines Limited. *Antimicrobial hypersensitivity.* 2019. www.tg.org.au

45. Teoh L. *Dental therapeutic guideline adherence in Australia.* PhD Thesis. University of Melbourne; 2020. http://hdl.handle.net/11343/265857

46. Australian Dental Association. *The epidemic of over-reported penicillin allergy.* Accessed February 25, 2019. https://staging.ada.org.au/News-Media/News-and-Release/Latest-News/The-epidemic-of-over-reported-penicillin-allergy

47. Encyclopedia Britannica. *Type IV hypersensitivity.* https://www.britannica.com/science/immune-system-disorder/Type-IV-hypersensitivity

48. Shenoy E, Macy E, Rowe T, Blumenthal K. Evaluation and Management of Penicillin Allergy: A Review. *JAMA.* 2019;321(2):188–199.

49. Aronson JK. Ferner RE. Clarification of terminology in drug safety. *Drug Saf.* 2005;28:851–870.

ANTIMICROBIALS

4

KEY POINTS

- The most important measure in managing dental infections is active dental treatment to address the underlying cause (e.g. extraction of the tooth or root canal treatment). Antibiotics are only adjunctive to dental treatment and are appropriate where the infection shows signs of systemic spread for an otherwise healthy patient.
- Narrow-spectrum antibiotics have been shown to be as effective as broad-spectrum antibiotics for empirical management of non-severe odontogenic infections in otherwise healthy patients, as long as dental treatment is also carried out to address the underlying cause.
- An Australian study showed that 55% of antibiotics prescribed by dentists were unnecessary, which demonstrated that antibiotic stewardship is required in dentistry.
- Antibiotic stewardship involves strategies to improve the use of antibiotics, including prescribing antibiotics with the narrowest but most appropriate spectrum, for the right indication, in the right dose, at the right frequency, and for the right duration.
- Prevention of infective endocarditis should be focused on maintaining good oral hygiene to reduce gingival inflammation, as the cumulative bacteraemia caused by daily activities such as toothbrushing is far greater than the bacteraemia generated during dental procedures.

4.1 Introduction

An antimicrobial is defined as a drug that kills, prevents, or inhibits the growth of any type of microorganism (1). These drugs originate from a variety of sources, including microorganisms, plants, animals, and can be semi-synthetic or synthetic. Antimicrobials can be antibacterial, antimycobacterial, antifungal, antiparasitic and antiviral (2). Strictly speaking, the term 'antibiotic' refers to an agent produced by a microorganism that kills another microorganism; it does not include synthetic substances (3). However, this specific meaning is often not emphasised in clinical practice. Therefore, in this book, the terms 'antibacterial' and 'antibiotic' will be used interchangeably.

4.2 General principles of antibiotic use in dentistry

Antibiotic use in dentistry is generally limited to a narrow range of circumstances. The fundamental principle of managing a dental infection is to address the source of infection by drainage, endodontics, exodontia or periodontal treatment. To manage dental infections, an accurate diagnosis is needed, followed by treatment of the source of infection (4). In general, the use of antibiotics in dentistry is adjunctive to active dental treatment when infections have spread from their localised area or if the person is immunocompromised.

Antimicrobial therapy is employed in one of three ways: prophylaxis, empirical therapy and directed therapy (4).

1. **Prophylaxis:** Antimicrobial prophylaxis in dentistry is used either to prevent infection at a distant site, such as the cardiac valves, or to prevent infection at a surgical site (5).

2. **Empirical therapy:** The most common method of prescribing antimicrobials in dentistry is empirical therapy. Here, the choice of antimicrobial is made by following prescribing guidelines recommending antimicrobials targeting the microorganisms most likely to cause that specific dental infection (4). Dentists rarely conduct microbiological investigation of bacterial isolates, although this practice does take place in specialist practices and hospitals. While identification of specific pathogens in community-based dental practice would be ideal prior to antimicrobial prescription, current systems take 2–3 days to provide this information, so empirical treatment is necessary to treat the infection as soon as possible.

3. **Directed therapy:** Directed antimicrobial therapy occurs when the specific causative pathogen and its antimicrobial sensitivities have been identified for a particular infection (4). From this, the most appropriate antimicrobial can be directed to target the precise cause of the infection. Directed therapy is usually only required in hospital settings to treat resistant or severe spreading infections.

4.3 Antimicrobial resistance

Antimicrobial resistance (AMR) occurs where pathogens (bacteria, fungi, viruses, parasites, helminths) develop the capability to survive or grow despite the presence of antimicrobials, making the antimicrobial ineffective (1). The microbial genes that code for antimicrobial resistance can then be passed and spread to other microorganisms promoting further resistance.

AMR is a well-known major public health issue, responsible for 700,000 deaths worldwide annually (6). Widespread use of antimicrobials is the main driver of the development and selection of AMR—the more antimicrobials are used, the greater the contribution towards AMR. Broader-spectrum antimicrobials contribute more towards resistance than narrow-spectrum, and longer durations of therapy contribute more than shorter durations. All prescribers have a professional responsibility to use and prescribe antimicrobials judiciously and only when necessary to minimise their contribution to AMR. The most common antimicrobials prescribed in dentistry are antibacterials.

4.3.1 Ecology of antibacterial resistance

The ability of bacteria to acquire resistance is a natural consequence of antibacterial use and developed as an evolutionary attribute of bacteria for survival purposes (7, 31). Bacteria develop resistance by selective pressure. With increased exposure to antibiotics, resistant strains are more likely to survive, develop, and multiply (7, 8). When exposure to antibiotics is reduced, resistant strains are eventually diluted out and susceptible strains repopulate. The degree of selective pressure, and thus the magnitude of formation of resistant bacteria, is directly influenced by the density of antibacterial use (7–9). Broad-spectrum antibiotics and prolonged duration of antibacterial therapy are therefore more likely to promote resistant strains, as they select for a wider range of bacteria and allow more time for the bacteria to develop AMR (10).

4.3.2 Mechanisms of antibiotic resistance

There are two ways in which bacteria become resistant to antibiotics: by intrinsic or acquired resistance (Table 4.1). Intrinsic resistance occurs where the entire species of bacteria possess a property that renders the antibiotic ineffective to bacteria (11). An example is mycobacteria's resistance to penicillins. Penicillin antibiotics target the penicillin-binding proteins on bacterial cell walls. Bacteria without a cell wall, such as *Mycoplasma* spp., are therefore not susceptible to this action and are naturally resistant.

Table 4.1 Mechanisms of resistance (9).

Type of resistance	Features
Intrinsic	• Characteristic property of the microorganism that renders the antibiotic resistance • Entire species will be resistant

Acquired	• Does not affect the entire species and will only be seen in some strains
	• Can occur by two methods:
	  1. Spontaneous chromosomal mutation
	    • Changes to the DNA occur as a spontaneous event
	    • Chromosomal mutations passed down to daughter cells (i.e. transferred vertically)
	  2. Horizontal gene transmission
	    • Transformation
	    • Transduction
	    • Conjugation

In contrast, acquired resistance does not occur in the entire species of bacteria but only in those which have acquired drug resistance genes either spontaneously or by vertical or horizontal transmission. Spontaneous chromosomal mutations of bacterial DNA can occur independent of the presence of antibiotics but rendering affected bacteria resistant to certain antibacterials. The chromosomal mutations encoded for resistant genes can be passed down to daughter cells as the bacterium divides. This form of resistance is therefore transferred vertically and the rate of transfer is reliant on how fast the bacteria can multiply.

The second method is where bacteria acquire resistant genes from other bacteria by horizontal gene transfer. They can either be transferred between the same or different species by transformation, transduction and conjugation—all of which result in the transfer of DNA-resistant gene segments (7). Horizontal gene transfer is thought to be the most concerning method, as it does not rely on the multiplication rate of bacteria and allows the development of multidrug-resistant bacteria.

4.3.3 Types of resistance

There are four methods by which bacterial gene expression confers resistance to antibiotics. These are:

1. Alteration of the bacteria's binding site for the antibiotic.
2. Changes to the porin channels which restrict the antibiotic from entering the cell.
3. Active extrusion of the antibiotic from the interior of a bacterial cell by an efflux pump.
4. Enzymatic inactivation or destruction of the antibiotic (12).

Figure 4.1 Resistance mechanisms of bacteria.

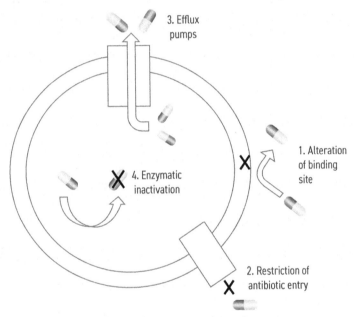

In dentistry, penicillins are the most commonly prescribed antibiotics (13–15). Penicillins and cephalosporins are known as β-lactam antibiotics, as they both possess a four-membered β-lactam ring central to their structure (see Section 4.7.1). The main type of resistance to β-lactam antibiotics occurs when bacteria produce β-lactamase enzymes. These enzymes catalyse breakage of the β-lactam ring, rendering the β-lactam antibiotic ineffective (3, 9). In a South Australian study, penicillin-resistant organisms were found to be present in approximately 11% of patients hospitalised for treatment of severe odontogenic infections (16). Penicillin-resistant odontogenic infections are associated with longer hospital stays, increased healthcare costs and poorer clinical outcomes (16, 17).

4.4 Antimicrobial stewardship

Antimicrobial stewardship has several definitions, including a 'coherent set of actions that promote the responsible use of antimicrobials' (2) and an Australian definition of 'the safe and appropriate use of antimicrobials to reduce harm while also curtailing the incidence of antimicrobial resistance' (1). With a declining number of new antibiotics in development, the focus in practice is on appropriate, judicious and prudent use of existing antibacterials.

Antibiotic stewardship (ABS) programs aim to promote appropriate prescribing of antibiotics. As overprescribing is common, reducing inappropriate prescribing often correlates with a reduction in antibiotic use (18, 19). The key steps to ABS are establishing legitimate need for an antibiotic for a patient's clinical condition, followed by appropriate selection of the antibacterial and its regimen (including dose, duration and frequency) according to evidence-based guidance.

Antibiotic prescribing by dentists account for approximately 10% of all prescribed antibiotics worldwide (20). In Australia, approximately 55% of dental antibiotic prescriptions are unnecessarily prescribed (21). In the US and UK, it has been reported that up to 80% of antibiotics prescribed in dentistry are unnecessary or not in accordance with guidance for both prophylactic and therapeutic purposes respectively (22, 23). As a result, it is recommended that dentists are included in ABS programs.

It is recognised that many factors, both clinical and non-clinical, influence inappropriate dental antibiotic prescription. Clinical factors include prescribing for localised infections where dental treatment alone would be sufficient, or prescribing for scenarios where antibiotics are unnecessary, such as for alveolar osteitis (21, 24). Non-clinical factors that influence dental antibiotic prescription include medico-legal concerns, clinical time pressure and patient expectations (21, 24).

While most antimicrobial stewardship programs are implemented in hospital settings, most dental antibiotic prescribing occurs in the community. Some examples of ABS programs in dentistry include clinical audit and feedback, implementation of clinical decision-making support tools, and targeted education to both prescribers and patients. While some factors that influence antibiotic overprescribing in medicine and dentistry are similar, there are some that are specific to dentistry, mostly because dentistry is primarily a surgical discipline where procedures are almost always needed to resolve infections (25). ABS programs therefore need to be designed for the specific dental context (20).

4.5 Antibiotics

4.5.1 Microbiology of dental infections

The oral cavity is inhabited by about 700 different species of bacteria, being a combination of commensal and pathogenic organisms. Microbial growth is sustained by sugars and amino acids derived from food and saliva (26). Odontogenic infections are polymicrobial in composition consisting of aerobes, facultative anaerobes and strict anaerobes. Examples of pathogenic species identified include *Fusobacterium, Peptostreptococcus, Porphyromonas, Prevotella* spp., and *Streptococcus* (27, 28). Periodontal infections tend to be dominated by anaerobic bacteria, including *Fusobacterium, Porphyromonas*, and *Prevotella* spp.

4.5.2 Bactericidal versus bacteriostatic

Bactericidal antibiotics kill bacteria, whereas bacteriostatic antibiotics prevent bacterial replication. In clinical practice, however, antibiotics are not chosen based on their bactericidal or bacteriostatic ability. The aim of using antibiotics is to make it easier for the patient's immune system to overcome the infection. Antibiotic choice in dentistry is based on the appropriate spectrum, the need for antibiotics in the specific clinical scenario, and recommendations from local guidelines (3).

4.5.3 Duration of antibiotic use

The most appropriate duration of antibiotic use in dentistry has not been established, although several studies show that shorter courses (three days) are as effective as longer courses for non-severe primary space odontogenic infections, provided that drainage has been established (27). Various guidelines recommend five days of antibiotic treatment of odontogenic infections (4, 29). As mentioned previously, the most important factor in controlling dental infections is addressing the cause, either by drainage through the root canal, soft tissue or by extraction.

4.6 Antibiotic prophylaxis

4.6.1 Principles of antibiotic prophylaxis for infective endocarditis

Infective endocarditis (IE) is a rare but serious condition with high morbidity and mortality of up to 25% (30, 31). The pathophysiology of infective endocarditis involves the entry of microorganisms into the blood stream which then adhere to a pre-existing defect on the surface of the endocardium of the cardiac valve, leading to formation of platelet-fibrin vegetation on the surface of cardiac tissue due to the turbulent flow of blood over the tissue (31, 32). Major complications of IE include stroke, pulmonary embolus and heart failure from the combination of thrombus formation and valvular dysfunction, and the incidence is reported to be 5–10 people per 100,000 per annum (33). Emboli in the brain, lung, spleen or extremities occur in up to 30% of patients and can be the presenting sign (34). Strains of oral microorganisms most commonly implicated in the development of IE are *Streptococci*, *Staphylococci* and *Enterococci*. The most common individual bacteria associated with IE in non-intravenous drug users are viridans *Streptococci*, which are also a well-known commensal of the gingival crevice. Intact oral epithelium normally prevents entry of bacteria into the circulation; however, a breach in the mucosal layer can allow the entry of oral bacteria into the blood stream.

Because of this, it is thought there may be a link between bacteria entering the systemic circulation during a dental procedure and the subsequent development of IE. Guidelines have been developed recommending the use of high-dose prophylactic antibiotics given to a high-risk patient prior to a dental procedure to reduce the risk of developing IE. The benefit of antibiotic prophylaxis (AP) to prevent IE is unknown, as it is based on expert opinion rather than evidence from controlled trials (30). A Cochrane Collaboration systematic review concluded that there is no evidence to demonstrate whether AP to prevent bacterial endocarditis from a dental procedure is effective (35). Other reviews also have found no benefit (36), although a further study concluded it was unclear as to whether AP is effective but appears that it may have a small impact (33).

It is recognised in dentistry that bacteraemia can also occur during daily activities such as chewing food and toothbrushing. Focusing on dental procedures as the sole source of oral pathogen bacteraemia is not evidence-based. Poor oral hygiene with the presence of plaque and gingival inflammation significantly increases the prevalence of bacteraemia after toothbrushing (37). Thus, the emphasis in IE prevention has been on maintaining good oral hygiene to reduce gingival inflammation.

4.6.2 Guidelines for IE worldwide

Due to inconsistent evidence for the effectiveness of AP, high prevalence of unnecessary antibiotic use and the need to reduce risk of adverse drug reactions, most antibiotic prophylaxis guidelines for IE prevention have shifted towards targeting high-risk patients and high-risk procedures. For example, the procedure-related risk of developing IE has been determined to be around 1:14,000,000 for dental procedures in the general population compared to 1:95,000 in patients who have had previous IE (31, 38).

Guidelines for AP differ worldwide. The American Heart Association recommends the use of prophylactic antibiotics for high-risk patients and high-risk procedures (39). The Australian *Therapeutic Guidelines Oral and Dental (Version 3)* similarly only recommend the use of prophylactic antibiotics for a specific set of high-risk patients undergoing high-risk procedures, with some differences for the Australian context; specifically, Indigenous people with rheumatic heart disease undergoing certain high-risk procedures (4).

Utilising the same principles, the European Society of Cardiology produced similar guidelines where prophylaxis is limited to high-risk patients (31, 38). The National Institute for Health and Care Excellence guidelines in the UK are markedly different from the rest of the world: IE antibiotic prophylaxis is not recommended for any patient, although dentists can exercise their own clinical judgement for certain high-risk cases (31, 40). All guidelines incorporate the principles of the frequency and cumulative bacteraemia from normal daily activities and emphasise the importance of maintaining oral hygiene and preventive care (4, 38, 39).

4.6.3 Principles of surgical antibiotic prophylaxis

AP for surgery is the use of antibiotics to prevent development of infection at a surgical site where no established bacterial infection is present (5). Surgical AP is indicated if the patient has an increased risk of developing a postoperative infection or would experience increased morbidity if postoperative infection developed (41). The need for antibiotics should be balanced against the risk of allergic and adverse reactions, toxicity and increased bacterial resistance (42).

In general, surgical AP is rarely required for dental procedures. Surgical antibiotic prophylaxis is determined on an individual patient basis depending on the procedure and the patient's risk factors, which should be discussed with the relevant medical team (4). For example, AP for patients with orthopaedic joint replacements is not warranted (43); AP would only be required if prophylaxis is indicated for the procedure or other risk factors rather than the joint replacement (4).

A Cochrane Review of antibiotic prophylaxis to prevent complications following tooth extractions found that antibiotic prophylaxis probably reduces infection risk, but 12 patients needed to be treated with antibiotics prior to impacted third molar extractions to prevent one postoperative infection (42). Therefore, clinicians should consider carefully whether treating 12 healthy patients with antibiotics to prevent one infection is likely to do more harm than good (42). This should discourage the use of routine AP in low-risk patients. This review also found that AP in patients who have undergone impacted third molar extractions does not prevent the development of fever, swelling or trismus one week after the procedure (42).

Current guidelines do not recommend the routine use of antibiotics for surgical prophylaxis; rather, complex cases should be assessed individually and discussed with the treating medical physician, with careful consideration of both procedural and patient risk factors (4). Antibiotics can be considered in cases where the risk of antibiotic adverse effects is outweighed by the risk of infections and/or consequences of the infection. Examples of such cases are a patient with immune compromise, or a patient with a reduced or impaired bone healing ability undergoing a complicated extraction with a difficult bone impaction (5).

With the exception of some major surgical procedures and medical conditions, a course of postoperative antibiotics (intravenous or oral) following extractions is not beneficial and only increases the risk of adverse effects (e.g. *C. difficile* infections) and bacterial resistance (41).

4.6.4 Principles of antibiotic prophylaxis for MRONJ

AP has not been shown to be effective in prevention of medication-related osteonecrosis of the jaw (MRONJ) for low-risk patients. Active infections should be treated, but the role of bacteria in the pathogenesis of MRONJ is still unclear.

The International Task Force on MRONJ recognises that bacteria are present in the necrotic MRONJ tissue and biofilms, but it is unclear if necrosis precedes or follows infection; the exact role of bacteria in the pathophysiology of MRONJ is unclear (44). Various studies trialling the use of antibiotic prophylaxis for MRONJ were reviewed and the authors concluded that antibiotic prophylaxis was beneficial (45, 88). However, there was no consensus on the most appropriate antibiotic and dosage, and the authors stated that sparse clinical data and lack of randomised controlled trials make it difficult to definitely identify the most appropriate protocol, with poor quality evidence available (45). Lastly, a Cochrane Review showed that prophylactic antibiotics may be beneficial but evidence supporting this was low, and this referred to only one trial of MRONJ in men with prostate cancer being treated with zoledronic acid; other medications associated with MRONJ were not included (46). Therefore, there is a lack of good quality clinical data to support the effectiveness of AP for prevention of MRONJ. AP would only be required if prophylaxis is indicated for the procedure or other risk factors (4).

4.6.5 Principles of AP for implant placement

AP prior to placing implants to prevent infection at the surgical site and reduce implant failure is controversial, and further research is still required to ascertain the benefit.

Evidence from studies in a Cochrane Review in 2013 showed that while it was unknown if postoperative antibiotics had any efficacy in reducing implant failures, there may be some benefit with prophylactic antibiotics. However, the studies showed that giving 25 patients prophylactic antibiotics was required to prevent failure of an implant in one patient (47). Several systematic reviews have found that prophylactic antibiotics in healthy subjects undergoing implant placement do not appear to improve clinical outcomes, and do not recommend the use of antibiotics routinely in healthy patients (48, 49). In addition, there is no standardised guide for the use of AP or the most effective regimen (50).

4.6.6 Duration, timing and doses for AP

The timing and route of administration of AP is crucial to achieve effective plasma and tissue concentrations at the time of procedure (41).

The recommended doses for commonly used antibiotics in dentistry for prophylaxis are shown in Table 4.2.

Table 4.2 Doses, timing and administration of commonly used antibiotics for prophylaxis in dentistry. Based on (4, 14).

Antibiotic	Route of administration	
	Oral	Intravenous
Amoxicillin	Adult: 2g, 1 hour prior to the procedure Child: 50mg/kg up to 2g, 1 hour prior to the procedure	Adult: 2g, within 1 hour prior to the procedure Child: 50mg/kg up to 2g, within 1 hour prior to the procedure
Cefalexin	Adult: 2g, 1 hour prior to the procedure Child: 50mg/kg up to 2g, 1 hour prior to the procedure	Not applicable
Cephazolin*	Not applicable	Adult: 2g, within 1 hour prior to the procedure Child: 30mg/kg up to 2g, within 1 hour prior to procedure
Clindamycin	Adult: 600mg, 1–2 hours prior to the procedure Child: 20mg/kg up to 600mg, 1–2 hours prior to the procedure	Adult: 600mg, within 2 hours prior to the procedure Child: 20mg/kg up to 600mg, within 2 hours prior to the procedure

Note:

* Can be used when oral administration is not possible, and the patient has a hypersensitivity reaction to penicillin but not cephalosporins.

For most dental procedures requiring AP only a single preoperative dose is needed. AP is considered effective from the time peak concentrations are reached, which is around one hour after administration for most antibiotics used in dentistry. AP efficacy lasts for two half-lives of the antibiotic, measured from the time the dose is administered, not from the time the procedure starts (41).

As timely management of these patients is crucial, it is incumbent on dentists to schedule the procedure at a time that ensures the patient takes the AP dose appropriately. To ensure appropriate AP timing, it is often recommended the antibiotic be administered to the patient at the dental practice under supervision.

Using amoxicillin as an example, its onset of peak plasma levels occurs one hour after oral administration and its half-life is one hour (see Table 4.3). Effective prophylaxis will last two half-lives, which for amoxicillin is two hours. Thus, if amoxicillin is administered at 9am, the procedure should take place between 10am and 11am as this is when plasma concentrations will be optimal for prophylaxis.

Table 4.3 Optimal timing for effective AP after administration based on the antibiotic half-life.

Antibiotic	Half-life (41, 51)	Optimal time *after administration* for effective AP levels (41)
Amoxicillin	1 hour	1–2 hours
Cephalexin	1 hour	1–2 hours
Cephazolin	1.2–2.2 hours	1–4 hours
Clindamycin	2.4–3 hours	1–6 hours

Note: These optimal times after administration apply to patients with normal kidney function.

While clindamycin has a longer half-life than amoxicillin, this antibiotic is not routinely recommended for longer procedures unless the patient is hypersensitive to penicillin, as clindamycin has a higher rate of adverse effects, including *C. difficile* infections (52).

For delayed or longer procedures during which the dose of AP would wear off, it is recommended that a second AP dose is not given, but multiple short appointments be arranged instead. If the procedure is inadvertently extended where the AP will become ineffective, it is strongly recommended that the procedure be stopped, the situation temporised, and the patient can either return at another time to complete the procedure or be referred to a practitioner who can complete the procedure within the effective time of AP.

4.6.7 Exceptional circumstances: where patients are already taking an antibiotic

Various situations arise in clinical practice where patients may already be taking an antibiotic or have recently taken a course of antibiotics. The following provides some guidelines as to how to address these circumstances.

- Patients who require prolonged dental procedures over multiple appointments on different days can be given the same antibiotic each time if prophylaxis is required, regardless of the time in between appointments (4).
- Patients who have recently taken a short course of a similar antibiotic within the previous month (e.g. amoxicillin) do not need a different antibiotic prescribed (i.e. amoxicillin can be given again as prophylaxis, if it is the drug of choice) (4).
- Patients taking continuous antibiotics for another indication (e.g. rheumatic heart disease) may require a different antibiotic for prophylaxis due to the likely bacterial resistance. In addition, the low regular doses of benzylpenicillin used are unlikely to give the steady-state concentration required for prophylaxis. Seek medical advice as to which antibiotic is advised for the specific patient (4).
- Patients who have already been taking an antibiotic with an appropriate spectrum immediately prior to their dental procedure do not require a new or additional AP dose as they would have already reached steady state (after five half-lives) and a prophylaxis dose would not provide additional benefit.

4.7 β-lactam antibiotics: penicillins and cephalosporins

4.7.1 Chemistry

Penicillins belong to the β-lactam family of antibiotics that possess a 4-membered β-lactam ring linked to a thiazolidine ring in their chemical structure. The side chains (R1, R2 and R3) give each penicillin its individual pharmacological properties (see Figure 4.2). The β-lactam ring is the target of one type of resistance as the hydrolysis of the β-lactam ring by β-lactamase enzymes renders the antibacterial ineffective.

Cephalosporins have a similar structure to penicillins but the 4-membered β-lactam ring is fused to a di-hydrothiazine ring. Side chains at R1 and R2 give each cephalosporin their individual properties.

Figure 4.2 Basic chemical structure of penicillins and cephalosporins.

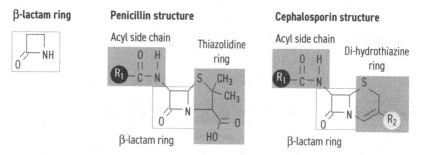

4.7.2 Pharmacodynamics

Penicillins and cephalosporins exert their bactericidal effect by binding to penicillin-binding proteins on the bacterial cell wall (3). After binding, they inhibit the formation of the peptidoglycan that forms the bacterial cell wall structure by targeting the transpeptidase enzyme, leading to lysis and bacterial cell death (3).

4.7.3 Spectrum of activity

4.7.3.1 Narrow-spectrum

Phenoxymethylpenicillin, dicloxacillin and flucloxacillin are narrow-spectrum penicillins and have activity against *Streptococcus* spp. and other oral anaerobes, including *Actinomyces, Fusobacterium* spp., *Peptostreptococcus* spp. and *Propionibacterium*. Dicloxacillin and flucloxacillin also have activity against *S. aureus* and coagulase-negative staphylococci (53).

4.7.3.2 Moderate-spectrum

Amoxicillin is a moderate-spectrum penicillin and has activity against most *Streptococcus* spp. and other oral anaerobes, including *Actinomyces, Fusobacterium* spp., *Peptostreptococcus* spp. and *Propionibacterium* (53).

Cephalexin is a moderate-spectrum cephalosporin, active against *Staphylococci* and *Streptococci*, with sensitivity to some anaerobes, including *Fusobacterium* spp.

4.7.3.3 Broad-spectrum

Clavulanic acid is a β-lactamase inhibitor that, when given in combination with amoxicillin, extends the antibacterial spectrum to cover β-lactamase producing microorganisms. Co-amoxiclav (amoxicillin with clavulanic acid) has activity against gram-positive *Staphylococcus aureus*, coagulase-negative *staphylococci*, most *Streptococcus* spp., and many oral anaerobes including *Bacteroides fragilis* group, *Fusobacterium* spp., *Peptostreptococcus* spp., *Prevotella* spp. and *Propionibacterium* (53).

4.7.4 Adverse effects

- Common adverse effects (>1%): Diarrhoea, nausea, vomiting, candidosis (53)
- Co-amoxiclav: *C. difficile*-overgrowth associated disease (see Practice points, Section 4.7.6) (54). If prescribed for >14 days, hepatic function should be monitored due to association with cholestatic hepatitis (53)

4.7.5 Drug interactions with β-lactam antibiotics

Table 4.4 Clinically relevant drug interactions with β-lactam antibiotics. Based on (53, 55–58).

β-lactam antibiotic	Interacting drug	What to do
Amoxicillin Phenoxymethylpenicillin (Penicillin V) Co-amoxiclav	Methotrexate: penicillins block methotrexate renal clearance	Avoid if patient on daily methotrexate. For patients on once-weekly methotrexate, penicillins can be safely taken on the other days of the week, avoiding the methotrexate day. Alternatively, an appropriate cephalosporin antibiotic can be prescribed
	Mycophenolate: co-amoxiclav interrupts mycophenolate enterohepatic recycling	Avoid co-amoxiclav
	Allopurinol: penicillins associated with increased risk of allopurinol-induced rash	If rash occurs, change antibiotic
	Warfarin: all penicillins linked with destabilising INR levels	Monitor INR at least every 3 days during antibiotic treatment and have warfarin dose adjusted accordingly
Cefalexin	Warfarin: may alter INR levels	Monitor INR at least every 3 days during antibiotic treatment and have warfarin dose adjusted accordingly

Note: INR: international normalised ratio.

4.7.6 Doses, formulations and practice points

Table 4.5 Spectrum of activity, doses and formulations of commonly used antibacterials in dentistry. Based on (4, 53, 59–61).

Antibacterial	Spectrum of activity	Doses for therapeutic use*	Formulations	Dose adjustment in renal impairment‡	Dose adjustment in hepatic impairment‡
Phenoxymethyl penicillin (Penicillin V)	Narrow-spectrum	Adult: 500mg orally, every 6 hours Child >1 month: 10–12.5mg mg/kg (maximum 500mg) orally, every 6 hours*	500mg capsules/tablets; 250mg capsules/tablets; 250mg/5mL suspension 100mL; 150mg/5mL suspension 100mL	Dose as per normal renal function	No significant hepatic risk
Dicloxacillin (for acute suppurative sialadenitis)	Narrow-spectrum	Adult: 500mg orally every 6 hours Child: 12.5–25mg/kg (maximum 500mg) orally every 6 hours*	500mg capsules; 250mg capsules	Reduce dose if CrCl <10mL/minute. Seek medical advice	Patients with a history of penicillin-induced cholestatic hepatitis should not be prescribed co-dicloxacillin Patients aged >55 years, or patients taking prolonged courses of >2 weeks are at increased risk of hepatitis
Flucloxacillin (for acute suppurative sialadenitis)	Narrow-spectrum	Adult: 500mg orally every 6 hours Child: 12.5–25mg/kg (maximum 500mg) orally every 6 hours*	500mg capsules; 250mg capsules; 250mg/5mL liquid 100mL; 125mg/5mL liquid 100mL.	Reduce dose if CrCl <10mL/minute. Seek medical advice	Patients with a history of penicillin-induced cholestatic hepatitis should not be prescribed co-flucloxacillin Patients aged >55 years, or patients taking prolonged courses of >2 weeks are at increased risk of hepatitis
Amoxicillin	Moderate-spectrum	Adult: 500mg orally every 8 hours Child: 15–25 mg/kg (maximum 500mg) orally every 8 hours*	500mg capsules; 250mg capsules; 500mg/5mL liquid 100mL; 250mg/5mL liquid 100mL; 125mg/5mL liquid 100mL; 100mg/mL liquid 20mL	Reduce dose or frequency if CrCl <30mL/minute. Seek medical advice	No significant hepatic risk

Table 4.5 (cont.)

Antibacterial	Spectrum of activity	Doses for therapeutic use*	Formulations	Dose adjustment in renal impairment‡	Dose adjustment in hepatic impairment‡
Co-amoxiclav	Broad-spectrum	Adult: 875mg/125mg orally every 12 hours Child >2 months: 22.5mg/3.2mg/kg (maximum 875mg/125mg) orally, every 12 hours	875mg/125mg tablets; 500mg/125mg tablets; 400mg/57mg/5mL suspension 60mL; 125mg/31.25mg/5mL suspension 75mL	Dosage reduction required if CrCl <30mL/minute. Seek medical advice	Patients with a history of penicillin-induced cholestatic hepatitis should not be prescribed co-amoxiclav Patients aged >55 years, or patients taking prolonged courses of >2 weeks are at increased risk of hepatitis
Cefalexin	Moderate-spectrum	Adult: 500mg every 6–12 hours, maximum of 4g/daily Child: 12.5mg/kg (maximum 500mg) every 6 hours*	500mg capsules; 250mg capsules; 250mg/5mL liquid 100mL; 125mg/5mL liquid 100mL	Reduce dose or frequency if CrCl <30mL/min. Seek medical advice	No significant hepatic risk

Notes:

* Paediatric dosage ranges are provided. Clinical judgement is required as to which dose to choose; for milder infections the lower end of the dosage range can be used, and conversely for more serious infections the higher end.

‡ Seek specialist advice regarding the dose reduction required.

CrCl: creatinine clearance.

Practice points

- Dicloxacillin, flucloxacillin and phenoxymethylpenicillin should be taken on an empty stomach (either 30 minutes before food or 2 hours after food) (53, 62).
- Amoxicillin may be given without food.
- Pseudoallergic reactions are common (maculopapular rash) with amoxicillin and tend to occur after >7 days treatment (53). Pseudo-allergic reactions do not exclude future use of the drug, but allergy testing is recommended before another penicillin exposure (53).
- Addition of metronidazole is not required for additional anaerobic coverage with co-amoxiclav (53).
- Co-amoxiclav is best tolerated and absorbed with food. If prescribed for >14 days, hepatic function should be monitored due to association with cholestatic hepatitis (53).
- Cefalexin may be given without food.
- All broad-spectrum antibiotics are associated with causing *Clostridioides difficile* disease. *C. difficile* produces a toxin that is damaging to the gut wall and can cause GI adverse effects ranging from mild diarrhoea to life-threatening pseudomembranous colitis (3, 53). In general, the broader spectrum antibiotics have a higher association, including cephalosporins, lincosamides (clindamycin) and co-amoxiclav (41, 54, 63, 64). In addition to colonic symptoms, other signs of *C. difficile*-associated disease include fever (>38.5° Celsius), haemodynamic instability and elevated creatine (65). If severe diarrhoea occurs, seek medical attention.

4.7.7 Pregnancy and lactation recommendations for commonly used β-lactam antibiotics in dentistry

See Table 14.2.

4.8 Metronidazole

4.8.1 Drug class

Nitroimidazole.

4.8.2 Pharmacodynamics

Metronidazole is a pro-drug and is inactive until taken up into the bacterial cell. Once in the cell, the nitro group is reduced by reductive activation, resulting in fragmentation of the imidazole ring and the generation of oxygen radicals that are cytotoxic to the anaerobic and microaerophilic bacteria (66–68). Bactericidal activity is derived from the production of toxic metabolites which cause DNA strand breakage and bacterial cell death (67).

4.8.3 Spectrum of activity

As metronidazole works by producing toxic oxygen products in the interior of the bacterial cell, it is effective against strict anaerobes and microaerophilic bacteria. It is not effective against aerobic or facultatively anaerobic bacteria. In dentistry, it is of most use in acute periodontal infections or where anaerobic bacteria predominate.

4.8.4 Contraindications/precautions

- Metronidazole should not be prescribed to patients with a history of blood dyscrasias, as they are more at risk of leukopenia and neutropenia with this drug (51).
- Nitroimidazoles should not be prescribed for patients with a history of neurological disorders as neurotoxic side effects including seizures, peripheral neuropathy and optic neuropathy have been reported (53, 68). Pre-existing neurological disease can be worsened. Peripheral neuropathy is most common in patients who receive >42g of metronidazole or over a 4-week period (69).

4.8.5 Adverse effects

- Common adverse effects (>1%): Metallic taste, gastrointestinal upset, loss of appetite, dizziness, headache (53)
- High dose/long treatment duration: Leukopenia, peripheral neuropathy, serious neurological adverse effects (e.g. cerebellar toxicity, seizures) (53)
- Oral adverse effects: Metallic taste, furry tongue, tongue discolouration, glossitis, stomatitis (51, 70)

4.8.6 Drug interactions with metronidazole

Table 4.6 Clinically relevant drug interactions with metronidazole. Based on (53, 71).

Antibiotic	Interacting drug	Mechanism	What to do
Metronidazole	Warfarin	Metronidazole can inhibit warfarin metabolism, increase INR and bleeding risk	Monitor INR every 3 days during treatment
	5-Fluorouracil	Metronidazole increases 5-fluorouracil concentration and increased risk of toxicity	Avoid combination by using an alternative anti-infective agent
	Alcohol	Metronidazole inhibits the metabolism of alcohol, causing acetaldehyde accumulation and symptoms of nausea, vomiting, flushing, headache and palpitations	Alcohol should be avoided during treatment and for 24 hours after the last dose. Be aware of alcohol in cough syrups and liquid herbal remedies.
	Disulfiram	Mechanism unknown	Combination may cause acute confusion or psychosis. Avoid combination. Do not use metronidazole within 2 weeks of disulfiram.
	Phenytoin	Phenytoin metabolism is reduced by metronidazole, and metronidazole metabolism is induced by phenytoin	Avoid metronidazole. Use alternative antibiotic

4.8.7 Doses, formulation and practice points

Table 4.7 Spectrum of activity, doses and formulations of metronidazole. Based on (4, 53, 61).

Antibacterial	Doses for therapeutic use	Formulations	Dose adjustment in renal impairment	Dose adjustment in hepatic impairment
Metronidazole	Adult: 200–400mg orally every 8–12 hours Child >1 month: 7.5 mg/kg orally (maximum 400mg) every 8 hours or 10mg/ kg (maximum 400mg) every 12 hours	200mg tablet; 400mg tablet; 200mg/5mL liquid 100 mL	Dose as per normal renal function	Dose reduction or avoidance required for patients with severe liver disease or impairment. Seek medical advice.

There are geriatric considerations for older people. Older patients are more vulnerable to gastrointestinal and neurological adverse effects. Metronidazole metabolites may accumulate in renal impairment and increase risk of adverse effects.

While metronidazole is most commonly prescribed at a frequency of three times per day, pharmacokinetic studies show that a 12-hourly dosage regimen maintains therapeutic plasma concentrations sufficiently (72). This is because metronidazole exhibits concentration-dependent rather than time-dependent bactericidal activity, and its relatively long half-life of 6–12 hours supports sustained serum concentrations (51, 67, 73).

Practice points

- Metronidazole tablets should be taken with food to improve GI tolerability. However, metronidazole liquid is best absorbed on an empty stomach (one hour before or two hours after food). Avoid alcohol during treatment and for 24 hours after the last dose. Metronidazole inhibits the metabolism of alcohol and can cause vomiting, flushing and headache (53).
- Metronidazole should be stopped if numbness, paraesthesia or weakness in the hands or feet develop; seek medical advice if this occurs (53).
- Full blood count is recommended for treatment >10 days in order to monitor for potential leukopenia (53).

4.8.8 Pregnancy and lactation recommendations for metronidazole

See Table 14.2.

4.9 Clindamycin

4.9.1 Drug class

Lincosamides.

4.9.2 Pharmacodynamics

Clindamycin is a bacteriostatic antibacterial that works by inhibiting the peptidyl transferase reaction on the 50S subunit of the bacterial ribosome, thereby inhibiting peptide bond formation, ribosome assembly and protein synthesis (3, 53).

4.9.3 Spectrum of activity

Clindamycin is active against some gram-positive, aerobic bacteria; for example, *Staphylococcus aureus*, many *Streptococcus* spp., as well as many oral anaerobes, including *Actinomyces, Bacteroides fragilis, Fusobacterium* spp., *Peptostreptococcus* spp., *Prevotella* spp. and *Propionibacterium* (53).

Clindamycin has good antimicrobial activity against facultative and strict anaerobes and is effective against β-lactamase-producing bacteria as well as having good alveolar bone penetration (31, 53, 63, 74). It is generally used for acute odontogenic infections or antibiotic prophylaxis in patients with penicillin allergy.

4.9.4 Contraindications/precautions

Clindamycin is associated with causing *Clostridioides difficile* overgrowth in the bowel, causing infection at an incidence of 0.1–1% (53). Two exotoxins, toxin A and toxin B, are produced from overgrowth of *C. difficile*. These toxins cause inflammation of the colon and damage the mucosa. Signs of *C. difficile*-associated disease can range from being asymptomatic or mild diarrhoea to a severe pseudomembranous colitis (3, 53, 75).

In general, all antibiotics, but especially broad-spectrum antibiotics, are associated with causing *C. difficile* overgrowth, including cephalosporins, lincosamides (including clindamycin) and co-amoxiclav (54, 63, 64). In addition to colonic symptoms, other signs of *C. difficile*-associated disease include fever (>38.5°C), haemodynamic instability and elevated creatine (65). If diarrhoea occurs in patients taking clindamycin, medical attention should be sought without delay.

Recent evidence has shown clindamycin is associated with causing acute kidney injury, with warnings about this now included in the manufacturers' information (76, 77). Clindamycin should therefore not be prescribed to people with a history of or current renal disease, renal impairment or renal transplant.

4.9.5 Adverse effects

- Common adverse effects (>1%): Diarrhoea, nausea, vomiting, abdominal pain (53)
- Uncommon adverse effects (0.1–1%): *C. difficile*-infection (see Section 4.9.4), acute kidney injury including acute renal failure (76, 77)
- Oral adverse effects: Taste disturbance (rare, <0.1%) (53, 78)
- Geriatric considerations: Older patients are more susceptible to gastrointestinal side effects of clindamycin and serious and fatal outcomes of *C. difficile* infection

4.9.6 Drug interactions with clindamycin

Table 4.8 Clinically relevant drug interactions with clindamycin. Based on (53, 71).

Antibiotic	Interacting drug	What to do
Clindamycin	Non-depolarising neuromuscular blockers (e.g. atracurium, cisatracurium, pancuronium, rocuronium, vecuronium) Clindamycin can exacerbate degree of muscle paralysis	Avoid clindamycin prior to administration of general anaesthetic involving neuromuscular blockers Advise anaesthetist of clindamycin use so neuromuscular blocker may be avoided or dose reduced
	CYP3A4 blockers (e.g. verapamil, diltiazem, clarithromycin, ketoconazole). Clindamycin is a CYP3A4 substrate; diltiazem is a moderate inhibitor of CYP3A4	Concomitant use of clindamycin and CYP3A4 inhibitors reduces clindamycin clearance, increases serum levels and increases the risk of adverse reactions Monitor closely for adverse effects if these drugs are used together
	CYP3A4 inducers (e.g. carbamazepine, corticosteroids, phenytoin, phenobarbital, rifampicin) Concomitant use of clindamycin and CYP3A4 inducers promotes clindamycin clearance, decreases clindamycin serum levels and reduces chance of therapeutic efficacy	Monitor for reduced therapeutic effect and if present, change antibiotic

4.9.7 Doses, formulations and practice points

Table 4.9 Spectrum of activity, doses and formulations of clindamycin. Based on (4, 53, 61, 77).

Antibacterial	Doses for therapeutic use	Formulations	Dose adjustment in renal impairment	Dose adjustment in hepatic impairment
Clindamycin	Adult: 300mg orally every 8 hours* Child >1 month: 5–10mg/kg (maximum 300 mg) every 8 hours‡	150mg capsules	Due to the risk of acute kidney injury, clindamycin should be avoided by patients with kidney disease. Seek medical advice regarding an alternative antibiotic.	Dosage interval should be prolonged in patients with moderate to severe hepatic impairment. Seek medical advice for patients with liver disease.

Notes:

* The quantity required for a 5-day course of clindamycin at a dose of 300mg three times a day is 30 × 150mg capsules, but only 24 capsules are funded on the Pharmaceutical Benefits Scheme (PBS) in Australia. In order to prescribe the full quantity on one prescription, a non-PBS 'private' prescription for 30 x 150mg capsules can be written instead.

‡ Solution to be made by dissolving contents of capsule with water as per the most recent edition of *Australian Medicines Handbook* or *Therapeutic Guidelines Oral and Dental*. If parents struggle with preparing paediatric doses from clindamycin capsules, it may be preferable to prescribe a different antibiotic such as cefalexin, which is readily available as a paediatric suspension, if the patient does not have cefalexin hypersensitivity.

Practice points

- Advise patients to take clindamycin with a full glass of water to reduce risk of oesophageal discomfort.
- Stop clindamycin immediately if diarrhoea or signs of renal impairment develops and seek urgent medical advice (53).
- Avoid concomitant use of proton pump inhibitors if diarrhoea begins as they may worsen the outcome if a *C. difficile* infection develops.
- Avoid use of antidiarrheal medication if diarrhoea begins, as the bowel relaxant effect will retain the toxin. If a *C. difficile* infection develops, seek medical advice (53).

4.9.8 Pregnancy and lactation recommendations for clindamycin

See Table 14.2.

4.10 Macrolides

4.10.1 Antibacterials

- Azithromycin
- Erythromycin
- Roxithromycin

4.10.2 Pharmacodynamics

Macrolide antibiotics are bacteriostatic and work by reversibly binding to the 50S subunit on the bacterial ribosomes. This leads to suppression of RNA-dependent bacterial protein synthesis (3, 51).

In addition to its bacteriostatic action, azithromycin is also thought to have anti-inflammatory effects. In gingiva, the drug is known to concentrate in fibroblasts and phagocytes and decrease pro-inflammatory cytokines, such as TNF-α and some interleukins, which is beneficial in the treatment of periodontal disease (79).

4.10.3 Spectrum of macrolide activity

Azithromycin has been used as a treatment for periodontitis as an adjuvant to non-drug dental treatment. Azithromycin is active against aerobic and anaerobic gram-positive and gram-negative bacteria, such as *Streptococcus* and some anaerobes such as *Actinomyces* (53, 79). Azithromycin carries some drug interaction risk, as it is an inhibitor of the drug transporter p-glycoprotein.

Erythromycin is not recommended in Australia for use in dentistry due to increasing patterns of resistance, high frequency of adverse reactions (especially GI) and great risk of significant drug interactions. GI symptoms including nausea, abdominal cramps, vomiting and diarrhoea are common (up to 30%) (53). This is due to erythromycin's chemical structure being similar to the prokinetic gut hormone called motilin.

Roxithromycin is often used as the macrolide of choice for treatment of odontogenic infections in paediatric patients who are hypersensitive to penicillins and cephalosporins.

It is effective against *Streptococcus* and some anaerobes such as *Actinomyces* (53). Roxithromycin is available in convenient paediatric dosage forms, and is also devoid of the GI risks and drug interactions associated with erythromycin.

4.10.4 Contraindications/precautions

Avoid all macrolides in patients at risk of prolonged QT interval, with congenital QT syndrome or are being treated with other drugs associated with QT prolongation (53).

4.10.5 Adverse effects

- Common adverse effects (>1%): Nausea, vomiting, diarrhoea, abdominal pain and cramps; GI adverse effects occur in up to 30% of patients taking erythromycin (53)
- Rare adverse effects: Deafness, tinnitus may occur with high or prolonged doses of all macrolides (53)
- Oral adverse effects: Hairy tongue may occur in patients taking erythromycin (70)

4.10.6 Drug interactions with macrolides

Roxithromycin and azithromycin are the preferred macrolides used in clinical practice due to their superior GI tolerability and reduced risk of drug–drug interactions.

Table 4.10 Clinically relevant drug interactions with macrolide antibiotics. Based on (53, 71).

Macrolide	Interacting drug/s	Mechanism	What to do
Azithromycin Erythromycin	Other drugs that prolong QT interval	Anti-arrhythmics, antipsychotics, anti-infectives, antidepressants antineoplastic agents	Check the cumulative risk of QT prolongation for the individual patients and avoid azithromycin and erythromycin if high risk
Azithromycin	PGP substates (e.g. dabigatran, rivaroxaban, apixaban, digoxin)	Azithromycin is a PGP inhibitor and can increase levels of PGP substrates	Avoid azithromycin use with PGP substrate drugs. Use different antibacterial agent.
Erythromycin	Many drugs, particularly those metabolised via CYP3A4 enzymes or transported via PGP	Inhibition of CYP3A4 and PGP blockade or both will increase intracellular and serum levels of substrate drugs increasing risk of side effects and toxicity	Do not prescribe erythromycin for patients on medications metabolised by CYP3A4 or transported via PGP
Roxithromycin	CYP3A4 substrates. Many drugs, including midazolam	As a weak CYP3A4 inhibitor, roxithromycin may increase substrate drug levels by up to two-fold	Use alternative antibiotic in patients taking CYP3A4 substrates with narrow therapeutic index
Roxithromycin	Digoxin	Likely due to PGP inhibition. Increased risk of digoxin toxicity.	Use alternative antibiotic in patients taking digoxin

Note: PGP = p-glycoprotein.

In general, erythromycin should be avoided wherever possible due to its poor tolerability and risk of drug interactions.

4.10.7 Doses, formulations and practice points

Table 4.11 Doses and formulations of commonly used macrolide antibiotics in dentistry. Based on (53, 61, 79).

Macrolide	Dose	Formulations	Dose adjustment in renal impairment[‡]	Dose adjustment in hepatic impairment[‡]
Azithromycin	Adult: 500mg orally daily for 3 days	500mg tablets	No dose reduction required in renal disease or impairment	Reduce dose in severe liver impairment. Seek medical advice for patients with liver disease
Erythromycin Clarithromycin	Not recommended for use in dentistry in Australia			
Roxithromycin	Adult: 300mg orally daily or 150mg orally twice daily Child: 6–40kg: 2.5–4mg/kg (maximum 150 mg) orally twice daily	50mg dispersible tablets; 150mg tablets; 300mg tablets	No dose reduction required in renal disease or impairment	Reduce dose in severe liver impairment Seek medical advice for patients with liver disease

Note:
[‡] Seek specialist advice regarding the dose reduction required.

Practice points

- Azithromycin has potential use in some periodontal disease under specialist care.
- Food decreases absorption of roxithromycin. It is best administered on an empty stomach (30 minutes before or 2 hours after food).
- All broad-spectrum antibiotics are associated with causing *C. difficile* overgrowth. *C. difficile* produces a toxin that is damaging to the gut wall and can cause GI adverse effects ranging from mild diarrhoea to life-threatening pseudomembranous colitis (3, 53). In addition to colonic symptoms, other signs of *C. difficile*-associated disease include fever (>38.5°C), haemodynamic instability and elevated creatine (65). If severe diarrhoea occurs, seek medical attention urgently.

4.10.8 Pregnancy and lactation recommendations for macrolide antibiotics

See Table 14.2.

4.11 Doxycycline

4.11.1 Drug class

Tetracyclines.

4.11.2 Pharmacodynamics

Doxycycline is taken up into the bacterial cell by active transport and subsequently reversibly binds to the 30S subunit on the bacterial ribosome, inhibiting the bacterial mRNA ribosome complex and thereby inhibiting protein synthesis (3, 51, 53).

Doxycycline is recommended in the Australian *Therapeutic Guidelines Oral and Dental (Version 3)* to prevent healing complications after tooth avulsion due to clinical experience with its use (4, 80, 81).

4.11.3 Spectrum of activity

Tetracyclines are broad-spectrum antibiotics, targeting many gram-positive and gram-negative bacteria, including *Enterococcus faecalis*, *Staphylococcus* spp., *Streptococcus* spp. and some anaerobes including *Actinomyces* (53).

4.11.4 Precautions

Symptoms of systemic lupus erythematous (SLE) may worsen during treatment with doxycycline. Avoid doxycycline use if possible or seek medical advice (53).

4.11.5 Adverse effects

- Common adverse effects (>1%): Nausea (risk can be mitigated if taken with a large glass of water in the middle of a meal), epigastric burning, photosensitivity (risk can be minimised with reduced sun exposure and applying sunscreen) (53)
- Rare: Raised intracranial pressure, oesophageal ulceration, liver toxicity, *C. difficile* overgrowth, exacerbation of SLE (53)
- Oral adverse effects: Doxycycline chelates with the calcium in teeth undergoing odontogenesis, forming a calcium orthophosphate complex, and is associated with permanent staining of the dentine and enamel (see Section 15.7). It should be avoided in pregnant women >18 weeks gestation and children <8 years old. However, doxycycline is unlikely to cause dental staining when used for up to 3 weeks in children younger than 8 years old (53)

4.11.6 Drug interactions with doxycycline

Table 4.12 Clinically relevant drug interactions with doxycycline. Based on (53, 71).

Drug	Interacting drug	Mechanism	Management
Doxycycline	Oral retinoids: isotretinoin, acitretin	Increased risk of benign intracranial hypertension	Contraindicated; avoid combination. Use alternate antibiotic
	Other phototoxic drugs (e.g. griseofulvin, azithromycin, amiodarone, isotretinoin)	Duplication of phototoxic effect	Avoid sun exposure, use sunscreen
	CYP3A4 inducers: carbamazepine, phenytoin, rifampicin, phenobarbital, St John's wort	Reduced doxycycline levels, reduced efficacy	Avoid combination
	Warfarin	Tetracyclines may increase warfarin's anticoagulant effect, occasionally causing bleeding	Check INR within the first 3 days of tetracycline treatment and decrease warfarin dose if necessary

4.11.7 Doses, formulations and practice points

Table 4.13 Doses and formulations of doxycycline in dentistry. Based on (53, 60).

Antibacterial	Doses for tooth avulsion (4)	Formulations	Dose adjustment in renal impairment	Dose adjustment in hepatic impairment
Doxycycline	Adult: 100mg orally daily for 7 days. Child: ≥8 years and <26kg: 50mg orally daily for 7 days Child: ≥8 years and between 26–35kg: 75mg orally daily for 7 days Child: ≥8 years and >35kg: 100mg orally daily for 7 days	100mg tablet; 100mg capsule; 50mg tablet; 50mg capsule	No dosage reduction required in renal disease or impairment	Avoid using high doses (200mg/day or more) in patients with liver disease Treatment with other hepatotoxic drugs may increase the risk of hepatotoxicity Seek medical advice

Practice points

- Absorption of doxycycline is affected by metal ions (calcium, aluminium, iron, zinc) and antacids; they chelate when given concurrently and prevent absorption of doxycycline. Foods/supplements containing these ions should be given 2 hours apart (53).
- Doxycycline causes an increased incidence of sensitivity to sunlight; minimise sun exposure and use sun protection (e.g. sunscreen) (53).
- Take doxycycline with food and a full glass of water to minimise stomach irritation and epigastric burning. (53)

4.11.8 Pregnancy and lactation recommendations for doxycycline

See Table 14.2.

4.12 Antivirals

4.12.1 Structure of viruses

Viruses are small intracellular parasites that infect host cells in order to produce virus particles (3, 82). They consist of fragments of DNA or RNA packaged in a protein coat, or capsid, that consists of repeating protein units in either a helical or icosahedral form (3). The genome and capsid are together called the nucleocapsid. Their DNA or RNA can either be single- or double-stranded and linear or circular in configuration (28). Viruses are generally classified according to their nucleic acid content.

Some viruses also possess an external lipid bilayer called the lipoprotein envelope that is attained by budding from the host cell membrane that it infects (3).

The lipoprotein envelope contains proteins that span the membrane that is responsible for receptor binding and fusion to the host cell. Viruses without an envelope use proteins attached to the capsid for receptor binding and entry into the host cell (3).

Viral nucleic acid can encode structural proteins such as the proteins in the nucleocapsid as well as non-structural proteins or enzymes to assist with viral replication, such as polymerases (28).

4.12.2 Herpes viruses

In dentistry, the most common virus encountered by dentists is the herpes simplex virus, which is categorised into two types: herpes simplex virus type 1 and type 2 (HSV-1 and HSV-2). HSV-1 causes predominately oral herpes, transmitted by oral contact, but can also cause genital herpes. HSV-2 causes genital herpes and is transmitted by sexual contact (83).

HSV are double-stranded DNA viruses in an icosahedral capsid, contain a lipid envelope and infect epithelial cells (26). For oral infections, they are also able to undergo cellular latency where the virus remains dormant in the trigeminal ganglion with no virion production (26). With appropriate stimuli, such as sunlight or immune compromise, the virus can be reactivated and infect host cells (26).

4.13 Guanine analogues

4.13.1 Antivirals

- Aciclovir (topical)
- Famciclovir

4.13.2 Pharmacodynamics

Aciclovir and famciclovir are pro-drugs that, when taken up into the viral-infected cells, undergo phosphorylation by viral-induced thymidine kinase to the monophosphate derivative, with subsequent activation to the triphosphate metabolite by the host cell enzymes. The active metabolite inhibits viral DNA polymerase and viral DNA synthesis. Aciclovir also has a second mechanism of action as it is incorporated in the viral DNA chain and causes DNA chain termination (3, 82, 84). These drugs are used in dentistry to treat recurrent oral mucocutaneous herpes simplex.

4.13.3 Adverse effects

- Common adverse effects (>1%): Famciclovir (single dose oral): headache, diarrhoea, vomiting (53)
- Uncommon adverse effects (0.1–1%): Famciclovir (single dose oral): dizziness (53)
- Topical aciclovir is very well tolerated

4.13.4 Drug Interactions with famciclovir

The short duration of famciclovir (a single 1500mg dose) means drug interactions are unlikely to arise or be of clinical significance.

4.13.5 Doses, formulation and practice points

Table 4.14 Doses and formulations of medications for recurrent oral mucocutaneous HSV. Based on (4, 53).

Medication	Dose and frequency	Formulation	Dose adjustment in renal impairment	Dose adjustment in hepatic impairment
Aciclovir	Adults and children >3 months: 5% cream applied topically to the lesions 5 times a day for 5 days	5% cream, 2g	None required	None required
Famciclovir	Adult: 3 × 500mg tablets (=1500mg) given orally as a single dose	500mg tablet	Reduce dose and/ or frequency in renal impairment. Seek medical advice.	No significant hepatic risk

Practice points

- Aciclovir cream should be applied at the first sign of recurrent herpes stomatitis or during the prodromal stage (4, 53).
- Famciclovir tablets should be started at the first sign of recurrent herpes stomatitis or the prodromal stage (4, 53).

4.13.6 Treatment courses of oral guanine analogues

Therapeutic courses of oral aciclovir, famciclovir and valaciclovir are often prescribed by oral medicine specialists for the treatment of widespread herpes labialis, intra-oral herpes stomatitis, herpes zoster affecting the trigeminal nerve, as well as herpes simplex-related erythema multiforme. They can also be used prophylactically in haematology-oncology patients, particularly in patients undergoing stem cell transplants.

Doses and duration of these medications depend on the indication for use and the specific patient cohort. Adverse effects of orally administered guanine analogues include neurological adverse effects, such as vertigo, confusion, hallucinations, delirium, and dizziness especially in high dose or in patients with renal impairment (53). Seek specialist advice for prescribing.

4.13.7 Pregnancy and lactation recommendations for guanine analogues

See Table 14.2.

4.14 Antifungals

4.14.1 General principles of antifungal medicines

Fungi are eukaryotic cells and fungal infections are common in the community. Human fungal infections are primarily classified according to the location and extent of their spread (i.e. superficial, subcutaneous or systemic) (82). Systemic fungal infections, especially in individuals with immune compromise, can have significant morbidity and mortality (3). Oral candidosis is the most common fungal infection seen in dental practice.

There are three main groups of fungi (3):

1. Yeasts (single cells)
2. Moulds (multicellular fungi in filamentous forms called hyphae, where the strands are interwoven together)
3. Dimorphic fungi that can exist as both yeast (blastophore), or mould (mycelial phase) depending on the growth conditions

Fungal cells contain a cell membrane that is predominately comprised of sterols, glycerophospholipids and sphingolipids. Ergosterol is the main component of the cell membrane, and both ergosterol and the enzymes involved in its biosynthesis are the main target for drugs since ergosterol is characteristic of fungal cells but not human cells (85).

Oral candidosis is caused by the dimorphic yeast species *Candida* and has a variety of clinical presentations. *Candida* spp. is present as a normal commensal in 25–75% of the population in the skin, mucous membranes of the oral cavity and GI tract (86). Pathogenicity usually occurs due to immune compromise, reduced saliva or a breach in the oral mucosa, with *Candida* eliciting disease by producing toxins or by direct tissue invasion (86, 87). While there are more than 200 *Candida* species, *Candida albicans* is most commonly implicated in oral candidosis and accounts for the vast majority of isolates (86).

4.15 Polyene antifungals

4.15.1 Antifungals

- Amphotericin (or Amphotericin B)
- Nystatin

4.15.2 Pharmacodynamics

The target site for the polyene antifungals is the fungal cell membrane where they irreversibly bind to ergosterol. This alters the permeability of the fungal cell wall, causing disruption of the ion balance and leakage of intracellular contents (3, 53). Antifungal drugs have little effect on human cells as ergosterol is found only in fungal cells and not in mammalian cells (3).

4.15.3 Doses, formulation and practice points

See Table 4.12.

4.15.4 Pregnancy and lactation recommendations for polyene antifungals

See Table 14.2.

4.16 Azole antifungals

4.16.1 Antifungals

- Clotrimazole
- Fluconazole
- Miconazole

4.16.2 Pharmacodynamics

Azole antifungals are fungistatic agents that bind to and impair the synthesis of ergosterol in the cell wall. By inhibiting fungal CYP3A enzyme, they inhibit the conversion of lanosterol to ergosterol, leading to fungal cell leakage and death (3, 53).

4.16.3 Contraindications/precautions

- Fluconazole can increase the risk of arrythmia by prolonging the QT interval and is contraindicated for use with other drugs that prolong the QT interval or in patients at risk of QT prolongation.

- Fluconazole is contraindicated from use with drugs metabolised by CYP3A4 and should be avoided with drugs metabolised by CYP2C9 or CYP2C19, such as clopidogrel, ibuprofen, warfarin, antidepressants, and oral hypoglycaemic agents (53).
- Miconazole is contraindicated by the manufacturer for use with drugs that are substrates of CYP3A4 or CYP2C9 (or both), such as warfarin, alprazolam, rivaroxaban, atorvastatin and simvastatin (51).

4.16.4 Drug interactions with azole antifungals

Significant drug interactions can occur with all azole antifungals as they are inhibitors of drug metabolizing enzymes CYP3A4, CYP2C9 and CYP2C19 in the gut wall and liver. Once absorbed, the azole antifungals can block these metabolic enzymes and increase serum concentrations of the substrate drugs, increasing the chance of side effects or toxicity. These interactions occur in a dose-dependent fashion, depending on how much azole antifungal and substrate drug are administered and absorbed.

Tiny doses dabbed onto small areas such as the corners of the mouth will not reach high enough serum concentrations to cause significant drug interactions. However, larger doses applied all over dentures, on large areas of oral mucosa or ingested orally can deliver systemic concentrations high enough to cause significant drug interactions.

Miconazole, which is used as a topical gel in dentistry, is extremely well absorbed through oral mucosa from this formulation and can reach serum concentrations that cause drug interactions. Miconazole is a moderate inhibitor of CYP2C9 and CYP3A4 and interacts with a wide range of drugs. Of note, miconazole inhibits the metabolism of the active isomer of warfarin, increasing its serum concentrations and raising the patient's international normalised ratio (INR). If this drug combination is used, more frequent monitoring of INR and dose adjustment is required.

Fluconazole is a strong inhibitor of CYP2C9, and moderate inhibitor of CYP2C19 and CYP3A4, lending it to many drug interactions. Giving fluconazole with drugs that are metabolised by these enzymes can increase their plasma concentrations and lead to significant side effects or toxicity (53). Expert advice on managing these drug–drug interactions should be sought.

4.16.5 Doses, formulations and practice points

Table 4.15 Doses and formulations of topically applied antifungals in dentistry. Based on (4, 53).

Medication	Dose	Formulations
Polyene antifungals		
Amphotericin	For oral candidosis: Adult, child ≥2 years: Suck one lozenge (10mg) 4 times daily for 1–2 weeks. Continue treatment for 3 days after signs of infection have resolved.	10mg lozenge
Nystatin	For oral candidosis: Adult and child: oral liquid 100,000 units (1mL) topically 4 times daily for 1–2 weeks. Continue treatment for 3 days after signs of infection have resolved.	100,000 units/ mL liquid, 24 mL

Table 4.15 (cont.)

Medication	Dose	Formulations
Azole antifungals		
Clotrimazole 1% cream	For angular cheilitis: Apply at the angles of the mouth twice daily for a minimum of 2 weeks. Continue for another 2 weeks after signs of infection have resolved.	1% cream 20g, 50g.
Miconazole 2% gel	For oral candidosis: Adult, child ≥2 years: 2.5mL 4 times daily for 1–2 weeks. Continue treatment for 1 week after signs of infection have resolved. Birth–2 years: 1.25mL 4 times daily for 1–2 weeks. Continue treatment for 1 week after signs of infection have resolved.	2% oral gel, 15g, 40g

Practice points

- Amphotericin lozenges are best administered after food or drink.
- Nystatin oral liquid is best administered after a meal or drink, and the liquid held in the mouth prior to swallowing to contact the candidosis-infected areas.
- Miconazole gel is used topically then swallowed. The gel is best used after food or drink; for young babies or for people with difficulty swallowing, the gel is best placed at the front of the mouth in small amounts or smeared onto the oral lesions (53).

4.16.6 Pregnancy and lactation recommendations for azole antifungals

See Table 14.2.

FURTHER READING

Teoh L, Thompson W, Suda K. Antimicrobial stewardship and dental practice. *Journal of the American Dental Association.* 2020; 151(8):589–595.

Thompson W, Williams D, Pulcini C et al. *FDI White Paper: The essential role of the dental team in reducing resistance.* FDI World Dental Federation; 2020.

REFERENCES

1. Australian Government Department of Health. *Australia's National Antimicrobial Resistance Strategy: 2020 and Beyond.* Report. 2020.
2. World Health Organization. *Antimicrobial stewardship programmes in health-care facilities in low- and middle-income countries: a WHO practical toolkit.* WHO; 2019.
3. Ritter J, Flower R, Henderson G, Loke YK, MacEwan D, Rang H. *Rang and Dale's Pharmacology.* 9th edition. Elsevier; 2020.
4. Oral and Dental Expert Group. *Therapeutic Guidelines Oral and Dental (Version 3).* Therapeutic Guidelines Pty Ltd; 2019.
5. Lawler B, Sambrook PJ, Goss AN. Antibiotic prophylaxis for dentoalveolar surgery: is it indicated? *Aust Dent J.* 2005;50(4 Suppl 2):S54–S59.

6. Interagency Coordination Group on Antimicrobial Resistance. *No Time to Wait: Securing the Future from Drug-resistant Infections.* WHO; 2019.

7. Al-Haroni M. Bacterial resistance and the dental professionals' role to halt the problem. *J Dent.* 2008;36(2):95–103.

8. Levy SB, Marshall B. Antibacterial resistance worldwide: causes, challenges and responses. *Nat Med.* 2004;10(12 Suppl):S122–S129.

9. Teoh L, Stewart K, Marino R, McCullough M. Antibiotic resistance and relevance to general dental practice in Australia. *Aust Dent J.* 2018;63(4):414–421.

10. Australian Commission of Safety and Quality in Health Care. *AURA 2016: first Australian report on antimicrobial use and resistance in human health.* ACSQHC; 2016.

11. Handal T, Olsen I. Antimicrobial resistance with focus on oral beta-lactamases. *Eur J Oral Sci.* 2000;108(3):163–174.

12. Andersson DI. The ways in which bacteria resist antibiotics. *International Journal of Risk and Safety in Medicine.* 2005;17(3–4):111–116.

13. Teoh L, Stewart K, Marino RJ, McCullough MJ. Part 1. Current prescribing trends of antibiotics by dentists in Australia from 2013 to 2016. *Aust Dent J.* 2018;63(3):329–337.

14. Smith A, Al-Mahdi R, Malcolm W et al. Comparison of antimicrobial prescribing for dental and oral infections in England and Scotland with Norway and Sweden and their relative contribution to national consumption 2010–2016. *BMC Oral Health.* 2020;20(1):172.

15. Durkin MJ, Hsueh K, Sallah YH et al. An evaluation of dental antibiotic prescribing practices in the United States. *J Am Dent Assoc.* 2017;148(12):878–886 e1.

16. Liau I, Han J, Bayetto K et al. Antibiotic resistance in severe odontogenic infections of the South Australian population: a 9-year retrospective audit. *Aust Dent J.* 2018;63(2):187–192.

17. World Economic Forum. *Global Risks 2013.* 8th edition. WEF; 2013.

18. Khadem TM, Dodds Ashley E, Wrobel MJ, Brown J. Antimicrobial stewardship: a matter of process or outcome? *Pharmacotherapy.* 2012;32(8):688–706.

19. Teoh L, Sloan AJ, McCullough MJ, Thompson W. Measuring Antibiotic Stewardship Programmes and Initiatives: An Umbrella Review in Primary Care Medicine and a Systematic Review of Dentistry. *Antibiotics (Basel).* 2020;9(9)607. doi:10.3390/antibiotics9090607

20. Thompson W, Williams D, Pulcini C, Sanderson S et al. *FDI White Paper: The essential role of the dental team in reducing resistance.* FDI World Dental Federation; 2020.

21. Teoh L, Marino RJ, Stewart K, McCullough MJ. A survey of prescribing practices by general dentists in Australia. *BMC Oral Health.* 2019;19(1):193.

22. Cope AL, Francis NA, Wood F, Chestnutt IG. Antibiotic prescribing in UK general dental practice: a cross-sectional study. *Community Dent Oral Epidemiol.* 2016;44(2):145–153.

23. Suda KJ, Calip GS, Zhou J et al. Assessment of the Appropriateness of Antibiotic Prescriptions for Infection Prophylaxis Before Dental Procedures, 2011 to 2015. *JAMA Netw Open.* 2019;2(5):e193909.

24. Teoh L, Stewart K, Marino RJ, McCullough MJ. Perceptions, attitudes and factors that influence prescribing by general dentists in Australia: A qualitative study. *J Oral Pathol Med.* 2019;48(7):647–654.

25. Thompson W, Tonkin-Crine S, Pavitt SH et al. Factors associated with antibiotic prescribing for adults with acute conditions: an umbrella review across primary care and a systematic review focusing on primary dental care. *J Antimicrob Chemother.* 2019;74(8):2139–2152.

26. Lamont R, Jenkinson HF. *Oral Microbiology at a Glance.* Wiley-Blackwell; 2010.

27. Teoh L, Cheung MC, Dashper S et al. Oral Antibiotic for Empirical Management of Acute Dentoalveolar Infections—A Systematic Review. *Antibiotics (Basel).* 2021;10(3)240; doi:10.3390/antibiotics10030240

28. Lamont R JH. *Oral Microbiology and Immunology.* 2nd edition. ASM Press; 2014.

29. Palmer N. *Antimicrobial Prescribing for in Dentistry—Good Practice Guidelines.* FGDP(UK), FDS; 2021.

30. Robinson AN, Tambyah PA. Infective endocarditis—an update for dental surgeons. *Singapore Dent J.* 2017;38:2–7.

31. Teoh L. *Dental Therapeutic Guideline Adherence in Australia.* The University of Melbourne; 2021.

32. Farbod F, Kanaan H, Farbod J. Infective endocarditis and antibiotic prophylaxis prior to dental/oral procedures: latest revision to the guidelines by the American Heart Association published April 2007. *Int J Oral Maxillofac Surg.* 2009;38(6):626–631.

33. Dayer M, Thornhill M. Is antibiotic prophylaxis to prevent infective endocarditis worthwhile? *J Infect Chemother.* 2018;24(1):18–24.

34. Infective Endocarditis Queensland. *Infective Endocarditis Clinician Information.* University of Queensland; 2020.

35. Glenny AM, Oliver R, Roberts GJ, Hooper L, Worthington HV. Antibiotics for the prophylaxis of bacterial endocarditis in dentistry. *Cochrane Database Syst Rev.* 2013(10):CD003813.

36. Cahill TJ, Harrison JL, Jewell P et al. Antibiotic prophylaxis for infective endocarditis: a systematic review and meta-analysis. *Heart.* 2017;103(12):937–944.

37. Tomas I, Diz P, Tobias A et al. Periodontal health status and bacteraemia from daily oral activities: systematic review/meta-analysis. *J Clin Periodontol.* 2012;39(3):213–228.

38. Habib G, Hoen B, Tornos P et al. Guidelines on the prevention, diagnosis, and treatment of infective endocarditis (new version 2009). *Eur Heart J.* 2009;30(19):2369–2413.

39. Wilson W, Taubert KA, Gewitz M et al. Prevention of infective endocarditis. *J Am Dent Assoc.* 2008;139 Suppl:3S-24S.

40. National Institute of Health and Care Excellence. Prophylaxis against infective endocarditis: antimicrobial prophylaxis against infective endocarditis in adults and children undergoing interventional procedures. *NICE Clinical Guidelines.* 2016;64.

41. Expert Group for Antibiotic Guidelines. 16th edition. *Therapeutic Guidelines: Antibiotic.* Therapeutic Guidelines Pty Ltd; 2019.

42. Lodi G, Figini L, Sardella A et al. Antibiotics to prevent complications following tooth extractions. *Cochrane Database Syst Rev.* 2012;11:CD003811.

43. Sollecito TP, Abt E, Lockhart PB et al. The use of prophylactic antibiotics prior to dental procedures in patients with prosthetic joints: Evidence-based clinical practice guideline for dental practitioners—a report of the American Dental Association Council on Scientific Affairs. *J Am Dent Assoc.* 2015;146(1):11–6 e8.

44. Khan AA, Morrison A, Hanley DA et al. Diagnosis and management of osteonecrosis of the jaw: a systematic review and international consensus. *J Bone Miner Res.* 2015;30(1):3–23.

45. Bermudez-Bejarano EB, Serrera-Figallo MA, Gutierrez-Corrales A et al. Prophylaxis and antibiotic therapy in management protocols of patients treated with oral and intravenous bisphosphonates. *J Clin Exp Dent.* 2017;9(1):e141–e149.

46. Beth-Tasdogan NH, Mayer B, Hussein H, Zolk O. Interventions for managing medication-related osteonecrosis of the jaw. *Cochrane Database Syst Rev.* 2017;10:CD012432.

47. Esposito M, Grusovin MG, Worthington HV. Interventions for replacing missing teeth: antibiotics at dental implant placement to prevent complications. *Cochrane Database Syst Rev.* 2013(7):CD004152.

48. Park J, Tennant M, Walsh LJ, Kruger E. Is there a consensus on antibiotic usage for dental implant placement in healthy patients? *Aust Dent J.* 2018;63(1):25–33.
49. Lund B, Hultin M, Tranaeus S et al. Complex systematic review—Perioperative antibiotics in conjunction with dental implant placement. *Clin Oral Implants Res.* 2015;26 Suppl 11:1–14.
50. Kim AS, Abdelhay N, Levin L et al. Antibiotic prophylaxis for implant placement: a systematic review of effects on reduction of implant failure. *Br Dent J.* 2020;228(12):943–951.
51. AusDI. *Independent Drug Monographs.* 2022. https://ausdi.hcn.com.au/browseDocuments .hcn?filter=PRODUCTS_WITH_MONGRAPH
52. Thornhill MH, Dayer MJ, Prendergast B et al. Incidence and nature of adverse reactions to antibiotics used as endocarditis prophylaxis. *J Antimicrob Chemother.* 2015;70(8):2382–2388.
53. Editorial Advisory Committee. *Australian Medicines Handbook.* AMH Pty Ltd; 2022.
54. Mullish BH, Williams HR. *Clostridium difficile* infection and antibiotic-associated diarrhoea. *Clin Med (Lond).* 2018;18(3):237–241.
55. MIMS Australia. *eMIMS.* 2021. https://emims.com.au
56. Invitae. *YouScript.* 2022. https://youscript.com/
57. Borrows R, Chusney G, Loucaidou M et al. The magnitude and time course of changes in mycophenolic acid 12-hour predose levels during antibiotic therapy in mycophenolate mofetil-based renal transplantation. *Ther Drug Monit.* 2007;29(1):122–126.
58. Bhagat V, Pandit RA, Ambapurkar S et al. Drug Interactions between Antimicrobial and Immunosuppressive Agents in Solid Organ Transplant Recipients. *Indian J Crit Care Med.* 2021;25(1):67–76.
59. Australian Medicines Handbook Children's Dosing Companion. *Australian Medicines Handbook Pty Ltd*; 2021. https://childrens.amh.net.au/auth
60. IBM Corporation. *IMB Micromedex Clinical Evidence Packages.* IBM Watson Health; 2021.
61. Ashley C, Dunleavy A. *The Renal Drug Handbook.* CRC Press; 2018.
62. Mylan. *Aspecillin VK: Australian Product Information.* 2020.
63. Brook I, Lewis MA, Sandor GK et al. Clindamycin in dentistry: more than just effective prophylaxis for endocarditis? *Oral Surg Oral Med Oral Pathol Oral Radiol Endod.* 2005;100(5):550–558.
64. Trubiano JA, Cheng AC, Korman TM et al. Australasian Society of Infectious Diseases updated guidelines for the management of *Clostridium difficile* infection in adults and children in Australia and New Zealand. *Intern Med J.* 2016;46(4):479–493.
65. Australian Commission of Safety and Quality in Health Care. *Clostridium difficile infection. Monitoring the national burden of Clostridium difficile.* ACSQHC; 2018.
66. Dingsdag SA, Hunter N. Metronidazole: an update on metabolism, structure-cytotoxicity and resistance mechanisms. *J Antimicrob Chemother.* 2018;73(2):265–279.
67. Lamp KC, Freeman CD, Klutman NE, Lacy MK. Pharmacokinetics and pharmacodynamics of the nitroimidazole antimicrobials. *Clin Pharmacokinet.* 1999;36(5):353–373.
68. Hernandez Ceruelos A, Romero-Quezada LC, Ledezma JC et al. Therapeutic uses of metronidazole and its side effects: an update. *Eur Rev Med Pharmacol Sci.* 2019;23(1):397–401.
69. Goolsby TA, Jakeman B, Gaynes RP. Clinical relevance of metronidazole and peripheral neuropathy: a systematic review of the literature. *Int J Antimicrob Agents.* 2018;51(3):319–325.
70. Teoh L, Moses G, McCullough MJ. A review and guide to drug-associated oral adverse effects—Dental, salivary and neurosensory reactions. Part 1. *J Oral Pathol Med.* 2019;48(7):626–636.

71. eMIMS. 2021. www.emims.com.au. [Subscription only]

72. Earl P, Sisson PR, Ingham HR. Twelve-hourly dosage schedule for oral and intravenous metronidazole. *J Antimicrob Chemother.* 1989;23(4):619–621.

73. Lloyd CJ, Earl PD. Metronidazole: two or three times daily—a comparative controlled clinical trial of the efficacy of two different dosing schedules of metronidazole for chemoprophylaxis following third molar surgery. *Br J Oral Maxillofac Surg.* 1994;32(3):165–167.

74. Kuriyama T, Karasawa T, Nakagawa K et al. Bacteriologic features and antimicrobial susceptibility in isolates from orofacial odontogenic infections. *Oral Surg Oral Med Oral Pathol Oral Radiol Endod.* 2000;90(5):600–608.

75. Kelly CP, LaMont JT. *Clostridium difficile* infection. *Annu Rev Med.* 1998;49:375–390.

76. Clifford KM, Selby AR, Reveles KR et al. The Risk and Clinical Implications of Antibiotic-Associated Acute Kidney Injury: A Review of the Clinical Data for Agents with Signals from the Food and Drug Administration's Adverse Event Reporting System (FAERS) Database. *Antibiotics (Basel).* 2022;11(10):1367. doi:10.3390/antibiotics11101367

77. Sarwal A, Chiu CY, Feinstein A. Does Clindamycin Induce Acute Kidney Injury? *Am J Med Sci.* 2020;359(5):303.

78. de Groot MC, van Puijenbroek EP. Clindamycin and taste disorders. *Br J Clin Pharmacol.* 2007;64(4):542–545.

79. Muniz FW, de Oliveira CC, de Sousa Carvalho R et al. Azithromycin: a new concept in adjuvant treatment of periodontitis. *Eur J Pharmacol.* 2013;705(1–3):135–139.

80. Hinckfuss SE, Messer LB. An evidence-based assessment of the clinical guidelines for replanted avulsed teeth. Part II: prescription of systemic antibiotics. *Dent Traumatol.* 2009;25(2):158–164.

81. Day PF, Flores MT, O'Connell AC et al. International Association of Dental Traumatology guidelines for the management of traumatic dental injuries: 3. Injuries in the primary dentition. *Dent Traumatol.* 2020;36(4):343–359.

82. Brenner G, Stevens C. *Brenner and Stevens' Pharmacology.* 5th edition. Elsevier; 2018.

83. World Health Organization. *Herpes Simplex Virus.* 2020. https://www.who.int/news-room/fact-sheets/detail/herpes-simplex-virus

84. King DH. History, pharmacokinetics, and pharmacology of acyclovir. *J Am Acad Dermatol.* 1988;18(1 Pt 2):176–179.

85. Sant DG, Tupe SG, Ramana CV, Deshpande MV. Fungal cell membrane-promising drug target for antifungal therapy. *J Appl Microbiol.* 2016;121(6):1498–1510.

86. Telles DR, Karki N, Marshall MW. Oral Fungal Infections: Diagnosis and Management. *Dent Clin North Am.* 2017;61(2):319–349.

87. Muzyka BC, Epifanio RN. Update on oral fungal infections. *Dent Clin North Am.* 2013;57(4):561–581.

88. Bermúdez-Bejarano EB, Serrera-Figallo MA, Gutiérrez-Corrales A et al. Prophylaxis and antibiotic therapy in management protocols of patients treated with oral and intravenous bisphosphonates. *J Clin Exp Dent.* 2017;9(1):e141–149.

ANALGESICS AND ANTI-INFLAMMATORIES

5

KEY POINTS

- Dental pain management involves providing the most appropriate diagnosis, prompt dental treatment, and, if using medications, tailoring the choice of drug to the type of pain (e.g. inflammatory, neuropathic and nociceptive) to patient factors and preferences.
- Most dental pain is nociceptive inflammatory pain, for which non-steroidal anti-inflammatory drugs (NSAIDs) in combination with paracetamol are most effective.
- Optimal administration of NSAIDs and paracetamol includes being taken simultaneously and on an empty stomach in order to optimise the rate and extent of absorption.
- If the combination of NSAIDs and paracetamol have been adequately trialled but ineffective, revisiting the diagnosis and trying a different NSAID is the next step.
- Opioids have a limited role in the management of dental pain as they are relatively ineffective and should also not be prescribed for chronic or neuropathic pain.

5.1 Introduction

Managing oral pain is a daily task for dental practitioners. Understanding the type of pain, accurately diagnosing the cause and being able to choose the most appropriate drug regimen (if required) is a fundamental skill for all dentists. This chapter describes the medicines commonly used for pain management in dentistry, their mechanism of action, appropriate doses, adverse effects, common drug interactions and their place in therapy.

5.2 Definition of pain

Pain is defined by the International Association for the Study of Pain (IASP) as 'an unpleasant sensory and emotional experience associated with, or resembling that associated with actual or potential tissue damage' (1).

Pain is subjective and is influenced by biological, psychological, emotional and social factors, as well as by coping strategies and past pain experience. It can be expressed both verbally and non-verbally and, while pain serves an adaptive role, it can negatively affect an individual's quality of life (1). While most dental and orofacial pain in dentistry is nociceptive and inflammatory in nature, patients can also present with other types of pain, including chronic or neuropathic pain and combinations thereof. The type and duration of pain needs to be determined in order to formulate the most appropriate treatment plan and choose the right medication.

5.3 Classification of pain

Pain can be classified in many ways, including by location, duration, circumstance, and the underlying pathological process. The location of pain in patients presenting to a dentist is expected to be in the orofacial region, but this location may extend from the scalp, face, neck, and jaws, to anywhere in the mouth and oropharynx.

Pain classified by duration falls into two main types: acute and chronic pain. This differentiation is made because pain changes overtime, both in its nature and quality.

Acute pain is the sharp, intense pain of recent onset resulting from a noxious stimulus such as injury or infection that serves as a warning sign of real or potential physical harm. Most acute pain is short-lived but may persist longer depending on the situation.

Chronic pain, also referred to as persistent pain, is pain that has lasted for three months or longer (2). Over this time, the original stimulus for the pain has often resolved and its pathology is no longer present. However, changes to the body's neuro-hormonal response to pain have resulted in alteration of pain sensation causing adaptation that may result in hyperalgesia, allodynia (pain due to a non-painful stimulus) and central sensitisation. Biopsychosocial factors also contribute to a person's experience of chronic pain over time, such as anxiety, depression, social functioning, sleep quality and quality of life. Thus, a multidisciplinary approach to pain management is recommended (3).

Acute-on-chronic pain is the term given to acute pain experienced on a background of chronic pain from a planned insult such as elective surgery or unplanned injury such as trauma.

5.4 Types of pain

Nociceptive pain arises from actual or threatened tissue damage by activation of nociceptors: receptors in the peripheral somatosensory nervous system sensitive to noxious stimuli (1, 4).

Neuropathic pain is defined by the IASP as 'pain caused by a lesion or disease of the somatosensory nervous system' (1). It usually manifests as burning, paraesthesia or shooting pains along the distribution of the nerve. Diagnostic tests and imaging are rarely helpful in diagnosing neuropathic pain, so diagnosis is based on clinical presentation, location and nature of the pain instead (1).

Nociplastic pain is pain due to central sensitisation. Examples include the pain of fibromyalgia, sciatica and chronic back pain (5). Common drugs used for different types of pain are shown in Table 5.1.

Table 5.1 Drugs commonly used for different types of dental pain.

Type of pain	Drugs
Nociceptive pain	NSAIDs Paracetamol Opioids
Neuropathic pain*	Amitriptyline Carbamazepine Gabapentin Pregabalin

Note:

* Due to the complexity of these drugs, the management of neuropathic pain is preferably conducted by an oral medicine specialist or medical pain specialist (9).

5.5 Pain physiology

5.5.1 Primary nociceptive afferent neurons

Tissue injury is detected by peripheral sensory neurons called nociceptors that are activated by thermal, mechanic, and chemical stimuli. Molecular messengers such as substance P, bradykinin, serotonin, TNF-α, and IL-1β are released in the presence of inflammation and tissue injury that activate these primary nociceptive afferent neurons (6, 7). There are two types of primary afferent neurons—Aδ and C fibres—that carry pain signals from the periphery to the spinal cord. The Aδ fibres are myelinated so can transmit pain signals rapidly, and are responsible for producing the intense, sharp and well-localised sensation of most acute pain. In contrast, C fibres are not myelinated and transmit pain more slowly, producing a delayed pain that is often described as a diffuse, dull ache that follows after the initial pain wears off (7).

5.5.2 Ascending pain pathways

The cell bodies of the primary afferent ascending neurons are located in the dorsal root ganglia that project into the dorsal horn of the spinal cord. From there, they synapse with spinothalamic tract neurons to extend into higher centres of the brain including the thalamus, somatosensory cortex and prefrontal cortex where pain signals are received (7). Such signals tell the individual the location, severity and presence of the pain and also communicate with the limbic structures of the brain to generate the emotional components of pain, such as suffering and discomfort (6, 7).

5.5.3 Descending inhibitory controls

Descending pain pathways control sensory input into the dorsal horns to modulate activation of the spinothalamic neurons (6, 7). The neurotransmitters that fuel the descending pathways include serotonin (5HT), noradrenaline (NA) and enkephalins and cause an inhibition of pain transmission (7). Opioid receptors are located in all these areas as well and also switch off pain transmission through descending pathways (6, 7). It is thought that antidepressants and tramadol aid in pain management by increasing levels of NA and 5HT via this pathway (6).

Figure 5.1 Pain pathway and descending inhibitory controls (7).

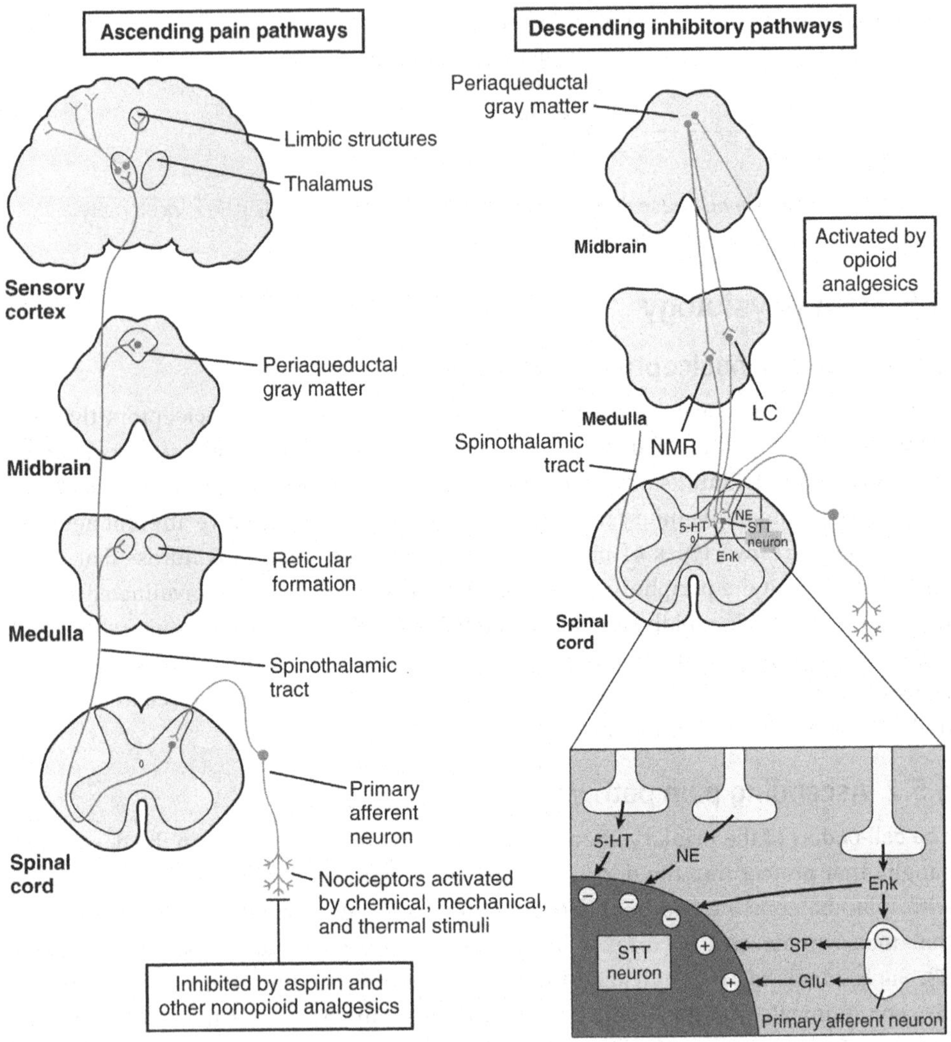

5.6 Pain management in dentistry

The vast majority of pain in dentistry is acute nociceptive inflammatory pain arising from pulpitis, abscesses, or postoperative wounds (e.g after extractions). The most effective and quickest way to treat pain due to infection is always by active dental treatment to address the cause; analgesia should only play an adjunctive role.

Modern pain management in dentistry is based on the concept of multimodal analgesia, which is managing pain using multiple therapeutic interventions or medicines, each with different mechanisms of action (1). Research and experience have shown that relying on a single drug, often in high doses, is less effective than using multiple drugs together. Several combinations of drugs can have additive effects, enabling lower doses of these medications to be used (8). In dentistry, an example is the use of paracetamol and a NSAID for acute nociceptive pain.

For some patients experiencing complex pain syndromes, a multidisciplinary team is most effective in managing their care. For example, management of orofacial pain may involve an oral medicine specialist and a medical pain specialist; a physiotherapist for management of jaw and shoulder movement; and a psychologist for management with cognitive and behavioural treatment.

5.7 Anti-inflammatories

5.7.1 NSAIDs and COX-2 inhibitors

5.7.1.1 Pharmacodynamics

Aspirin was the first NSAID ever used in clinical practice, having been developed from the bark of the willow tree in the 1700s. Aspirin was one of the first drugs to relieve inflammation, which was revolutionary at the time. It works by inhibition of the of cyclo-oxygenase (COX) enzymes that catalyse the first step in the production of prostaglandins from arachidonic acid, a precursor fatty acid in cell membranes (10).

Aspirin's main disadvantages are its short duration of action (3–4 hours) and high risk of adverse effects, mainly bleeding, GI irritation and ulceration. Modern NSAIDs such as diclofenac and ibuprofen were developed in the 1960s to 1980s as inhibitors of COX enzymes but with prolonged duration of action and reduced risk of GI-adverse effects. Nevertheless, all conventional NSAIDs remain plagued by the risks of bleeding and GI ulceration.

Selective COX-2 inhibitors were developed in the 1990s from the discovery that the COX enzyme was present in two different forms: COX-1 and COX-2.

Table 5.2 Differences between COX-1 and COX-2 enzymes.

COX-1	COX-2
• Constitutively expressed in most cells • Produces prostaglandins involved in housekeeping functions (e.g. maintaining the mucosal layer of the gut with PGE2, promoting platelet aggregation)	• Mostly produced in times of acute inflammation • Produces prostaglandins (PGs) and inflammatory cytokines (e.g. interleukin-1 (IL-1) and TNF-α) • Clinical effects are pain, swelling, fever, hyperalgesia, vasodilation and increased capillary permeability (6)

The discovery of COX-2 and the establishment of its chemical structure rapidly 'led to the development of selective inhibitors of this enzyme, such as celecoxib and rofecoxib', that have 'potent anti-inflammatory actions with reduced gastrotoxic effects' (88).

Interestingly, both COX-1 and COX-2 are involved in dilation of blood vessels in the kidneys that promotes renal perfusion as a homeostatic function.

5.7.1.2 NSAIDs in dentistry

NSAIDs are the most commonly used medicines for pain relief in dentistry and are recommended as first-line treatment of acute inflammatory pain in patients for whom these drugs are safe. As explained above, NSAIDs are divided into two main groups: non-selective and selective.

Non-selective NSAIDS inhibit both cyclo-oxygenase enzymes COX-1 and 2 that are responsible for the production of prostaglandins (PGs) and thromboxanes (see Table 5.2 and Figure 5.2). Selective NSAIDs preferentially inhibit COX-2 more than COX-1.

Figure 5.2 Mechanism of action of NSAIDs.

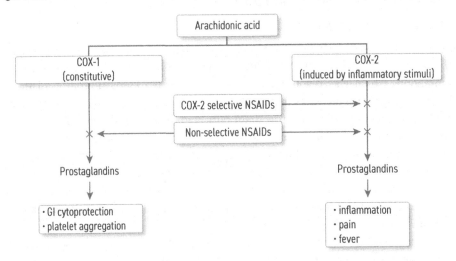

With the exception of aspirin, inhibition of COX-1 and COX-2 by non-selective NSAIDs is reversible. Aspirin, however, is an irreversible inhibitor as its acetyl group binds irreversibly to the COX-1 enzyme on platelets, leading to a permanent anti-platelet effect from the impairment of that platelet's coagulation ability for the rest of its lifespan.

By inhibition of COX-2, three primary effects of NSAIDs occur:

1. **Anti-inflammatory effect**: a reduction in the inflammatory PGs subsequently leads to a decrease in oedema and swelling, and a reduction in capillary permeability (6, 10).
2. **Analgesic effect**: the inhibition of COX in the periphery leads to a reduced sensitisation of nociceptors due to inflammatory cytokines and other mediators. In addition, the inhibition of inflammatory PGs (PGE2 and PGI2) centrally are also responsible for the analgesic effect (6).

3. **Anti-pyretic effect:** the production of Interlukin-1 (IL-1) in the hypothalamus stimulated by bacterial endotoxins goes on to produce PGs that alter the thermo-regulatory control of the hypothalamus to increase the set temperature to above 37°C, inducing fever. Inhibition of COX leads to a reduction in prostaglandins cen-trally, and therefore has an anti-pyretic effect (6).

5.7.1.3 Contraindications/precautions

- Active or recent history of peptic ulcer disease or GI bleeding
- Moderate to severe renal impairment (eGFR <30mL/min), renal impairment, severe hepatic impairment and cirrhosis
- Advanced age, due to the chance of increased risk of renal and cardiovascular impairment
- Heart failure or significant cardiovascular risk (35)
- NSAID-induced asthma/bronchospasm (see below)

5.7.1.4 Adverse effects

Due to the inhibition of COX enzymes, three primary types of adverse effects are associ-ated with non-selective NSAIDs: GI, renal and cardiovascular (CV).

GI complications

COX-1 produces PGs in the gastroduodenal mucosa that are responsible for cytopro-tection, including a reduction in gastric acid production, and an increased produc-tion of mucous and bicarbonate to protect the stomach lining from acid. Inhibition of COX-1 in the GI system leads to an increased risk of GI erosions, bleeding, ulcerations and perforation. Dose and duration of the NSAID is directly proportional to the risk of GI complications, increasing by 2.5–5.0% in people who have a previous history of GI ulceration (12).

In addition, people who are on other medications that carry a GI risk, such as contin-uous corticosteroids or selective serotonin reuptake inhibitors (SSRI) antidepressants, will be at an increased cumulative GI risk. Certain other factors also predispose patients to an increased GI risk, including smoking, older age, and high alcohol consumption (4, 13).

COX-2 selective inhibitors, such as celecoxib, have the primary advantage of reducing the risk of GI bleeding and ulceration, and therefore are preferentially used in patients with a history or who are at risk of adverse GI effects.

Renal complications

Physiological regulation of renal function
In the kidney, both COX-1 and COX-2 are constitutively expressed to maintain renal blood flow (perfusion) as well as electrolyte and fluid balance. COX-1 is responsible for dilation of afferent blood vessels that bring in blood for filtration through the glomerulus, thus maintaining the glomerular filtration rate. Expression of COX-1

will increase in times of renal hypoperfusion, low blood volume or fluid depletion. COX-2 is responsible for maintaining sodium, water retention, and electrolyte and fluid balance (10, 12).

The renin–angiotensin system in the kidney is responsible for producing renin and angiotensin II which cause the vasoconstriction of the renal efferent arterioles, creating a back pressure which forces blood through the filtration apparatus of the glomerulus. In addition, angiotensin II promotes sodium retention in exchange for potassium (due to its effect on aldosterone) (14).

Table 5.3 GI, kidney and CV effects of COX-1 and COX-2.

GI mucosa	Kidney	Cardiovascular
Effects of cox-1: • gastric cytoprotection • increased bicarbonate production • increased mucous secretion	**Effects of cox-1 and cox-2:** • vasodilatation of afferent arterioles • increased renal blood flow and filtration rate • increased sodium and water excretion	**Effects of cox-1:** • vasoconstriction • platelet aggregation **Effects of cox-2:** • vasodilatation • inhibition of platelet aggregation
Effects of cox-1 inhibition: • decreased mucous secretion and cytoprotection • gastric/duodenal ulcers • gi bleeding	**Effects of cox-1 and cox-2 inhibition:** • sodium and water retention • increased workload on kidney • acute kidney injury • exacerbation of ckd	**Effects of cox-1 and cox-2 inhibition** • increased blood pressure • increased risk of stroke and myocardial infarction **Effect of cox-2 inhibition only** • increased platelet aggregation and risk of thrombosis

Note: CKD: chronic kidney disease.

NSAIDs and renal impairment

NSAIDs are associated with both acute kidney injury (AKI) and exacerbation of CKD. AKI is seen mostly in patients taking high doses of NSAIDs or in the presence of other risk factors such as diabetes or medications like angiotensin converting enzyme inhibitors (ACEIs) and diuretics. NSAID use is associated with approximately 15% of cases of AKI (12). Manifestations of AKI include acute interstitial nephritis, papillary necrosis, electrolyte imbalance, renal tubular acidosis, hyponatremia, hyperkalaemia and acute hypertension (12). Inhibition of renal PGs and increased aldosterone levels also cause sodium and fluid retention, which contributes to hypertension and fluid overload, exacerbating heart failure and/or CKD. For this reason, NSAIDs are contraindicated in patients with heart failure (12).

Interaction between NSAIDs and ACEIs/ARBs

In situations of low blood volume or reduced serum sodium concentrations, renin is released from the juxtaglomerular cells into the circulation (15). Renin converts angiotensinogen to angiotensin 1 (AT1), which is then converted by an angiotensin converting enzyme (ACE) to angiotensin 2 (AT2), a potent vasoconstrictor. AT2 also increases sympathetic output, increases arterial pressure and cardiac output, and stimulates the release of aldosterone, which in turn increases sodium and water retention (15).

There are two types of drugs that can reduce the effects of AT2 and thereby lower blood pressure and reduce the effects of fluid overload on the heart and kidneys. These are ACEIs, which impair the conversion of of AT1 to AT2, and those called AT2 receptor blockers (ARBs), which block the tissue receptors that AT2 would bind to.

The 'triple whammy' effect

Diuretic medicines are often used with ACEIs and ARBs to treat hypertension and heart failure but need to be managed carefully to avoid compromising kidney function. Adding NSAIDs to this combination creates the so called 'triple whammy' of drugs that block the effects of AT2, diuretics and NSAIDs, and can sometimes trigger acute renal failure.

When a NSAID is administered in addition to an ACEI/ARB, blood pressure and autoregulatory mechanisms to maintain renal perfusion are disturbed. NSAIDs impair the PG-induced vasodilation of the afferent arterioles and maintenance of electrolyte balance. ACEIs/ARBs impair the renin–angiotensin system and the vasoconstriction of the efferent arterioles to maintain renal homeostasis and blood pressure (15). If diuretics are also added in, they cause relative hypovolaemia. These three drug classes work on different parts of the kidney to compromise renal function; and the kidney is unable to maintain homeostasis, resulting in a drop in GFR and blood pressure (15) (see Figure 5.3).

Since both COX-1 and COX-2 are involved in renal homeostasis, the COX-2 inhibitor drugs also cause renal adverse effects and can be involved in triple whammy combinations.

Cardiovascular complications

Myocardial infarction and thrombotic stroke are the main CV complications of NSAID use due to increased risk of vasoconstriction and thrombogenesis arising from the disturbed balance between COX-1 and COX-2. COX-1 normally promotes formation of thromboxane A2 (TXA2) in platelets favouring platelet aggregation. COX-2 in the vascular endothelium normally promotes formation of PGI2 (also known as prostacyclin) which has a vasodilatory and anti-aggregatory effect. Relative inhibition of these enzymes shifts the vascular homeostatic balance towards vasoconstriction and thrombus formation, and thus the increased risk of CV events due to blood clotting.

Figure 5.3 The 'triple whammy' effect is the combination of all three factors that can cause acute kidney injury.

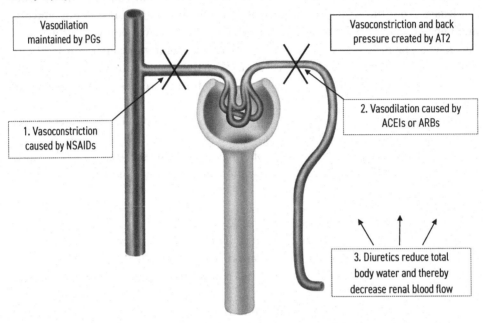

In general, the more COX-2 inhibition, the greater the shift towards thrombogenesis, as seen with the highly selective COX-2 inhibitor rofecoxib, which was withdrawn from the worldwide market in 2004 due to thrombogenic CV events. Of the non-selective NSAIDs, diclofenac has the most COX-2 inhibition and the highest CV risk profile (16, 17). Of the non-selective NSAIDs, naproxen has relatively less COX-2 inhibition, so a slightly better CV risk profile. However, all NSAIDs, including naproxen, are associated with an increased risk of CV events. Despite being a selective COX-2 inhibitor, celecoxib has a similar CV risk profile to the other NSAIDs (18, 19). This risk occurs in the first week of use for all NSAIDs; therefore, using a NSAID for the shortest possible duration is important.

NSAID-induced asthma/bronchospasm

Aspirin-induced asthma (AIA), also known as NSAID-exacerbated respiratory disease (NERD), affects between 3–11% of adults and 2% of children (20). The average age of onset of this condition is 30 years, so children are infrequently affected (20). Those affected initially experience upper respiratory tract symptoms that mimic hay fever including a runny nose, nasal obstruction, facial flushing, sneezing, and watery eyes, usually within 20 minutes to 3 hours of taking a NSAID or aspirin. These symptoms may progress to shortness of breath and bronchospasm in patients with asthma. Risk factors include severe asthma (e.g. patients who have required hospitalisation due to asthma), long-term nasal congestion and nasal polyps (20). Prevalence data shows that approximately 80–90% of adults with asthma can safely tolerate aspirin and other NSAIDs, so it should not be assumed that a patient history of asthma necessitates NSAID avoidance (21). Instead, patients should be warned of the potential for development of NERD—particularly older patients with adult-onset asthma, nasal polyps and nasal congestion—and reminded to be familiar with their asthma management plan (20, 21).

As the mechanism of this syndrome is thought to be mediated via inhibition of COX-1, evidence suggests that COX-2 inhibitors can be safely tolerated in these patients. Therefore, if an anti-inflammatory is necessary, a COX-2 inhibitor could be trialled under medical supervision (22).

5.7.1.5 Common drug interactions with NSAIDs

Table 5.4 Common drug interactions with NSAIDs. Based on (11, 23, 24).

Drugs prone to interaction with NSAIDs	Mechanism of interaction and outcome	Management
Lithium	NSAIDs impair renal clearance of lithium, resulting in elevated lithium serum levels	Avoid NSAIDs if possible. If unavoidable, use lowest NSAID dose for shortest time, and monitor patient for signs and symptoms of lithium toxicity. Reduce lithium dose if necessary
ACEI/ARB +/- diuretic	Combined effect of ACEI/ARB + diuretic + NSAID can cause rapid decline in renal perfusion and acute renal impairment	Combination may be used under close medical supervision. Do not use NSAIDs in patients with underlying moderate to severe renal impairment
Systemic corticosteroids	Additional risk of GI irritation, bleeding and ulceration	Use lowest corticosteroid and NSAID doses for shortest possible period of time
Antihypertensives	NSAIDs can increase blood pressure by 3–5mmHg within days	Monitor blood pressure if risk of slight elevation is clinically significant
SSRI or SNRI antidepressants	Serotonergic antidepressants have an antiplatelet effect, which will add to NSAID bleeding risk	Monitor and warn patient of increased bleeding risk. If bleeding occurs, cease NSAID (not antidepressant)

5.7.1.6 Analgesic doses and adjustment in renal/hepatic impairment

Table 5.5 Pharmacokinetic parameters, doses and formulations of commonly used NSAIDs in dentistry. Adapted from (4, 11, 25–28).

Drug	Half-life (hours)	Time to peak concentration after oral administration (hours)	Formulations available	Dose	Dose adjustment in renal impairment[‡]	Dose adjustment in hepatic impairment[‡]
Paracetamol	1–3	0.5–2	OTC: 500mg tablets, capsules, soluble tablets. 665mg bilayer tablets. Many formulations for children (e.g. liquid, suppositories)	Adult: 1000mg every 4–6 hours; maximum 4g/day. Maximum 3g per day if fasting, alcoholic, liver-impaired.	Dose reduction required if CrCl <10mL/minute. Seek medical advice	Increased risk of liver damage in patients with chronic liver disease. Seek medical advice
Ibuprofen	2	1–2	OTC: 200mg tablets Prescription: 400mg tablets	Adult: 400mg orally, every 6–8 hours, maximum 1200mg/day; maximum 5 days without review	Avoid where possible. Seek medical advice	Contraindicated in severe liver impairment. Seek medical advice for patients with liver disease
Diclofenac	1–2	IR tablet: 0.5 EC tablet: 2	OTC: 12.5mg tablets; 25mg tablets Prescription: 50mg EC tablets	Adult: 75–150mg daily in 2–3 divided doses, maximum 5 days without review	Avoid where possible. Seek medical advice	Contraindicated in severe liver impairment. Seek medical advice for patients with liver disease

Naproxen	14	2–4	OTC: 275mg tablets Prescription: 250mg tablets; 500mg tablets	250–500mg IR every 12 hours, maximum 5 days without review	Avoid where possible Seek medical advice	Contraindicated in severe liver impairment. Seek medical advice for patients with liver disease
Celecoxib	4–15	2–3 (fasting)	Prescription: 100mg capsules; 200mg capsules	Adult: 100mg orally every 12 hours, maximum 5 days without review	Avoid where possible. Contraindicated when CrCl is <30mL/minute. Seek medical advice	Contraindicated in severe liver impairment. Seek medical advice for patients with liver disease
Etoricoxib	22	1 (fasting)	Prescription: 30mg tablets; 60mg tablets; 120mg tablets	90mg orally once daily, maximum 5 days without review	Avoid where possible. Contraindicated when CrCl is <30mL/minute. Seek medical advice	Contraindicated in severe liver impairment. Seek medical advice for patients with liver disease

Notes:

‡ Seek specialist advice regarding the dose reduction required.

CrCl: creatinine clearance; EC: enteric coated; IR: immediate release; OTC: over the counter (without prescription).

5.7.1.7 Concurrent dosing

While NSAIDs are first line for those who can tolerate them, administering a NSAID concurrently with paracetamol achieves additive analgesia. The combination also achieves a longer-lasting duration of pain relief, compared to either drug alone, without an increase of adverse effects (29, 30). Often, similar levels of pain relief can be achieved with reduced dosages of each drug. Good evidence supports the use of ibuprofen or diclofenac with concomitant paracetamol (29, 31).

Practice points

- Paracetamol and NSAIDs should be taken on an empty stomach, as this has shown to produce a faster time to peak plasma concentrations, produce higher peak serum levels, and prolong pain relief (32). Explain to patients that taking NSAIDs or paracetamol on an empty stomach has not been shown to produce a greater incidence of adverse GI effects, or that taking these medications with food prevents adverse GI effects (32). These drugs can be taken with food if patients prefer, with the understanding that absorption will be slightly reduced. A COX-2 selective anti-inflammatory such as celecoxib can be offered to patients with persistent concerns of NSAID-induced GI irritation or ulceration.
- Current evidence does not show increased risk of acute kidney injury in patients taking occasional, short-term NSAIDs (e.g. for 1 or 2 days) while on ACEIs or ARBs with a diuretic (33). However, the risk is highest within the first month of taking the triple combination. Therefore, NSAIDs should be avoided if possible in patients taking an ACEI or ARB with a diuretic. But if an NSAID is essential, use for 1–2 days may be tolerated in most patients on this combination, depending on the patient's renal function (33). Alternatively, paracetamol alone can be prescribed.
- Etoricoxib is a selective COX-2 inhibitor registered in Australia for management of acute dental pain. The adult dose is 90mg given once daily without regard to meals (11). More frequent dosing provides no additional benefit. Safety and effectiveness have not been established for people younger than 16 years. Etoricoxib use has been associated with severe hypertension and increased risk of thrombotic cardiovascular disease (11). Therefore, avoid this drug in patients with high cardiovascular risk.
- The elderly are more susceptible to adverse effects of NSAIDs such as renal impairment, thrombosis and heart failure (11). A careful assessment must be made of potential benefit versus risk in these patients.

5.7.1.8 Pregnancy and lactation recommendations for NSAIDs

See Table 14.2.

5.7.2 Paracetamol

Paracetamol is the first line analgesia for dental pain for infants and children, as well as pregnant and breastfeeding women. It also can be used as monotherapy for patients who cannot tolerate NSAIDs but are able to take paracetamol. When used appropriately, it is safe and well tolerated, with few significant drug interactions.

5.7.2.1 Pharmacodynamics

Paracetamol's mechanism of action is subject to debate. Some authors claim it inhibits COX-1 and COX-2 centrally to reduce prostaglandin synthesis, which confers analgesic and antipyretic effects similar to the non-selective NSAIDs (6). Others suggest it works via inhibition of cannabidiol receptors in the CNS, therefore explaining why it has little or no peripheral anti-inflammatory action (36, 37). It also lacks GI adverse effects and antiplatelet activity (6).

5.7.2.2 Overdose of paracetamol

Frequency of hospital admissions due to paracetamol overdose has significantly increased in Australia over the past two decades, likely due to the ready availability of paracetamol in many different formulations (38). Accidental paracetamol overdoses are common in both adults and children, and toxic paracetemol doses are the most common source of severe acute liver injury in Australia (39).

Paracetamol poisoning can occur with either acute or chronic overdose. An acute dose of either 10g (20 tablets of 500mg) or 200mg/kg body weight (whichever is less) in a 24-hour period will cause toxic effects (39). Chronic overdose is considered whenever >4g paracetamol has been consumed per day for several days or more.

In an adult, ingestion of less than 4g of paracetemol per day is metabolised without causing liver injury. In overdose, paracetamol is shunted to a pathway where it is metabolised to the highly reactive and toxic metabolite N-acetyl-p-benzoquinone-imine. The hepatotoxicity of paracetamol is increased by the presence of the following factors:

- chronic/excessive alcohol use
- glucose-6-phosphate dehydrogenase (G6PD) deficiency
- hepatic impairment (26)

If an overdose is suspected, dentists should send the patient to hospital immediately due to the risk of irreversible hepatotoxicity. An antidote is available for the treatment of paracetamol poisoning but must be initiated as quickly as possible.

In hospital, overdoses are managed with activated charcoal to adsorb the paracetamol to prevent absorption, but, if hepatotoxicity has occurred, intravenous acetylcysteine is administered to increase glutathione synthesis to neutralise the toxic metabolite (39). Ensure the patient advises emergency staff exactly which paracetamol product/formulation was consumed, as management varies depending on the formulation.

5.7.2.3 Contraindications/precautions

- Severe liver or renal impairment
- Phenylketonuria (PKU): soluble paracetamol tablets contain aspartame which is converted in the body to phenylalanine. As people with PKU cannot breakdown phenylalanine, soluble paracetamol tablets should be avoided by these patients (11, 26)

5.7.2.4 Common drug interactions with paracetamol

Table 5.6 Common drug interactions with paracetamol. Based on (11, 23, 24).

Drug	Interaction	Management
Warfarin	Regular use of paracetamol may increase INR; occasional paracetamol use has no significant effect	More frequent warfarin monitoring and dose adjustment may be required
Excessive alcohol use*; liver enzyme inducers, hepatotoxic drugs	Increased risk of hepatotoxicity from paracetamol combined with other hepatotoxic substances	Use very short courses and low doses of paracetamol in patients at risk of cumulative hepatotoxicity

Notes:
* Seek expert medical advice regarding excessive alcohol use.
INR: international normalised ratio.

Practice points

- Paracetamol is best taken on an empty stomach, as food reduces its absorption and time to peak concentration. Simultaneous administration of paracetamol and NSAIDs is preferred (see Section 5.7.1.7)
- Oral administration of paracetamol is recommended wherever possible. Many liquid and soluble forms are available if tablets and capsules are inappropriate. Rectal administration may be used in emergencies or if oral route is unavailable (e.g. vomiting, difficulty swallowing). However, paracetamol absorption via the rectal route can be unpredictable and delayed (11).
- There is a risk of paracetamol overdose (>4g per day for several days, or ›10g taken in a 24-hour period) when this drug is accidentally taken from multiple different preparations. This risk can arise when paracetamol is taken from a variety of over-the-counter combination products or when people are taking paracetamol regularly for conditions such as osteoarthritis. Ensure the correct formulation and dose form is prescribed, and make sure the patient is not taking multiple paracetamol-containing products as this raises the risk of paracetamol overdose (11).

5.7.2.5 Pregnancy and lactation recommendations for paracetamol

See Table 14.2.

5.8 Opioids

Morphine, derived from the resin of the opium poppy, is the original opium alkaloid from which the term 'opioid' is derived. Although morphine has been used for pain management for centuries, it was not isolated from opium until 1806 and its chemical structure determined in 1847 (40). Codeine was isolated from the opium resin decades later and its chemical structure found to be very similar to morphine, as 3-methylmorphine, soon after.

Opioid is the broad term given to any drug which binds to opioid receptors in the body. Therefore, this term includes opiates, semi-synthetic and synthetic opioids, as shown in Table 5.7.

Table 5.7 Classification of opioids by their derivation.

Opiates (naturally occurring opioids)	Semi-synthetic opioids (derived from natural opiates)	Synthetic opioids
Codeine	Buprenorphine	Fentanyl
Morphine	Diethylmorphine (heroin)	Methadone
Papaverine	Hydromorphone	Tapentadol
Thebaine	Oxycodone	Tramadol

Opioids are not the first-line agents for the management of dental pain as they are not very effective and safer alternatives exist. Since most dental pain is acute, nociceptive pain of inflammatory origin, NSAIDs are most effective as they attenuate the inflammatory process, reducing the formation of the PGs responsible for the inflammation. Opioids block pain perception, but do not work on the inflammation. Many studies comparing NSAIDs and opioids, as well as systematic reviews, have demonstrated the superior effectiveness of NSAIDs compared with opioids for dental pain (41–43).

Opioids have a limited place in managing pain in dentistry. Opioids are also not effective for neuropathic pain and should be avoided in the management of chronic pain as they can contribute to the development of hyperalgesia (3). However, in some circumstances, short-term opioids may be needed in dentistry but the potential adverse effects, degree of benefit, as well as the risks of diversion and misuse should be considered carefully prior to prescribing.

5.8.1 Pharmacodynamics

Opioid drugs bind to opioid receptors that are distributed throughout the CNS and the periphery, including the GI tract, immune system and several other sites (40).

There are three types of opioid receptors that have been identified in the CNS: μ, δ and κ. More recently, a fourth opioid receptor has been identified: ORL1. (7). These receptors have now been renamed by the International Union of Pharmacology to MOP, DOP and KOP respectively, as shown in Table 5.8 (40). Activation of these receptors leads to the inhibition of adenylate cyclase and changes to the permeability of the K+ and Ca+ channels, leading to the inhibition of the pain signal. Opioids can act as agonists (such as morphine), antagonists (such as naloxone) or partial agonists (buprenorphine) at opioid receptors.

The binding of opioids as agonists at these receptors are responsible for the analgesic, as well as the adverse effects, of opioids such as respiratory depression, constipation and dependence.

Table 5.8 Functional effects associated with the opioid receptors (6).

Receptor (classical terminology)	μ	δ	κ	ORL$_1$
Receptor (recommended new terminology)	MOPr	DOPr	KOPr	NOPr

Analgesia:
  Supraspinal
  Spinal
  Peripheral
	+++
	++
	++
		– ?
		++
		–
			–
			+
			++
				Antiopioid*
				++
				–

Respiratory depression	+++	++	–	–
Pupil constriction	++	–	+	–
Reduced GI motility	++	++	+	–
Euphoria	+++	–	–	–
Dysphoria and hallucinations	–	–	+++	–
Sedation	++	–	++	–
Catatonia	–	–	–	++
Physical dependence	+++	–	–	–

Note:
* ORL$_1$ agonists were originally thought to produce nociception or hyperalgesia but it was later shown that they reverse the supraspinal analgesic effects of endogenous and exogenous μ opioid receptor agonists.

5.8.2 Main pharmacological effects of opioids

Since opioid receptors are present throughout the CNS, they have effects on all major organs as shown in Table 5.9. Adverse opioid effects are experienced by >90% of people taking opioids for both acute and chronic pain (50).

5.8.2.1 Analgesia and other CNS effects

The analgesic effects of all opioids are mediated by the agonism of μ opioid receptors located at the peripheral, spinal and supraspinal levels. At the spinal level, opioids inhibit the transmission of pain impulses from nociceptive afferent neurons through the dorsal horn ganglia, thereby preventing the pain signal from reaching supraspinal sites (6). They also inhibit the transmission of pain impulses via the activation of opioid receptors in the periductal grey area in the midbrain, nucleus magnus raphe and the locus coeruleus (7). Peripheral opioid receptors exist but are thought to undergo different regulation and expression compared with central opioid receptors (44). Recent research has shown that they are upregulated in the presence of inflammation, both in the dorsal root ganglion but also the terminals of sensory neurons (45).

Opioid-induced euphoria is also mediated by activation of μ receptors and dysphoria is mediated via activation of κ receptors (6).

Hyperalgesia is a side effect of the prolonged use of opioids, where they paradoxically increase a patient's sensitivity to pain (46). Clinically, this can present as a reduced effectiveness to the same dose of opioid (6).

Table 5.9 Main pharmacological effects of opioids. Adapted from (7).

Body system	Pharmacological effect
CNS	Analgesia Euphoria Dysphoria Miosis ('pinpoint pupils') Hyperalgesia Dependence and tolerance Sedation Nausea and vomiting (by stimulation of the CTZ) Confusion Delerium Hallucinations Dizziness
Gastrointestinal	Constipation (by decreasing intestinal peristaltic contractions) Nausea and vomiting Spasm of biliary sphincter of Oddi (biliary colic)
Oral	Dry mouth
Respiratory	Respiratory depression Inhibition of cough reflex
Genito-urinary	Urine retention
Cardiovascular	Reduced myocardial oxygen requirements Vasodilation and hypotension
Dermal	Flushing, pruritis Direct stimulation of histamine release (associated with the natural opioids, e.g. morphine and codeine)
Immune system	Suppression of the natural killer cells
Musculoskeletal	Myoclonus (longer term effect)

5.8.2.2 GI effects

Opioids have pronounced effects on the μ receptors of the gut (47). Constipation is the most commonly reported adverse GI effect of opioids, affecting up to 41% of people using opioids for non-cancer pain, and often experienced after the very first dose (48, 49). This effect is caused by the relaxation of longitudinal smooth muscle, causing slowed GI transit time, greater fluid reabsorption and decreased GI secretions. Narcotic bowel syndrome is a lesser-known adverse effect of prolonged opioid use, due to increased contraction of the circular muscle, characterised by severe abdominal pain (49).

Opioids are also frequently associated with nausea and vomiting due to stimulation of the chemoreceptor trigger zone (CTZ) in the brain and slowing of the gut. Nausea is experienced in up to 40% of people taking opioids and vomiting in 20% of subjects (50).

Opioid use, particularly with naturally occurring opiates such as codeine, is associated with spasm of the sphincter of Oddi in the gall bladder causing biliary colic. This adverse effect occurs early in treatment, most often with the first few doses. Opioids also cause spasm of the urinary sphincter causing urinary retention. Both conditions are very painful and can be avoided by ceasing or switching to a different opioid (51).

5.8.2.3 Respiratory

The respiratory depressant effect of opioids is mostly mediated by activation of μ receptors in the respiratory centre in the brain to cause a decreased sensitivity to arterial P CO_2, suppression of ventilatory response to hypercapnia, and a reduction in respiration rate and tidal volume (6, 7, 52). This respiratory depressant effect is generally seen with opioids in high dose or overdose.

5.8.2.4 Other adverse effects

Long-term use of opioids also has a wide range of effects on the human body. Opioids cause the inhibition of the hypothalamic–pituitary–gonadal axis, resulting in hypogonadism in males and females. In males, this results in testosterone deficiency and sexual dysfunction, affecting around 63% of males on chronic opioids (53). In females, this results in menstrual irregularities and menopausal symptoms, such as amenorrhoea and hot flushes (53). Patients on either acute but more likely long-term opioids, particularly morphine, may experience myoclonus and other involuntary muscle movements such as tics and twitching as a sign of opioid-induced neurotoxicity (54).

5.8.2.5 Opioid allergy versus pseudo-allergy

Opioid allergy is misdiagnosed in approximately 90% of people who claim an opioid allergy, as the affected patients are often found to have experienced an adverse effect or a pseudo-allergic reaction instead (55, 56). The incidence of true opioid allergy is rare, and literature is limited around its true incidence (57). It has generally been reported at approximately 2%, but this is not based on validated tests to confirm the hypersensitivity reaction (57).

True hypersensitivity reactions are mediated by IgE antibodies or a T-cell mediated reaction and are characterised by signs such as widespread maculopapular rash, hypotension, bronchospasm and angioedema (see Chapter 3).

The natural opiate derivatives, codeine and morphine, are able to directly stimulate the release of histamine from mast cell degranulation, causing signs mediated by histamine release, such as flushing, hives, sweating, and exacerbation of asthma (56). This is seen less commonly with the semi-synthetic and synthetic opioids (see Table 5.10). Drug provocation testing is the 'gold standard' to determine true allergy, which involves supervised and controlled administration of the suspected medication, using an individualised protocol with an allergist (57).

It has been shown that a person with a true allergy to one opioid can demonstrate cross-reactivity to other opioids regardless of the opioid class, so another opioid should not be tried without appropriate medical supervision. People who have experienced pseudo-allergic reactions, however, can be prescribed an opioid of a different class; for example, a patient with a pseudo-allergic reaction to codeine (from phenanthrene class) can be prescribed tramadol (from phenylpiperidine class). However, this reaction should be medically confirmed, as the pseudo-allergic reaction and a true allergic reaction (IgE or T-cell mediated) can be clinically indistinguishable.

Table 5.10 Chemical classification of opioids. Adapted from (57, 58).

Chemical class of opioid	Opioid	Source
Diphenylheptanes	Methadone	Synthetic
Phenanthrenes	Buprenorphine	Semi-synthetic
	Codeine	Opium alkaloid (natural)
	Heroin	Semi-synthetic
	Hydrocodone	Semi-synthetic
	Morphine	Opium alkaloid (natural)
	Naltrexone	Synthetic
	Oxycodone	Semi-synthetic
Phenylpiperidines	Fentanyl	Synthetic
	Tramadol	Synthetic
Benzenoid	Tapentadol	Synthetic

5.8.3 Comparative information and pharmacokinetics

The majority of opioids used in dentistry (codeine, tramadol, tapentadol and oxycodone) have good oral bioavailability, and after absorption are widely distributed throughout the body, crossing the blood–brain barrier to work in their primary site of action—the CNS. They cross into the CNS by active transport but may be ejected via p-glycoprotein efflux transporters. All opioids are extensively metabolised in the liver, which can dramatically alter their serum levels and interindividual response. Once broken down, most opioid metabolites are excreted renally. In the presence of impaired kidney function, these metabolites can accumulate and, in addition to prolonging the opioid benefits, may accumulate and cause toxic opioid effects (59). See Table 5.12 for a comparison of the different pharmacokinetic characteristics of commonly used opioids in dentistry.

5.8.3.1 Morphine

Morphine undergoes extensive first pass metabolism by glucuronidation to produce morphine-3-glucuronide (M3G) and morphine-6-glucuronide (M6G). While the M3G metabolite does not produce analgesic effects, the M6G metabolite is a potent μ receptor agonist and contributes to the analgesic efficacy of morphine itself.

5.8.3.2 Codeine

Codeine, also known as 3-methyl morphine, is a pro-drug which undergoes first pass metabolism by the enzyme CYP2D6 to morphine, the active metabolite (see Figure 5.4). Approximately 6–10% of Caucasians and 1–2% of Asians have defective or absent alleles in their genes to code for this enzyme, and therefore are unable to synthesise

CYP2D6 (11). These individuals are referred to as 'slow metabolisers' and their status results in little or no conversion of codeine to morphine and any other drug that requires CYP2D6 for conversion as well (11). Since morphine is responsible for the analgesic effect (binding to the μ opioid receptor), codeine provides little or no analgesic activity for these patients. However, codeine still confers adverse effects in these patients, such as sedation and constipation.

Figure 5.4 Metabolism of codeine.

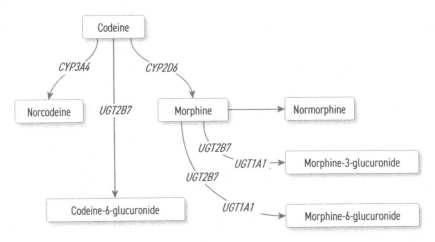

Pharmacogenomic variation in metabolism can also lead to a super-fast metabolism of drugs. Around 10% of Caucasians, 1–2% of Asians, up to 21% of Middle Eastern people and almost 30% of Ethiopians are ultra-rapid metabolisers and have multiple copies of the alleles that code for 2D6 enzymes (11). These patients make more CYP2D6 and, for them, codeine will be converted more quickly and efficiently to morphine, resulting in higher levels of morphine and potential toxicity (11).

In addition to genetic status, drug interactions that result in inhibition or induction of CYP2D6 or other relevant metabolic enzymes will further complicate the effects of codeine and morphine (see Section 5.8.4).

DNA testing that determines people's genetic status for various CYP enzymes is now available through many pathology companies in Australia.

5.8.3.3 Oxycodone

As oxycodone is not a pro-drug and the parent compound is the active form, it has more predictable pharmacodynamics and pharmacokinetics and its use is therefore generally preferred over codeine. Oxycodone is metabolised by CYP3A4/5 and CYP2D6 to metabolites noroxycodone and oxymorphone respectively (60) (see Figure 5.5). While these metabolites are active, their clinical contribution towards analgesia is insignificant. Although it is unclear if the pharmacogenomic variability of CYP2D6 and CYP3A4 status affects the plasma levels of oxycodone, drugs that are inducers or inhibitors of these enzymes can still cause significant interactions (60, 87).

Figure 5.5 Metabolism of oxycodone.

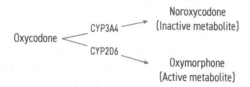

5.8.3.4 Tramadol

Tramadol is a pro-drug, converted to its active forms in a similar way to codeine via CYP2D6. However, tramadol is converted to two metabolites (see Figure 5.6). The mechanism of action of the parent compound tramadol is inhibition of reuptake of noradrenaline (NA) and serotonin (5HT) in the CNS (61). It is metabolised by CYP2D6 to the main metabolite, O-desmethyltramadol (M1), which is a μ opioid agonist that confers a weak opioid analgesic effect. The combined effect of parent tramadol and the M1 metabolite are useful in some specific kinds of pain; the N-desmethyltramadol (M2) metabolite is considered inactive.

Figure 5.6 Metabolism of tramadol.

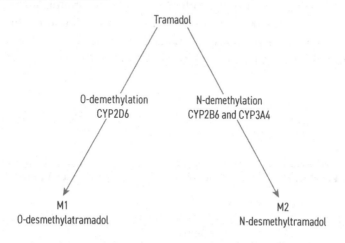

The pharmacogenomic variability of the enzyme CYP2D6 will alter the metabolism of tramadol to its active metabolites and therefore alter the effectiveness of tramadol exactly the way codeine's transformation to morphine is adversely affected (see Section 5.8.3.2).

Renal excretion accounts for 90% elimination of tramadol and the active M1 metabolite; therefore, the dose should be reduced or dosage interval prolonged in patients with reduced kidney function.

Due to tramadol's inhibition of serotonin reuptake, serotonin excess can occur from use of this drug. The risk of developing serotonin syndrome, which is a medical emergency, is low unless tramadol is used in the presence of other risk factors, such as concurrent medications that increase serotonin levels (e.g. antidepressants, antiemetics, antipsychotics), higher dosages, medications that inhibit CYP2D6, or the patient is a CYP2D6 poor metaboliser. These risk factors can lead to a reduced metabolism of tramadol to the active metabolite and increased levels of the parent compound (61). If a patient experiences troubling symptoms of serotonin excess, the dose of the culprit medication could be reduced or the drug gradually ceased, depending on the clinical circumstances and patient preference. Serotonin syndrome is characterised by increased levels of serotonin at the nerve synapses, and has three defining characteristics: altered mental status, autonomic dysfunction and neuromuscular hyperactivity (61). Clinically, this can present as hyperreflexia, tremor, incoordination, confusion, sweating, fever or diarrhoea. Serotonin toxicity warrants immediate discontinuation of the implicated drug and possible emergency care.

Tramadol also increases the risks of seizures in a dose-dependent manner; this is usually in the context of overdose, use with other serotonergic dugs, and with doses at the upper end of the therapeutic range (50–400mg/day). The mechanism is likely to be the same as the risk of seizures observed with serotonin toxicity (62).

5.8.3.5 Tapentadol

Tapentadol is a dual-action, centrally acting analgesic, with the parent compound acting as both an opioid-receptor agonist as well as inhibiting the reuptake of NA. Evidence to support its use in dental pain is poor, with one study demonstrating that varying doses of tapentadol (between 75–200mg) were inferior to 400mg of ibuprofen for dental pain after surgical third molar extractions (63). Tapentadol's main advantage is the improved GI adverse effect profile compared to conventional opioids (64).

Table 5.11 Pharmacokinetic characteristics of commonly used oral opioids in dentistry. Based on (26).

Opioid	Pro-drug?	Metabolism	Active metabolite	Half-life (hours)
Codeine	Yes	CYP2D6; then as per morphine	Yes: morphine	2–4
Morphine	No, but active metabolites	Glucuronidation primarily UGT2B7	Yes: morphine-3-glucuronide and morphine-6-glucuronide	2–3
Oxycodone	No	CYP3A4/5 and CYP2D6	No*	3–5

Table 5.11 (cont.)

Opioid	Pro-drug?	Metabolism	Active metabolite	Half-life (hours)
Tramadol	Yes (parent compound is active; inhibits reuptake of serotonin and noradrenaline)	CYP2D6 to the active metabolite; also via CYP2B6 and CYP3A4	Yes: M1 (O-desmethyltramadol; a weak opioid agonist)	5–7; M1 metabolite: 6–8
Tapentadol	No	Glucuronidation (UGT enzymes) (97%)	No	4 (IR)

Notes:

* metabolites of oxycodone are not considered to be pharmacologically active.

IR: immediate release.

5.8.4 Common drug interactions with opioid analgesics

Table 5.12 General classes of drugs with significant interactions with opioid analgesics. Based on (11, 23, 24).

Class of drug	Mechanism and outcome	Management
Sedatives/hypnotics (e.g. benzodiazepines, Z-drugs, sedative antihistamines, alcohol, gabapentinoids, tricyclic antidepressants, muscle relaxants)	Cumulative CNS and respiratory depression. May be life-threatening, especially in opioid naive patients. Also increased risk of hazardous behaviours	Avoid these drugs in combinations wherever possible. If unavoidable, use lowest dose for shortest period, preferably under medical supervision. Monitor for signs of respiratory/CNS depression.
Anticholinergic/antimuscarinic agents (e.g. atropine, belladonna alkaloids, hyoscyamine, propantheline, tolterodine, sedative antihistamines, prochlorperazine, clozapine, tricyclic antidepressants)	Increased risk of anticholinergic syndromes (e.g. delirium, sedation, dry mucous membranes, constipation, thermal dysregulation, and paralytic ileus)	Avoid combination or use drug with less anticholinergic burden
CYP2D6 inhibitors (e.g. amiodarone, chlorpheniramine, diphenhydramine, desvenlafaxine, prochlorperazine, paroxetine, olanzapine)	Impaired conversion of codeine and tramadol to active forms Impaired metabolism of tapentadol to inactive metabolites	Use opioids that do not solely rely on CYP2D6 for conversion (e.g. oxycodone, or no opioid at all)
CYP2D6 inducers (e.g. rifampicin, dexamethasone)	Increased conversion of codeine and tramadol to active metabolites. Increased efficacy and risk of toxicity	Use opioids which are not metabolised solely by CYP2D6

Table 5.12 (cont.)

Class of drug	Mechanism and outcome	Management
CYP3A4 inhibitors (e.g. clarithromycin, erythromycin, fluoxetine, ketoconazole, itraconazole, verapamil, diltiazem, voriconazole, grapefruit juice, turmeric, black pepper, star fruit, ritonavir)	Decreased conversion of oxycodone to inactive metabolites. Accumulation of oxycodone levels and potential for toxicity	Avoid interacting drugs where possible. Switch to different analgesic
CYP3A4 inducers (e.g. carbamazepine, phenytoin, rifabutin, rifampicin, St John's wort)	Increased conversion of oxycodone to inactive metabolites. Decreased efficacy of oxycodone	Avoid interacting drugs where possible. Switch to different analgesic

5.8.5 Doses of opioids used in dentistry

Table 5.13 Doses and equianalgesic doses of opioids commonly prescribed in dentistry. Adapted from (4, 11, 27).

Opioid	Dose in dentistry	Dose adjustment in renal impairment[‡]	Dose adjustment in hepatic impairment[‡]	Dose equivalent to codeine 60mg*
Oxycodone	5mg orally (immediate release) every 4–6 hours when required, for the minimum duration required (maximum 3 days)	Dose reduction required. Seek medical advice	Dose reduction required in moderate to severe liver impairment. Seek medical advice	5mg
Codeine	30–60mg (in combination with paracetamol 500–1000mg) every 4–6 hours to a maximum of codeine 240mg/ paracetamol 4000mg/24 hours when required, for the minimum duration required (maximum 3 days)	Avoid use. Seek medical advice	Dose reduction required in moderate to severe liver impairment. Seek medical advice	60mg

Table 5.13 (cont.)

Opioid	Dose in dentistry	Dose adjustment in renal impairment‡	Dose adjustment in hepatic impairment‡	Dose equivalent to codeine 60mg*
Tramadol	50mg IR every 4–6 hours when required, for the minimum duration required (maximum 3 days); maximum 400mg/day	Dose reduction required if CrCl <30mL/minute. Seek medical advice. Controlled release products are contraindicated in renal impairment	Dose reduction required in moderate to severe liver impairment. Seek medical advice	40mg

Notes:

* http://www.opioidcalculator.com.au/opioidtarget.html?total=8. These doses are not an equivalent but an estimate. When switching from one opioid to another, the dose would need to be decreased then titrated back up again.

‡ Seek specialist advice regarding the dose reduction required.

IR: immediate release; CrCl: creatine clearance.

Practice points

- Oxycodone is a potent opioid used for moderate–severe pain.
- Codeine is a pro-drug metabolised to morphine by CYP2D6. Be aware of variability with CYP2D6 metabolism and effectiveness of codeine. It is contraindicated in children <12 years and breast-feeding women.
- Dentists should not prescribe tramadol or tapentadol unless they have been specifically trained to do so competently.
- Tramadol is a complex pro-drug, with serotonergic, noradrenergic and opioid effects. It has un-predictable pharmacology and pharmacokinetics, which makes it difficult to use safely. Be aware of variability with CYP2D6 metabolism and effectiveness of tramadol. Avoid in people >75 years.
- Tapentadol has opioid and noradrenergic effects. It is a highly potent drug, with more linear kinetics than tramadol, but increased opioid effects.
- As synthetic opioids, both tramadol and tapentadol may be analgesic options for people who are allergic to other types of opioids. Seek medical advice (4, 11).

5.8.6 Appropriate use of opioids in dentistry

The quickest and most effective method of managing dental pain is by active dental treat-ment. When pain medication is needed, opioids are not very effective for dental pain; it is established that NSAIDs with/without paracetamol are far superior.

NSAIDs and paracetamol should always be tried first for dental pain for those who can tolerate them. There is inter-patient variability in the responsiveness of different NSAIDs, and so if one NSAID is not as effective (e.g. ibuprofen), a different one can be recommended (e.g. naproxen). Dentists should check that the administration of the NSAID and paracetamol is correct: appropriate doses, taken concurrently, on an empty stomach, with appropriate dosing intervals (see Section 5.7.1).

If an opioid needs to be prescribed, the lowest dose over the shortest time frame (maximum 3 days) is recommended (4). Minimal quantities should be prescribed to avoid leftover pills.

5.8.6.1 Check black box warnings before prescribing

Be aware that regulatory agencies around the world are increasingly discouraging the use of opioids for both acute and chronic pain management, due to their wide range of adverse effects, drug interactions and tendency for misuse. Before prescribing opioids, be sure to consult the manufacturer's prescribing information as many are now accompanied with black box warnings that prescribers must heed. In addition, the advent of Real Time Prescription Monitoring means prescribers must comply with state government prescribing rules and regulations for monitored medicines such as opioids. It is strongly recommended that prescribers who have not been trained to prescribe opioids avoid doing so as this practice will fall outside their area of competency.

5.8.7 Dependence, tolerance and substance abuse

Tolerance and dependence are associated with opioid use. Tolerance occurs when the patient experiences a reduced effect from the same dose of opioid, due to the desensitisation or down-regulation of the opioid receptors (6, 7). This is also known as tachyphylaxis, where continuous or repeated administration of a drug results in a loss of pharmacodynamic response (65). Dependence occurs when an individual continues to administer the drug to prevent an abstinence or withdrawal syndrome. Abrupt discontinuation can produce symptoms such as restlessness, irritability, diarrhoea and shivering (6). Opioids produce tolerance and dependence after repeated administration to varying degrees, depending on the context of use.

Substance abuse disorder is a behavioural syndrome in which individuals depend on and seek drugs for their CNS effects, despite adverse medical and/or social consequences (4). Drug abuse is not a pharmacological consequence of opioid use.

5.8.7.1 Potential for diversion and need for opioids in dentistry

Opioids and benzodiazepines are the most common drug classes associated with pharmaceutical misuse of drugs. People can be seeking opioids for non-medical use for themselves, a family member or friend, or for the purposes of diversion. The opioid crisis is a major public health issue, with harms from prescription opioid misuse and pharmaceutical opioid poisonings having far surpassed that of heroin (66).

Dental opioid prescribing has increased during the last decade, despite opioids not being particularly effective for dental pain (67). Studies from the US have also associated dental opioid prescriptions for third molar extractions with an increased risk of persistent opioid use in adolescents and young adults (68, 69).

It is established that the most common source of opioid for non-medical use is left-over pills from legitimate prescriptions, sourced through social networks (70). Often, patients are prescribed more opioids than necessary, rendering leftover pills (71).

A prospective cohort study of patients undergoing surgical third molar extractions showed that only 7% of the 81 patients included in the study needed oxycodone; ibuprofen and paracetamol provided sufficient pain relief for the remaining cohort (71). The authors concluded that the need for opioids for asymptomatic surgical third molar extractions was minimal.

It has been shown in dentistry that patient satisfaction and care is one factor that drives dental prescribing. A survey of patients to assess self-reported outcomes of satisfaction and care after surgical third molar extractions found that prescribing opioids was associated with higher levels of pain, and there were no reported differences in the levels of satisfaction perceived between patients who were and who were not prescribed opioids (72).

5.8.8 Pregnancy and lactation recommendations for opioid analgesics

See Table 14.2.

5.9 Drugs used for treatment of neuropathic pain in the orofacial region

Common diagnoses involving neuropathic pain in the orofacial region include trigeminal neuralgia, persistent idiopathic facial pain, and post-traumatic trigeminal neuropathic pain. Neuropathic pain arises from damaged nerves, often presenting with allodynia, hyperalgesia, hyperpathia (pain that increases after removal of the stimulus) or dysaesthesia. Imbalances between excitatory and inhibitory signalling in the somatosensory system, as well as modulation of the ion channels, are associated with the alteration of the pain messages in neuropathic pain (73). Opioids, paracetamol and NSAIDs are not very effective for neuropathic pain (6, 9). Drugs such as antidepressants and anticonvulsants are generally used, with varying degrees of evidence and effectiveness (9).

5.9.1 Amitriptyline

Tricyclic antidepressants amitriptyline.

5.9.1.1 Pharmacodynamics

Amitriptyline is a tricyclic antidepressant that has been used for decades to treat neuropathic pain. Amitriptyline inhibits the reuptake of Na and 5HT, thought to work by promoting the descending pathways from the brain to the spinal cord that switch off pain signals from the periphery. Amitriptyline inhibits the reuptake of Na and 5HT, which promote the descending inhibitory pain pathways from the brain that switch off pain signals from the periphery. Na is also thought to exhibit an anti-allodynic action by acting on α-2A and β-2 adrenoceptors (74).

5.9.1.2 Contraindications/precautions

- Prostatic hypertrophy

- History of closed-angle glaucoma
- Epilepsy, history of seizures
- History or factors for QT prolongation including other drugs which prolong the QT interval
- Second- or third-degree heart block, severe ischaemic heart disease or myocardial instability
- Suicidal ideation; overdose carries a high risk of fatality
- Dementia, as potent anticholinergic effects exacerbate memory impairment
- Moderate-to-severe dry mouth or dry eyes due to anticholinergic effects
- Multiple other anticholinergic drugs, due to risk of cumulative anticholinergic toxicity (11)

5.9.1.3 Adverse effects

The main adverse effects of amitriptyline are:

- anticholinergic effects, including confusion, delirium, dry mouth, constipation, urinary retention and increased risk of falls
- sedation
- orthostatic hypotension
- CV adverse effects, causing prolonged QT interval, slowed cardiac conduction, T wave inversion arrhythmias, sinus tachycardia

5.9.1.4 Common drug interactions with amitriptyline

Amitriptyline is a CYP2D6 and CYP2C19 substrate. It is metabolised to its active metabolite of nortriptyline that also relies on CYP2D6 for its metabolism.

Table 5.14 Common drug interactions with amitriptyline. Based on (11, 23, 24).

Interacting drugs	Mechanism and outcome	Management
Serotonergic drugs	Combination of drugs that elevate serotonin levels in the CNS risk serotonin excess and/or serotonin syndrome	Avoid use with other serotonergic drugs
Anticholinergic drugs	AMT has strong anticholinergic effects (NTP less so). Use with other anticholinergic drugs risks anticholinergic syndromes, especially in the elderly	Be aware of cumulative anticholinergic burden. Avoid AMT use with other anticholinergic drugs where possible. Choose a less anticholinergic drug
Drugs which cause QT prolongation	AMT and NTP prolong QT interval. Concomitant use with other QT prolonging drugs, may result in acute ventricular arrhythmias including torsades de pointes and death	Check potential for this interaction. Consult expert resources before prescribing

Table 5.14 (cont.)

Interacting drugs	Mechanism and outcome	Management
CYP2D6 inhibitors (e.g. amiodarone, chlorpheniramine, diphenhydramine, desvenlafaxine, prochlorperazine, paroxetine, olanzapine)	Increased levels of AMT and NTP. Increased risk of side effects and toxicity	Avoid CYP2D6 inhibitors
CYP2C19 inhibitors (e.g. clarithromycin, fluconazole, fluoxetine, fluvoxamine, omeprazole, ketoconazole)	Increased levels of AMT (but not NTP). Increased risk of AMT side effects and toxicity	Avoid CYP2C19 inhibitors
CYP2D6 inducers (e.g. rifampicin, dexamethasone)	Decreased levels of AMT and NTP. Reduced efficacy	Monitor for clinical efficacy. If efficacy declines, cease the interacting drug rather than increasing the amitriptyline dose.

Notes: AMT: amitriptyline; NTP: nortriptyline.

5.9.1.5 Doses in neuropathic pain

Table 5.15 Dose of amitriptyline for neuropathic pain. Based on (11, 13, 27).

Dose of amitriptyline for neuropathic pain	Dose adjustment in renal impairment	Dose adjustment in hepatic impairment[‡]
5–12.5mg at night initially; gradually increase every 7 days, depending on the response, up to a maximum of 50mg at night for orofacial pain management Older patients (>70 years) require a slower titration of the dose.	Dose as per normal renal function	Reduce dose or avoid in severe liver impairment. Seek medical advice

Note:
[‡] Seek specialist advice regarding the dose reduction required.

Practice points

- Amitriptyline can increase the CNS effects of alcohol; avoid alcohol while undergoing treatment (11).
- The anticholinergic side effects of amitriptyline can be debilitating, especially in combination with other anticholinergic drugs. Monitor patient for such side effects in case the drug should be ceased (11).
- Orthostatic hypotension may put patients at increased risk of falls and fractures. Ensure the patient is warned of this, and to rise from lying or sitting position slowly to prevent falls (11).

- On cessation, the dose of amitriptyline should be reduced slowly to avoid withdrawal effects (11).
- Avoid use in the elderly due to their greater vulnerability to anticholinergic effects (11).

5.9.1.6 Pregnancy and lactation recommendations for amitriptyline

See Table 14.2.

5.9.2 Carbamazepine and oxcarbazepine

Carbamazepine is an anti-epileptic drug, with a range of other actions including anticholinergic, antineuralgic, antidiuretic, muscle relaxant, antimanic, antidepressive, and anti-arrhythmic properties. In dentistry, it is recommended as a first-line drug treatment of trigeminal neuralgia. Its mechanism of action is thought to be elicited by inhibiting voltage-gated sodium and calcium channels to produce a neuronal membrane stabilising effect, leading to a decrease in neuronal hyperexcitability, reduced seizure potential and less pain transmission (75). Oxcarbazepine is an analogue of carbamazepine with a very similar mechanism of action, but has a reduced risk of adverse reactions and drug interactions.

5.9.2.1 Contraindications/precautions

- Heart failure, atrioventricular conduction abnormalities
- History of bone marrow depression, hyponatraemia, porphyria (11)
- Epilepsy unless under medical supervision due to high risk of drug interactions and increased risk of absence or myoclonic seizures (11)
- Hypersensitivity to carbamazepine, phenytoin, phenobarbitone or oxcarbazepine
- Patients positive for the HLA-B*1502 and/or HLA-A*3101 alleles in at-risk populations (see Section 5.9.2.2) or only under close medical supervision where benefits outweigh risks (26)

5.9.2.2 Severe skin reactions, SJS and TEN

Patients with the HLA-B*1502 allele have a significantly increases the risk of severe skin reactions, including Stevens-Johnson syndrome (SJS) and toxic epidermal necrolysis (TEN) (89). Certain subgroups of the population, including people of Han Chinese, Thai and Malay ancestry, have an increased expression of this polymorphism (76). Testing for this allele is recommended in at-risk groups prior to commencing carbamazepine or oxcarbazepine.

The HLA-A*3101 allele is associated with milder skin reactions and multi-organ sensitivity. At-risk people tend to be those of Northern European and Japanese descent (11).

It is therefore recommended to conduct genetic testing prior to commencing carbamazepine for people who are most likely to have these variant HLA types (77).

5.9.2.3 Adverse effects

Up to 40–60% of patients experience adverse effects from carbamazepine (75). These include:

- hyponatremia: manifesting as confusion, seizures and coma (78). Low sodium may also be caused by carbamazepine-induced syndrome of inappropriate antidiuretic hormone
- CNS depression with impaired memory, inattention, confusion, ataxia, dizziness, blurred vision, headache (11, 78). It may also involve mental health changes such as emotional lability and depression
- weight gain
- osteomalacia and osteoporosis, due to induction of vitamin D metabolism. Calcium and vitamin D supplementation is usually required
- bone marrow suppression. Monitor regularly for leukopenia and thrombocytopenia
- oral adverse effects: dry mouth, taste changes, orofacial dyskinesia (11)
- severe skin reactions: multi-organ hypersensitivity syndrome, also known as drug rash with eosinophilia and systemic symptoms (DRESS) syndrome, is rare. Carbamazepine is one of the more common inducers of DRESS, accounting for between 5–20% of cases (78). It has a 2–6-week latency period after commencing carbamazepine, and can lead to kidney and liver failure. Early symptoms include fever, rash, bruising/bleeding (11)

5.9.2.4 Common drug interactions with carbamazepine

Carbamazepine is a CYP3A4 substrate but also potent inducer of CYP enzymes and p-glycoprotein transport. It also induces its own metabolism.

Oxcarbazepine is a substrate for glucuronidation enzymes, but inhibits CYP2C19 and induces CYP3A4/5.

Table 5.16 Common drug interactions with carbamazepine and oxcarbazepine. Based on (11, 23, 24, 26).

Interacting drug	Mechanism and outcome	Management
Clozapine	Both carbamazepine and clozapine can cause bone marrow suppression. Increased risk when used together Carbamazepine also induces the CYP3A4 metabolism of clozapine, resulting in reduced clozapine serum levels Oxcarbazepine and clozapine carry increased of seizures	Avoid use of clozapine with either carbamazepine or oxcarbazepine
Levothyroxine	Carbamazepine induces the liver metabolism of levothyroxine resulting in reduced free T4 levels and increased dosage requirements. Oxcarbazepine does not interact in this way	Do not use carbamazepine in patients on levothyroxine unless undergoing regular monitoring of T4 and TSH levels. Oxcarbazepine may be used

Table 5.16 (cont.)

Interacting drug	Mechanism and outcome	Management
CYP3A4/5 inhibitors (e.g. amiodarone, ciclosporin, clarithromycin, erythromycin, fluconazole, miconazole, verapamil, posaconazole, ritonavir, voriconazole)	Increased carbamazepine levels, with increased risk of side effects and toxicity	Avoid these drug combinations. Seek expert advice
CYP3A4/5 inducers (e.g. armodafinil, bosentan, corticosteroids, modafinil, phenobarbital, rifabutin, St John's Wort)	Reduced carbamazepine levels, and reduced efficacy	Avoid these drug combinations. Seek expert advice
CYP3A4/5 substrates (e.g. alprazolam, amlodipine, amitriptyline, atorvastatin cannabidiol, diltiazem, fluoxetine, ethinyl oestradiol, prednisone, progesterone, quetiapine, simvastatin, tramadol, warfarin, zolpidem)	Carbamazepine induces CYP3A4/5 synthesis, and therefore, can increase metabolism of CYP3A4/5 substrates. The latter drug's serum levels can decline and efficacy wane	Seek expert advice before prescribing
CYP2C19 substrates	Oxcarbazepine inhibits CYP2C19, and therefore can increase levels of substrates for this enzyme	Seek expert advice before prescribing

Note: TSH: thyroid stimulating hormone.

5.9.2.5 Doses in trigeminal neuralgia

Table 5.17 Doses of carbamazepine and oxcarbazepine for trigeminal neuralgia. Based on (11, 26, 27, 29, 79).

Drug	Dose for trigeminal neuralgia	Dose adjustment in renal impairment	Dose adjustment in hepatic impairment
Carbamazepine	Adult: 100mg modified release tablets orally twice daily. Titrate up gradually if required every 7 days to maximum of 400mg twice daily	Dose as per normal renal function	Avoid in liver impairment. Seek medical advice
Oxcarbazepine	Adult: 300mg tablets orally twice daily. Titrate up gradually if required every 7 days to 600mg twice daily	Reduce dose if CrCl <30 mL/minute. Seek medical advice for patients with renal impairment	Seek medical advice for patients with liver impairment

It should be noted that oxcarbazepine is not registered for treatment of trigeminal neuralgia in Australia or New Zealand, and therefore its use for this indication would be off-label.

Practice points

Carbamazepine and oxcarbazepine

- The effects of alcohol are increased, and drowsiness, dizziness or blurred vision is common on commencement of therapy. Tolerance to drowsiness does develop over time (11).
- Monitor for skin reactions (e.g. exfoliative dermatitis, SJS).
- Monitor for DRESS syndrome: if rash, sore throat, fever, bruising/bleeding occurs, seek medical advice.
- Oxcarbazepine has a lower incidence of severe skin reactions, hepatic impairment, CNS adverse effects and fewer drug interactions compared with carbamazepine (11, 80).

Carbamazepine only

- Avoid grapefruit juice which inhibits the CYP3A4 mediated metabolism of carbamazepine (11).
- Full blood counts are needed prior to starting treatment and regularly thereafter; stop treatment if bone marrow depression occurs (11).

5.9.2.6 Pregnancy and lactation recommendations for carbamazepine and oxcarbazepine

See Table 14.2.

5.9.3 Gabapentinoids: gabapentin and pregabalin

Gabapentin and pregabalin exhibit structural similarity to the endogenous neurotransmitter (GABA); however, their mechanism of action is thought to be related to the modification of voltage-gated calcium channels and reduced neurotransmitter release at the supraspinal and spinal levels to regulate pain processing and reduce neuronal hyperexcitability (6, 81, 82).

A review demonstrated that use of gabapentin for 4–12 weeks in people with moderate–severe chronic neuropathic pain due to post-herpetic neuralgia or diabetic neuropathy can substantially reduce pain (83). It is used in trigeminal neuralgia, and other chronic neuropathies (81).

Pregabalin has been shown to be effective for treatment of some neuropathic pain symptoms, including post-herpetic neuralgia and diabetic neuropathies, although significantly more likely to be associated with adverse effects (84). While a small proportion of people will experience moderate to substantial benefit from pregabalin, many will have no little or benefit (85).

5.9.3.1 Contraindications/precautions

Gabapentin and pregabalin are best avoided in patients with a history of absence seizures, and who are on drugs that increase the risk of seizures, due to possible aggravation of epilepsy (11).

5.9.3.2 Adverse effects

The main adverse effects of gabapentinoids are:

- fatigue, sedation, dizziness, diplopia, nystagmus, tremor, memory impairment, somnolence
- weight gain
- neuropsychiatric effects (including suicidal ideation)
- dry mouth
- ataxia
- peripheral oedema
- euphoria
- increased risk of falls (11, 84)

5.9.3.3 Common drug interactions with gabapentinoids

Gabapentin and pregabalin are such small molecules that they are not metabolised and are both excreted unchanged via the kidney. Therefore, there are no pharmacokinetic interactions of concern; however, there are several key pharmacodynamic interactions.

Table 5.18 Common drug interactions with gabapentinoids. Based on (11, 23, 24).

Interacting drug	Mechanism and outcome	Management
Alcohol	Gabapentinoids will enhance the CNS effects of alcohol	Advise patient to avoid alcohol if possible or drinking only in moderation
CNS depressants (e.g. sedative antihistamines, benzodiazepines, Z-drugs)	Gabapentinoids will enhance the CNS effect of other CNS depressants. Combination will have effects on sleep, mood and behaviour.	Avoid combination wherever possible

5.9.3.4 Doses for treatment of trigeminal neuralgia

Table 5.19 Doses of gabapentin and pregabalin for trigeminal neuralgia. Based on (11, 79).

Gabapentinoids	Dose for trigeminal neuralgia	Doses for elderly patients	Dose adjustment in renal impairment
Gabapentin	300mg daily, taken orally at night. The dose can be slowly increased every 3–7 days up to 600–1200mg orally, 3 times a day, if required	Start with lower initial doses. Slower dose increases may be required. Seek medical advice	Reduce dose in renal impairment. Seek medical advice
Pregabalin	75mg daily, taken orally at night. The dose can be slowly increased every 3–7 days up to 150–300mg twice daily, if required	Start with lower initial doses (e.g. 25mg daily, orally at night). Slower dose increases may be required. Seek medical advice	Reduce dose in renal impairment. Seek medical advice

Practice points

- The CNS depressant and disinhibitory effects of alcohol may be increased in combination with gabapentinoids.
- These drugs are associated with increasing risk of suicidal ideation. If patient displays these symptoms, ensure the gabapentinoid is promptly ceased. Doses should be ceased gradually; seek medical advice.
- The efficacy of gabapentin and pregabalin for neuropathic pain has been studied in controlled trials of only up to 12 and 13 weeks respectively; consider re-assessment for treatment duration of longer than 12 weeks.
- When gabapentinoids are stopped, taper the dose slowly over at least 1 week; seek medical advice.
- Pain relief may take several weeks to achieve with gabapentinoids: minimal or no benefit is shown in most patients, so treatment should be stopped (with slowing dose tapering) if no improvement is seen or if adverse effects cannot be tolerated (11).

5.9.3.5 Misuse and abuse of gabapentinoids

Increasing evidence has shown widespread misuse and abuse of gabapentinoids in the community, thought to be due to their anxiolytic and dissociative effects through modulatory effects on GABA and glutamate (82). High doses are often used to produce euphoric effects (86). Gabapentinoid abuse often occurs in high-risk populations, including those with a history of substance abuse and psychiatric co-morbidities (86). Prescribers should be aware of this potential especially when gabapentinoids are requested by the patient. Since pain is a multi-factorial disease, one property that both opioids and gabapentinoids have in common is their ability to reduce anxiety and produce the dissociative effects (82).

5.9.3.6 Pregnancy and lactation

See Table 14.2.

FURTHER READING

Best AD, De Silva RK, Thomson WM, Tong DC, Cameron CM, De Silva HL. Efficacy of Codeine When Added to Paracetamol (Acetaminophen) and Ibuprofen for Relief of Postoperative Pain After Surgical Removal of Impacted Third Molars: A Double-Blinded Randomized Control Trial. *J Oral Maxillofac Surg.* 2017;75(10):2063–2069.

Moore PA, Ziegler KM, Lipman RD, Aminoshariae A, Carrasco-Labra A, Mariotti A. Benefits and harms associated with analgesic medications used in the management of acute dental pain: An overview of systematic reviews. *J Am Dent Assoc.* 2018;149(4):256–265 e3.

REFERENCES

1. International Association for the Study of Pain. *Terminology.* 2017. https://www.iasp-pain .org/Education/Content.aspx?ItemNumber=1698

2. Treede RD, Rief W, Barke A et al. Chronic pain as a symptom or a disease: the IASP Classification of Chronic Pain for the International Classification of Diseases (ICD-11). *Pain.* 2019;160(1):19–27.

3. NPS MedicineWise. *Chronic Pain.* 2015. https://www.nps.org.au/news/chronic-pain#r7

4. Oral and Dental Expert Group. *Therapeutic Guidelines Oral and Dental (Version 3).* Therapeutic Guidelines Pty Ltd; 2019.

5. Cohen M. What is nociplastic pain? *Pain Management Today.* 2021;8(1):89–92.

6. Ritter J, Flower R, Henderson G, Loke YK, MacEwan D, Rang H. *Rang and Dale's Pharmacology.* 9th edition. Elsevier; 2020.

7. Brenner G, Stevens C. *Brenner and Stevens' Pharmacology.* 5th edition. Elsevier; 2018.

8. Chou R, Gordon DB, de Leon-Casasola OA et al. Management of Postoperative Pain: A Clinical Practice Guideline From the American Pain Society, the American Society of Regional Anesthesia and Pain Medicine, and the American Society of Anesthesiologists' Committee on Regional Anesthesia, Executive Committee, and Administrative Council. *J Pain.* 2016;17(2):131–157.

9. Murnion B. Neuropathic pain: current definition and review of drug treatment. *Aust Prescr.* 2018;41:60–63.

10. Bacchi S, Palumbo P, Sponta A, Coppolino MF. Clinical pharmacology of non-steroidal anti-inflammatory drugs: a review. *Antiinflamm Antiallergy Agents Med Chem.* 2012;11(1):52–64.

11. Editorial Advisory Committee. *Australian Medicines Handbook.* AMH Pty Ltd; 2022.

12. Bindu S, Mazumder S, Bandyopadhyay U. Non-steroidal anti-inflammatory drugs (NSAIDs) and organ damage: A current perspective. *Biochem Pharmacol.* 2020;180:114147.

13. Pain and Analgesia Expert Group. *Therapeutic Guidelines: Pain and Analgesia.* Therapeutic Guidelines Limited; 2020.

14. Horl WH. Nonsteroidal Anti-Inflammatory Drugs and the Kidney. *Pharmaceuticals (Basel).* 2010;3(7):2291–2321.

15. Prieto-Garcia L, Pericacho M, Sancho-Martinez SM et al. Mechanisms of triple whammy acute kidney injury. *Pharmacol Ther.* 2016;167:132–145.

16. McGettigan P, Henry D. Use of non-steroidal anti-inflammatory drugs that elevate cardiovascular risk: an examination of sales and essential medicines lists in low-, middle-, and high-income countries. *PLoS Med.* 2013;10(2):e1001388.

17. Perry A CM, Atkins A, Minehart M. Cardiovascular risk associated with NSAIDs and COX2 inhibitors. *US Pharm.* 2014;39:35–38.

18. Bally M, Dendukuri N, Rich B et al. Risk of acute myocardial infarction with NSAIDs in real world use: bayesian meta-analysis of individual patient data. *BMJ.* 2017;357:j1909.

19. Nissen SE, Yeomans ND, Solomon DH et al. Cardiovascular Safety of Celecoxib, Naproxen, or Ibuprofen for Arthritis. *N Engl J Med.* 2016;375(26):2519–2529.

20. National Asthma Council Australia. *Aspirin/NSAID-intolerant asthma: pharmacy notes.* National Asthma Council Australia Ltd; 2009.

21. Wan Y. *Can nonsteroidal anti-inflammatory drugs be used in adult patients with asthma?* NHS Specialist Pharmacy Service; 2020.

22. Woo SD, Luu QQ, Park HS. NSAID-Exacerbated Respiratory Disease (NERD): From Pathogenesis to Improved Care. *Front Pharmacol.* 2020;11:1147.

23. MedicinesComplete. *Stockley's Drug interactions.* 12th edition. Pharmaceutical Press; 2023.

24. IBM Corporation. *IMB Micromedex Clinical Evidence Packages.* IBM Watson Health; 2021.

25. What dose of paracetamol for older people? *Drugs and Therapeutics Bulletin.* 2018;56(6):69–72. doi:10.1136/dtb.2018.6.0636

26. AusDI. *Independent Drug Monographs.* 3 April 2021. https://ausdi.hcn.com.au/browseDocuments.hcn?filter=PRODUCTS_WITH_MONGRAPH

27. Ashley C, Dunleavy A. *The Renal Drug Handbook*. CRC Press; 2018.

28. Imani F, Motavaf M, Safari S, Alavian SM. The therapeutic use of analgesics in patients with liver cirrhosis: a literature review and evidence-based recommendations. *Hepat Mon.* 2014;14(10):e23539.

29. Ong CK, Seymour RA, Lirk P, Merry AF. Combining paracetamol (acetaminophen) with nonsteroidal antiinflammatory drugs: a qualitative systematic review of analgesic efficacy for acute postoperative pain. *Anesth Analg.* 2010;110(4):1170–1179.

30. Moore RA, Derry S, Aldington D, Wiffen PJ. Single dose oral analgesics for acute postoperative pain in adults—an overview of Cochrane reviews. *Cochrane Database Syst Rev.* 2015;(9):CD008659.

31. Derry CJ, Derry S, Moore RA. Single dose oral ibuprofen plus paracetamol (acetaminophen) for acute postoperative pain. *Cochrane Database Syst Rev.* 2013;(6):CD010210.

32. Moore RA, Derry S, Wiffen PJ, Straube S. Effects of food on pharmacokinetics of immediate release oral formulations of aspirin, dipyrone, paracetamol and NSAIDs—a systematic review. *Br J Clin Pharmacol.* 2015;80(3):381–388.

33. Best Practice Advocacy Centre New Zealand. *Avoiding the triple whammy in primary care.* BPAC NZ; 2018. https://bpac.org.nz/2018/triple-whammy.aspx

34. LaForge JM, Urso K, Day JM et al. Non-steroidal Anti-inflammatory Drugs: Clinical Implications, Renal Impairment Risks, and AKI. *Adv Ther.* 2023;40:2082–2096. doi:10.1007/s12325-023-02481-6

35. National Heart Foundation. *CVD risk calculators.* https://www.heartfoundation.org.au/bundles/heart-health-check-toolkit/cardiovascular-disease-risk-calculators

36. Klinger-Gratz PP, Ralvenius WT, Neumann E et al. Acetaminophen Relieves Inflammatory Pain through CB1 Cannabinoid Receptors in the Rostral Ventromedial Medulla. *J Neurosci.* 2018;38(2):322–334.

37. Ohashi N, Kohno T. Analgesic Effect of Acetaminophen: A Review of Known and Novel Mechanisms of Action. *Front Pharmacol.* 2020;11:580289.

38. Cairns R, Brown JA, Wylie CE et al. Paracetamol poisoning-related hospital admissions and deaths in Australia, 2004–2017. *Med J Aust.* 2019;211(5):218–223.

39. Chiew AL, Reith D, Pomerleau A et al. Updated guidelines for the management of paracetamol poisoning in Australia and New Zealand. *Med J Aust.* 2020;212(4):175–183.

40. Pathan H, Williams J. Basic opioid pharmacology: an update. *Br J Pain.* 2012;6(1):11–16.

41. Best AD, De Silva RK, Thomson WM et al. Efficacy of Codeine When Added to Paracetamol (Acetaminophen) and Ibuprofen for Relief of Postoperative Pain After Surgical Removal of Impacted Third Molars: A Double-Blinded Randomized Control Trial. *J Oral Maxillofac Surg.* 2017;75(10):2063–2069.

42. Aminoshariae A, Kulild JC, Donaldson M, Hersh EV. Evidence-based recommendations for analgesic efficacy to treat pain of endodontic origin: A systematic review of randomized controlled trials. *J Am Dent Assoc.* 2016;147(10):826–839.

43. Moore PA, Ziegler KM, Lipman RD, Aminoshariae A, Carrasco-Labra A, Mariotti A. Benefits and harms associated with analgesic medications used in the management of acute dental pain: An overview of systematic reviews. *J Am Dent Assoc.* 2018;149(4):256–265 e3.

44. Jeske NA. Dynamic Opioid Receptor Regulation in the Periphery. *Mol Pharmacol.* 2019;95(5):463–467.

45. Sehgal N, Smith HS, Manchikanti L. Peripherally acting opioids and clinical implications for pain control. *Pain Physician.* 2011;14(3):249–258.

46. Lee M, Silverman SM, Hansen H et al. A comprehensive review of opioid-induced hyperalgesia. *Pain Physician.* 2011;14(2):145–161.

47. Muller-Lissner S, Bassotti G, Coffin B et al. Opioid-Induced Constipation and Bowel Dysfunction: A Clinical Guideline. *Pain Med.* 2017;18(10):1837–1863.

48. Kalso E, Edwards JE, Moore AR, McQuay HJ. Opioids in chronic non-cancer pain: systematic review of efficacy and safety. *Pain.* 2004;112(3):372–380.

49. Smith HS, Laufer A. Opioid induced nausea and vomiting. *Eur J Pharmacol.* 2014;722:67–78.

50. Nicholson BD. Economic and clinical burden of opioid-induced nausea and vomiting. *Postgrad Med.* 2017;129(1):111–117.

51. Walker R, Whittlesea C. *Clinical Pharmacy and Therapeutics.* 4th edition. Churchill Livingstone; 2007.

52. Imam MZ, Kuo A, Ghassabian S, Smith MT. Progress in understanding mechanisms of opioid-induced gastrointestinal adverse effects and respiratory depression. *Neuropharmacology.* 2018;131:238–255.

53. de Vries F, Bruin M, Lobatto DJ et al. Opioids and Their Endocrine Effects: A Systematic Review and Meta-analysis. *J Clin Endocrinol Metab.* 2020;105(3).

54. Magnusson J MJ. *Opioid induced neurotoxicity.* College of Pharmacists of Manitoba; 2001.

55. Li PH, Ue KL, Wagner A, Rutkowski R, Rutkowski K. Opioid Hypersensitivity: Predictors of Allergy and Role of Drug Provocation Testing. *J Allergy Clin Immunol Pract.* 2017;5(6):1601–1606.

56. Saljoughian M. Opioids: Allergy vs Pseudoallergy. *US Pharm.* 2006;7:HS-5–HS-9.

57. Kalangara J, Potru S, Kuruvilla M. Clinical Manifestations and Diagnostic Evaluation of Opioid Allergy Labels—A Review. *J Pain Palliat Care Pharmacother.* 2019;33(3–4):131–140.

58. Langford RM, Knaggs R, Farquhar-Smith P, Dickenson AH. Is tapentadol different from classical opioids? A review of the evidence. *Br J Pain.* 2016;10(4):217–221.

59. Drewes AM, Jensen RD, Nielsen LM et al. Differences between opioids: pharmacological, experimental, clinical and economical perspectives. *Br J Clin Pharmacol.* 2013;75(1):60–78.

60. Kinnunen M, Piirainen P, Kokki H et al. Updated Clinical Pharmacokinetics and Pharmacodynamics of Oxycodone. *Clin Pharmacokinet.* 2019;58(6):705–725.

61. Beakley BD, Kaye AM, Kaye AD. Tramadol, Pharmacology, Side Effects, and Serotonin Syndrome: A Review. *Pain Physician.* 2015;18(4):395–400.

62. Nakhaee S, Amirabadizadeh A, Brent J et al. Tramadol and the occurrence of seizures: a systematic review and meta-analysis. *Crit Rev Toxicol.* 2019;49(8):710–723.

63. Kleinert R, Lange C, Steup A, Black P, Goldberg J, Desjardins P. Single dose analgesic efficacy of tapentadol in postsurgical dental pain: the results of a randomized, double-blind, placebo-controlled study. *Anesth Analg.* 2008;107(6):2048–2055.

64. Hartrick CT. Tapentadol immediate release for the relief of moderate-to-severe acute pain. *Expert Opin Pharmacother.* 2009;10(16):2687–2696.

65. Liu S. *Tachyphylaxis: Science Direct.* 2005. https://www.sciencedirect.com/topics/biochemistry-genetics-and-molecular-biology/tachyphylaxis

66. Roxburgh A, Hall WD, Dobbins T et al. Trends in heroin and pharmaceutical opioid overdose deaths in Australia. *Drug Alcohol Depend.* 2017;179:291–298.

67. Teoh L, Hollingworth S, Marino R, McCullough MJ. Dental opioid prescribing rates after the up-scheduling of codeine in Australia. *Sci Rep.* 2020;10(1):8463.

68. Schroeder AR, Dehghan M, Newman TB et al. Association of Opioid Prescriptions From Dental Clinicians for US Adolescents and Young Adults With Subsequent Opioid Use and Abuse. *JAMA Intern Med.* 2019;179(2):145–152.

69. Harbaugh CM, Nalliah RP, Hu HM et al. Persistent Opioid Use After Wisdom Tooth Extraction. *JAMA.* 2018;320(5):504–506.

70. Hulme S, Bright D, Nielsen S. The source and diversion of pharmaceutical drugs for non-medical use: A systematic review and meta-analysis. *Drug Alcohol Depend.* 2018;186:242–256.

71. Resnick CM, Calabrese CE, Afshar S, Padwa BL. Do Oral and Maxillofacial Surgeons Over-Prescribe Opioids After Extraction of Asymptomatic Third Molars? *J Oral Maxillofac Surg.* 2019;77(7):1332–1336.

72. Nalliah RP, Sloss KR, Kenney BC et al. Association of Opioid Use With Pain and Satisfaction After Dental Extraction. *JAMA Netw Open.* 2020;3(3):e200901.

73. Colloca L, Ludman T, Bouhassira D et al. Neuropathic pain. *Nat Rev Dis Primers.* 2017;3:17002.

74. Kremer M, Salvat E, Muller A et al. Antidepressants and gabapentinoids in neuropathic pain: Mechanistic insights. *Neuroscience.* 2016;338:183–206.

75. Gambeta E, Chichorro JG, Zamponi GW. Trigeminal neuralgia: An overview from pathophysiology to pharmacological treatments. *Mol Pain.* 2020;16:1744806920901890.

76. Chouchi M, Kaabachi W, Tizaoui K et al. The HLA-B*15:02 polymorphism and Tegretol®-induced serious cutaneous reactions in epilepsy: An updated systematic review and meta-analysis. *Rev Neurol (Paris).* 2018;174(5):278–291.

77. Amstutz U, Shear NH, Rieder MJ et al. Recommendations for HLA-B*15:02 and HLA-A*31:01 genetic testing to reduce the risk of carbamazepine-induced hypersensitivity reactions. *Epilepsia.* 2014;55(4):496–506.

78. Fricke-Galindo I, LLerena A, Jung-Cook H, Lopez-Lopez M. Carbamazepine adverse drug reactions. *Expert Rev Clin Pharmacol.* 2018;11(7):705–718.

79. Neurology Expert Group. *Therapeutic Guidelines Neurology (Version 5).* Therapeutic Guidelines Limited; 2018.

80. Peterson S, Benzon HT, Hurley RW. Membrane Stabilizers. In Benzon H, Srinivasa N, Fishman S et al (eds). *Essentials of Pain Medicine.* Elsevier/Saunders; 2018.

81. Kukkar A, Bali A, Singh N, Jaggi AS. Implications and mechanism of action of gabapentin in neuropathic pain. *Arch Pharm Res.* 2013;36(3):237–251.

82. Morrison EE, Sandilands EA, Webb DJ. Gabapentin and pregabalin: do the benefits outweigh the harms? *J R Coll Physicians Edinb.* 2017;47(4):310–313.

83. Moore A, Derry S, Wiffen P. Gabapentin for Chronic Neuropathic Pain. *JAMA.* 2018;319(8):818–819.

84. Onakpoya IJ, Thomas ET, Lee JJ et al. Benefits and harms of pregabalin in the management of neuropathic pain: a rapid review and meta-analysis of randomised clinical trials. *BMJ Open.* 2019;9(1):e023600.

85. Derry S, Bell RF, Straube S et al. Pregabalin for neuropathic pain in adults. *Cochrane Database Syst Rev.* 2019;1:CD007076.

86. Evoy KE, Morrison MD, Saklad SR. Abuse and Misuse of Pregabalin and Gabapentin. *Drugs.* 2017;77(4):403–426.

87. Fujiwara Y, Toyoda M, Chayahara N, Kiyota N, Shimada T, Imamura Y et al. Effects of Aprepitant on the Pharmacokinetics of Controlled-Release Oral Oxycodone in Cancer Patients. *PLoS ONE.* 2014;9(8):e104215.

88. Fields C, Drye L, Vaidya V, Lyketsos CG. Celecoxib or Naproxen Treatment Does Not Benefit Depressive Symptoms in Persons Age 70 and Older: Findings From a Randomized Controlled Trial. *The American Journal of Geriatric Psychiatry.* 2011;20(6):505–513.

89. Gonclaves, S. Dionne, RA. Moses, G. Carrozzo, M. Pharmacotherapeutic Approaches in Oral Medicine, Contemporary Oral Medicine. In Farah C, Balasubramaniam R, McCullough M (eds) *Contemporary Oral Medicine.* Springer, Cham; 2018. doi:10.1007/978-3-319-28100-1_11-1

6 ANXIOLYTICS

KEY POINTS

- Dental fear and phobia are common and can lead to stress and avoidance of dental procedures resulting in deterioration of oral health.
- Anxiolysis can improve patient comfort in order to complete the dental procedure.
- Safe and appropriate use of benzodiazepines or nitrous oxide can help anxious patients attend their dentist to the benefit of their oral health.

6.1 Introduction

Dental fear and phobia are common and affect around 1 in 6 Australian adults (1). Fear of dental care can lead to significant stress and avoidance resulting in neglect and deterioration of oral health (2). The aim of anxiolysis is to improve patient comfort in order to complete dental examination, investigations and procedures (3). This chapter will focus on the pharmacological measures used for anxiolysis in community dentistry.

6.2 Definition of anxiolysis

Anxiolysis, also known as 'minimal sedation', is defined as a reduction in anxiety achieved by pharmacological or non-pharmacological measures (4). When patients are minimally sedated, they are able to respond normally to verbal commands, 'cognitive function and co-ordination may be impaired, but no interventions are required to maintain a patent airway, spontaneous ventilation or cardiovascular function' (4, 5). Indications for the use of anxiolysis include dental phobia, pre-procedural anxiety, or a history of adverse dental experience which impairs the patient's ability to endure a dental procedure (2).

6.3 Definitions of sedation and sedation as a continuum

Levels of sedation occur on a continuum from minimal (anxiolysis) to general anaesthesia, as indicated in Table 6.1. There is no clear clinical distinction between the degrees of sedation. Further, using anxiolytic doses of sedative medicines does not guarantee the patient will not progress immediately to unconsciousness. For this reason, close and careful monitoring and use of very low dose oral anxiolytic medicines is recommended.

Table 6.1 Levels of sedation. Adapted from (3).

Level of sedation	Defining features
Minimal sedation (anxiolysis)	• Normal response to verbal commands • No interventions required to maintain a patent airway, ventilation is spontaneous • Cardiovascular function is not affected
Conscious sedation	• Drug-induced state. Patients can respond purposefully to verbal commands or light tactile sensation. • In some circumstances, interventions to maintain a patent airway, ventilation or cardiovascular function may be required
Deeper sedation	• Drug-induced state with a depression of consciousness that can progress to loss of consciousness • The patient is unable to maintain a patent airway, ventilate or maintain cardiovascular function without intervention • Similar risks are involved compared to general anaesthesia
General anaesthesia	• Drug-induced state, with the absence of purposeful response to any stimulus • Loss of protective airway reflexes • Depression of respiration

According to the Dental Board of Australia (DBA), dentists in general dental practice are competent to undertake minimal sedation (6). However, additional training and credentialing is required for the practitioner to be permitted to conduct conscious sedation (6). The DBA also stipulates that anxiolysis involves dosing of a single enteral (oral) drug that should not exceed the maximum recommended dose of a drug that is normally prescribed for unmonitored at-home use (7). In addition, minimal sedation does not include polypharmacy as the use of multiple drugs is only permitted for conscious sedation (6, 7).

6.4 Medications for anxiolysis

The medications recommended for anxiolysis in general dental practice are:

- for adults (≥18 years): oral benzodiazepines or nitrous oxide (but not together) (4)
- for children and adolescents (from 2–17 years): nitrous oxide only (4)

Oral benzodiazepines and nitrous oxide have been widely used to manage dental anxiety for many decades. Nitrous oxide was first used in dentistry in 1844 by Horace Wells, an American dentist who was administered nitrous oxide while having his own tooth extracted (8), and now is used commonly for analgesia and anxiolysis in dentistry. It is the first-line recommendation for pharmacological management of anxiety in children, and has been trialled and used extensively in children and adults for procedural sedation (9, 10) (see Section 6.6).

Anxiolysis involves administration of a single anxiolytic agent only. Use of more than one anxiolytic or sedative agent (i.e. multiple benzodiazepines or benzodiazepine plus nitrous oxide or methoxyflurane) fits the definition of conscious sedation and should only be used in the context of adequate training and monitoring due to the additive respiratory and central nervous system (CNS) depressant effects.

Safety and efficacy have not been established in children aged less than 16 years for lorazepam, oxazepam and temazepam (11).

6.5 Benzodiazepines

6.5.1 Drugs used for anxiolysis in general dentistry

- Diazepam
- Lorazepam
- Oxazepam
- Temazepam

6.5.2 Pharmacodynamics

Benzodiazepines potentiate the effect of the neurotransmitter gamma amino butyric acid (GABA) by enhancing the binding of GABA to the GABA-A receptor, increasing the depressant effects on the CNS, resulting in decreased neuronal activity (12, 13). Benzodiazepines can have multiple effects including anxiolytic, anticonvulsant, hypnotic, sedative and skeletal muscle relaxant effects. As such, they can be prescribed for many different reasons.

6.5.3 Evidence for use as oral sedation in dentistry

While benzodiazepines have been used extensively in dentistry for years, there is minimal evidence to support this practice and most are used off-label for preoperative anxiolysis (2). Only lorazepam is legally registered for this indication (13).

While midazolam is often used in dentistry for minimal sedation, it is only available in Australia as fluid for injection. Using this parenteral formulation for oral administration is not only considered off-label, but also inappropriate as there is no established oral dose for this formulation. Furthermore, midazolam is associated with rapid onset of action and profound sedation, especially in children, requiring careful up-titration of the dose that is virtually impossible to do with an oral liquid. In addition, the stability of midazolam mixed with a substance such as orange juice and/or paracetamol syrup has not been established, and distribution of the drug in the orange juice is impossible to determine, making dosing likely to be inaccurate. This drug also has a high incidence of adverse effects, including paradoxical excitation such as agitation, restless and disorientation in up to 1–15% of children (2, 5). For these reasons, midazolam is not recommended for oral sedation in dentistry in Australia, unless the dentist is endorsed to practice conscious sedation.

6.5.4 Contraindications/precautions

- Benzodiazepines are contraindicated in respiratory disease, sleep apnoea, myasthenia gravis, severe hepatic impairment (13).
- Benzodiazepines should be avoided in the elderly (>75 years) as they are more susceptible to the pharmacodynamic effects, increasing the risk of excessive sedation, delirium, memory impairment, confusion and falls (13).

Benzodiazepines should only be administered to children <17 years under the care of a paediatric dental specialist or special needs dentist. This is due to children in this age group having greater sensitivity to paradoxical excitation and CNS depressant effects, and the possibility of these children being on medications that may require specialist prescribing (13).

6.5.5 Adverse effects

- Common adverse effects (>1%): drowsiness, over-sedation, memory loss, slurred speech, blurred vision (13)
- Less common adverse effects (0.1–1%): paradoxical excitation, euphoria, aggression, respiratory depression (13)
- Paradoxical excitation: more common in children (3–19 years) (8). It manifests as restlessness, agitation and anxiety that may be misinterpreted as the drug being ineffective, prompting consideration of redosing. If this occurs, the procedure should not proceed and medical advice sought (8).

6.5.6 Drug interactions

Diazepam is broken down in the liver via CYP2C19 and CYP3A4 enzymes to several active metabolites, predominately desmethyldiazepam. Oxazepam and temazepam are other minor active metabolites (14). Therefore, potent inhibition of the CYP2C19 enzyme by drugs such as fluoxetine and omeprazole, as well as inhibition of the CYP3A4 enzymes by medications such as ritonavir, clarithromycin or erythromycin, can cause increased levels of diazepam. Therefore, diazepam should be avoided in patients on these medications (14). In contrast, inducers of CYP2C19 and CYP3A4, such as rifampicin and prednisone, topiramate, carbamazepine, St John's wort, phenytoin, or barbiturates, can cause lower levels of diazepam and diminish its effectiveness (14).

6.5.7 Doses, time of onset, half-life and practice points

Table 6.2 Doses, time of onset and half-life of commonly used benzodiazepines in dentistry. Based on (4, 11).

Benzodiazepine	Dose	Time to peak plasma concentrations (hours)	Half-life (hours)
Diazepam	5mg orally, 1 hour prior to the procedure	1–2	20–80
Lorazepam	1mg orally, 1–2 hours prior to the procedure	1–6	10–20
Oxazepam	7.5mg orally, 1–2 hours prior to the procedure	1–4	5–15
Temazepam	10mg orally, 1 hour prior to the procedure	0.5–2	5–15

Practice points

- Patients should be given the dose of the benzodiazepine in the clinic so they can be supervised once they are sedated (4).
- Drowsiness can occur with all benzodiazepines and can persist the following day (4).
- Diazepam has much longer half-life due to active metabolites compared to the other benzodiazepines; be aware of residual drowsiness (4).
- Patients should not drink any alcohol on the day of taking these medications (13).

6.5.8 Pregnancy and lactation recommendations for benzodiazepines

See Table 14.2.

6.5.9 Benzodiazepine abuse

Benzodiazepines are one of the most common drug classes associated with misuse in Australia (15). They are mostly associated with polydrug abuse, most often with opioids (16). In Australia, use of benzodiazepines in dentistry has increased in recent years, despite rates reducing in the US and at very low levels in the UK (17).

Benzodiazepines work in polydrug abuse by enhancing the euphoria from opioids, mitigating the dysphoria and withdrawal states between opioid or heroin doses, and enhancing the effects of alcohol (16, 17). Physiological and psychological dependence on benzodiazepines can develop within a week (18), where the patient continues to administer the benzodiazepine to prevent withdrawal symptoms, and has a reluctance to discontinue the benzodiazepine in fear of psychological symptoms such as anticipatory rebound anxiety (16). Short-acting benzodiazepines with a rapid onset of action, that are highly lipophilic and potent, and that cross the blood–brain barrier easily are more associated with producing reinforcing effects, such as alprazolam and lorazepam (16, 19). Alprazolam is one of the most commonly misused benzodiazepines in Australia and is not recommended for use in dentistry (20). Benzodiazepine-like agents, zolpidem and zopiclone, were introduced in the 1980s for the treatment of insomnia in the hope that they would be less prone to addiction and misuse; however, this has not been the case (18).

6.6 Nitrous oxide

6.6.1 Pharmacodynamics

Nitrous oxide has analgesic, anxiolytic and anaesthetic properties through its effect on receptors at the supraspinal and spinal levels (21). It stimulates the release of endogenous opioid peptides to activate specific subtypes of opioid receptors to cause antinociceptive effects (22). The anxiolytic effect is exerted by the drug binding to and activating GABA-A receptors (22).

6.6.2 The use of nitrous oxide in dentistry

Table 6.3 Doses and pharmacokinetic parameters of nitrous oxide. Based on (4, 5, 13).

Doses	Time to onset	Time to peak effect	Time to offset
Adult/child: 30–50% nitrous oxide/50–70% oxygen	30–60 seconds	3–5 minutes	Rapid; administer supplemental oxygen for 3–5 minutes after ceasing the flow of nitrous oxide

Practice points

- In dentistry, nitrous oxide is delivered by inhalation through a nasal mask. Nitrous oxide should always be administered with supplemental oxygen to prevent the development of hypoxia.
- Ensure there is no nasal obstruction prior to treatment as nitrous oxide is delivered by inhalation (e.g. the patient does not have a sinus infection).
- Patients need to be cooperative to have the mask placed.
- Nitrous oxide reduces the gag reflex: ensure the airway is protected during treatment.
- An appropriate gas scavenger system and effective ventilation are required to minimise air contamination; it is unknown if chronic low level occupational exposure is harmful to dental personnel (it has been associated with increased rates of spontaneous abortions) (5).
- When used for procedural sedation, patients usually have spontaneous respiration and intact protective airway reflexes, but monitoring is still required (5).

6.6.3 Contraindications/precautions

- Nitrous oxide displaces nitrogen and subsequently increases pressure within closed spaces due to its higher infusibility. Therefore, nitrous oxide is contraindicated in patients with closed-space conditions, such as small bowel obstruction, middle ear surgery, intraocular surgeries, pneumothorax (5, 21).
- Nitrous oxide is also contraindicated in patients with vitamin B12 deficiency, severe cardiac disease, psychiatric disorders and pulmonary hypertension (21).

6.6.4 Adverse effects

Adverse effects of nitrous oxide:

- nausea (a possible hazard if the mask is strapped over the patient's mouth), dizziness, voice change, euphoria and laughter (5, 13)
- effects relating to hypoxia: loss of consciousness, impaired cough and reduced gag reflex (4)
- In pregnancy, short-term exposure to nitrous oxide is considered safe. However, there is some evidence that repeated nitrous oxide inhalation during the first trimester of pregnancy, e.g. during occupational exposure or with abuse, has been

associated with abnormalities of the baby's CNS. Pregnant patients may use nitrous oxide for a single dental appointment; however, pregnant dental staff should avoid exposure as much as possible (23). (See Chapter 14, Table 14.2).

6.7 Methoxyflurane

Methoxyflurane is used in Australasia primarily as a self-administered analgesic for relief of severe pain associated with acute trauma, where the patient is managed by the emergency services and there is access to full resuscitation equipment. Its use in dentistry is controversial as this drug is registered as an analgesic and its action is a general anaesthetic. Therefore, its use as an anxiolytic is off-label and often not supported by practitioner training or a patient consent process.

The use of methoxyflurane in dentistry was initially for its analgesic and sedative properties (24). It is problematic that dentists use methoxyflurane as an anxiolytic as it is actually an inhalational anaesthetic. A randomised, prospective study comparing methoxyflurane to nitrous oxide for the sedation of patients undergoing extraction of third molars under local anaesthesia found that sedation produced by both agents were comparable (25). Like other inhaled anaesthetics, methoxyflurane is associated with significant adverse effects, such as liver toxicity and malignant hyperthermia which most dentists are not trained to manage and do not have the antidote (dantrolene) on hand. Given that there are many alternatives with fewer risks, methoxyflurane is not recommended for use in general dental practice.

6.7.1 Adverse effects

Methoxyflurane is associated with renal failure, correlated with total dose and frequency of exposure (26). Multiple low doses are also associated with cumulative renal and liver toxicity (27). The cause of renal failure is due to accumulation of fluoride ions in the kidney and is usually irreversible. Nephrotoxicity is also more likely in diabetic and elderly patients (26).

There have also been a number of reports of hepatotoxicity, with repeated exposure thought to be a risk factor (27).

Prolonged respiratory depression (especially in obese patients) is also a concern, as methoxyflurane can partition into fatty tissues to create a slow-release reservoir for days after the initial exposure (27).

FURTHER READING

Kingon A, Yap T, Bonanno C, Sambrook P, McCullough M. Methoxyflurane: a review with emphasis on its role in dental practice. *Aust Dent J.* 2016;61(2):157–162.

Knuf K, Manni CV. *Nitrous Oxide.* StatsPearls; 2021. https://www.ncbi.nlm.nih.gov/books/NBK532922/

Nielsen S. Benzodiazepines. *Curr Top Behav Neurosci.* 2017;34:141–159. doi:10.1007/7854_2015_425

Teoh L, Thompson W, Hubbard CC, Gellad W, Finn K, Suda KJ. Comparison of Dental Benzodiazepine Prescriptions From the U.S., England, and Australia From 2013 to 2018. *Am J Prev Med.* 2021;61(1):73–79.

REFERENCES

1. Armfield JM, Heaton LJ. Management of fear and anxiety in the dental clinic: a review. *Aust Dent J.* 2013;58(4):390–407; quiz 531.
2. Araujo JO, Bergamaschi CC, Lopes LC et al. Effectiveness and safety of oral sedation in adult patients undergoing dental procedures: a systematic review. *BMJ Open.* 2021;11(1):e043363.
3. Australia and New Zealand College of Anaesthetists. *Guideline on sedation and/or analgesia for diagnostic and interventional medical, dental or surgical procedures.* 2014. https://www .anzca.edu.au/getattachment/c64aef58-e188-494a-b471-3c07b7149f0c/PS09-Guideline-on-sedation-and-or-analgesia-for-diagnostic-and-interventional-medical,-dental-or-surgical-procedures
4. Oral and Dental Expert Group. *Therapeutic Guidelines Oral and Dental (Version 3).* Therapeutic Guidelines Pty Ltd; 2019.
5. Krauss B, Green SM. Procedural sedation and analgesia in children. *Lancet.* 2006;367(9512):766–780.
6. Dental Board of Australia. *Registration Standard: Endorsement for Conscious Sedation.* AHRPA; 2015.
7. Australian Dental Association. *Policy Statement 6.33—Relative Analgesia in Dentistry.* 2019. https://staging.ada.org.au/Dental-Professionals/Policies/Dental-Practice/Relative-Analgesia/PS6-33-Relative-Analgesia11-12Apr19_Approved.aspx
8. Robin C, Trieger N. Paradoxical reactions to benzodiazepines in intravenous sedation: a report of 2 cases and review of the literature. *Anesth Prog.* 2002;49(4):128–132.
9. Babl FE, Oakley E, Seaman C, Barnett P, Sharwood LN. High-concentration nitrous oxide for procedural sedation in children: adverse events and depth of sedation. *Pediatrics.* 2008;121(3):e528–e532.
10. Zier JL, Liu M. Safety of high-concentration nitrous oxide by nasal mask for pediatric procedural sedation: experience with 7802 cases. *Pediatr Emerg Care.* 2011;27(12):1107–1112.
11. AusDi Medical Director. *Benzodiazepines (Systemic): Independent Drug Monograph.* 2021. https://ausdi.hcn.com.au/productMonograph.hcn?file=0496
12. Ogle OE, Hertz MB. Anxiety control in the dental patient. *Dent Clin North Am.* 2012;56(1):1–16, vii.
13. Editorial Advisory Committee. *Australian Medicines Handbook* Australian Medicines Handbook Pty Ltd; 2021.
14. Dhaliwal JS, Rosani A, Saadabadi A. *Diazepam.* StatPearls Publishing LLC; 2022.
15. Hulme S, Bright D, Nielsen S. The source and diversion of pharmaceutical drugs for non-medical use: a systematic review and meta-analysis. *Drug Alcohol Depend.* 2018;186:242–256.
16. Longo LP, Johnson B. Addiction: Part I. Benzodiazepines—side effects, abuse risk and alternatives. *Am Fam Physician.* 2000;61(7):2121–2128.
17. Teoh L, Thompson W, Hubbard CC, Gellad W, Finn K, Suda KJ. Comparison of Dental Benzodiazepine Prescriptions From the U.S., England, and Australia From 2013 to 2018. *Am J Prev Med.* 2021;61(1):73–79.
18. Nielsen S. Benzodiazepines. *Curr Top Behav Neurosci.* 2017;34:141–159.
19. Rush CR, Higgins ST, Bickel WK, Hughes JR. Abuse liability of alprazolam relative to other commonly used benzodiazepines: a review. *Neurosci Biobehav Rev.* 1993;17(3):277–285.
20. Reynolds M, Fulde G, Hendry T. Trends in benzodiazepine abuse: 2007–2011. *Emerg Med Australas.* 2013;25(2):199–200.
21. Knuf K, Manni CV. *Nitrous Oxide.* StatsPearls; 2021. https://www.ncbi.nlm.nih.gov/books/NBK532922/

22. Emmanouil DE, Quock RM. Advances in understanding the actions of nitrous oxide. *Anesth Prog.* 2007;54(1):9–18.
23. Briggs GG, Freeman RK, Towers CV, Forinash AB. *Drugs in Pregnancy and Lactation.* 11th edition. Lippincott Williams & Wilkins; 2017.
24. Grainger JG, Harris NK. Methoxyflurane (penthrane) analgesia in dentistry. *Dent Anaesth Sedat.* 1973;2(2):10–13.
25. Abdullah WA, Sheta SA, Nooh NS. Inhaled methoxyflurane (Penthrox) sedation for third molar extraction: a comparison to nitrous oxide sedation. *Aust Dent J.* 2011;56(3):296–301.
26. Australian Product Information. *Methoxyflurane (Penthrox) Inhalation.* Medical Developments International Limited; 2019.
27. Kingon A, Yap T, Bonanno C, Sambrook P, McCullough M. Methoxyflurane: a review with emphasis on its role in dental practice. *Aust Dent J.* 2016;61(2):157–162.

LOCAL ANAESTHESIA

7

KEY POINTS

- Most local anaesthetics (LAs) used in dentistry are amides whose physiochemical properties, including pK_a, lipophilicity and degree of vasodilation, determine their individual differences.
- Reasons for decreased effectiveness of LA in the presence of infection include the acidic environment of an abscess, increased excitability of sensory nerves, and increased systemic LA absorption in the presence of inflammation.
- Vasoconstrictors are co-formulated in LA solutions as they reduce local blood flow, retain LA at the site, reduce the total dose of LA required to produce anaesthesia and improve operator visibility by reducing haemorrhage. There are very few contraindications to the use of vasoconstrictors.
- LAs have binding characteristics at many other channels and receptors other than those on nerve terminals, which give rise to their non-dental uses and systemic side effects.

7.1 Introduction

LAs are used to produce nerve blocks in a specific region of the body. The difference between anaesthesia and analgesia is that anaesthesia is defined by the loss of all sensation, whereas analgesia reduces pain sensation only.

In dentistry, the main aim of using LAs is to achieve local analgesia; that is, to avoid pain while other sensory elements such as touch and proprioception remain intact.

7.2 Chemistry: amide versus ester LAs

The chemical structure of LAs consists of two regions: a lipophilic, aromatic ring, and a hydrophilic, basic side-chain. These regions are linked by either an amide or ester bond, which gives rise to their classification (1) (see Figure 7.1). Most LAs used in contemporary dentistry are amides; however, some esters are used topically and articaine is a bit of both.

Amide compounds have evolved as the preferred LA choice for most dentists, as they are better tolerated and have longer durations of action than ester LAs. When ester LAs are metabolised they release para-aminobenzoic acid (PABA), which is believed to be responsible for their more frequent allergic reactions (2).

Figure 7.1 Structure of ester and amide LAs (58).

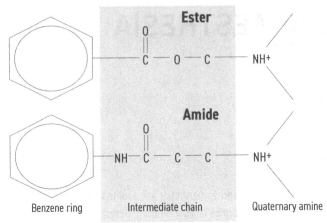

Benzene ring   Intermediate chain   Quaternary amine

7.3 Pharmacodynamics and physiochemical properties

LAs work by reversible inhibition of sodium channels on axonal membranes causing a conformational change of these channels, inhibiting the influx of sodium ions, thereby preventing initiation and propagation of action potentials. This prevents pain signals from being transmitted along an affected nerve fibre (1, 3, 4).

LAs inhibit nerve impulses transmitted by unmyelinated or lightly myelinated nerve fibres with a relatively small diameter (e.g. A delta and C-type pain fibres) more readily than myelinated, wider-diameter fibres (e.g. motor neurons) (1, 4, 5). However, sensory fibres can vary in their ion channel composition, electrophysiological properties and diameters, thus diminishing their response to LA and patients can often still feel pressure even when local analgesia is satisfactory (6).

LA compounds can bind to other target sites, including calcium channels, potassium channels, N-methyl-D-aspartate (NMDA) receptors and nicotinic acetylcholine receptors, which give rise to their other uses and systemic effects (5). In cardiology, lidocaine is used as an anti-arrhythmic drug due to its sodium channel blocking effect in the myocardium.

The physiochemical properties of each LA, such as their pK_a, lipophilicity, protein binding and vasodilating properties, give rise to their differentiating characteristics (5).

LA solutions are weak bases formulated as the hydrochloride salt in order to be dissolved in water (7). As it is only the uncharged form of a LA that exerts its effect by freely crossing the hydrophobic lipid bilayer of the axonal membrane, efficacy depends on the degree of ionisation, which in turn depends on the pK_a of the LA molecule and the pH of the solution (5). The pK_a is the pH at which the LA is present as the charged and uncharged forms in equal concentrations. As all LAs are weak bases, their pK_a is higher than physiological pH (7.4), ranging between 7.6–8.1 (see Table 7.1). The greater the pK_a compared with physiological pH, the more LA molecules will be in their ionised form. Conversely, the closer the pK_a to the physiological pH, the more LA will exist in the uncharged form and be able to diffuse through the membrane.

Table 7.1 Duration of action and pK$_a$ of commonly used LAs. Based on (1, 3, 5, 10).

Local anaesthetic	pK$_a$ of LA	Duration of action			
		Infiltration		Inferior alveolar nerve block	
		Pulpal	Soft tissue	Pulpal	Soft tissue
3% prilocaine with felypressin (0.03IU/mL)	7.9	40 minutes	150 minutes	90 minutes	210 minutes
4% articaine with with 1:100,000 adrenaline	7.8	60 minutes	170 minutes	90 minutes	220 minutes
0.5% bupivacaine with 1:200,000 adrenaline	8.1	40 minutes	340 minutes	240 minutes	440 minutes
2% lidocaine with 1:100,000 adrenaline	7.9	60 minutes	170 minutes	85 minutes	190 minutes
3% mepivacaine	7.6	25 minutes	90 minutes	40 minutes	165 minutes

Therefore, the pK$_a$ is the most important factor in determining the time of onset of a LA, as it determines how much of the drug will be unionised and able to diffuse across the neuronal membrane (8).

$$B + H_2O \leftrightarrow BH^+ + OH^-$$

The Henderson-Hasselbalch equation is utilised to determine the pH of buffer solutions:

$$pH = pK_a + \log\frac{[\text{base}]}{[\text{acid}]}$$

The rate of onset and effectiveness of a LA is influenced by other factors such as the lipid solubility, type of injection (e.g. infiltration or nerve block) and vasoconstrictor use (8).

Once the unionised LA molecules diffuse across the axonal membrane, they re-establish an equilibrium inside the axonal membrane. The subsequent ionised form binds to the interior of the open sodium channel, thus preventing initiation and propagation of action potentials and electrical impulses along the nerve fibre.

7.3.1 Use-dependent blockade

The target site for LAs is the voltage-gated sodium channel, which exists in either open, inactivated or closed states. A closed state occurs when there is no firing of the action potential (1). On depolarisation, an open state occurs when there is an influx of sodium ions into the cell. After the action potential passes, the sodium channel progresses to an inactivated state (1). Open and inactivated channels are the target for LA molecules, giving rise to the use-dependent block (1).

7.3.2 Lipid solubility and effect on vasculature

The degree of lipophilicity of the LA molecule directly influences its potency. Lipophilicity is mostly determined by the aromatic ring and substitutions in the chemical structure of the molecule. LAs with greater potency can also be used in a lower strength (3). For example, bupivacaine is more lipophilic and therefore more potent than lidocaine, which is why bupivacaine is presented in a 0.5% solution compared with 2% solution for lidocaine (3).

LAs vary in their ability to cause vasodilation. Lidocaine has a natural vasodilating ability, which leads to the sequestration of the drug away from the site of action and diminution of its effect (9). For this reason, vasoconstrictors such as adrenaline and felypressin are added to LA formulations to constrict local tissue vasculature and prolong the effect of the LA (see Section 7.6) (6).

7.3.3 Metabolism and elimination

The differing metabolism of ester and amide bonds determines the dissimilar durations of action and half-lives. The ester bond is metabolised by esterase enzymes in the plasma, and these LAs are generally metabolised faster than amide anaesthetics which are not metabolised until they reach the liver (1, 3). Articaine is a unique molecule as it has both an amide bond and an ester side chain, the latter determines its metabolism. This side chain is quickly hydrolysed by esterases in the plasma. As a result, articaine has a short half-life of around 20–40 minutes when formulated as the sole active ingredient, without a vasoconstrictor (6).

Table 7.2 Comparative information of commonly used LAs in dentistry.

Local anaesthetic	Comparative information
Prilocaine	• Prilocaine is a short-acting LA with vasodilating properties • When formulated with the vasoconstrictor felypressin, prilocaine provides an alternative for patients who prefer not have adrenaline or for whom adrenaline is inappropriate • Prilocaine is metabolised to o-toludine, a toxic metabolite that is associated with causing methaemoglobinaemia (see Section 7.11.3) • Prilocaine should not be used in children <12 months (especially if they are exposed to medicines or other substances that also cause methaemoglobinaemia), patients with hereditary methaemoglobinaemia, or in pre-term babies (11)
Articaine	• Superior efficacy of articaine over other LAs is debated. While some reviews show that articaine is more effective than lidocaine for inferior alveolar nerve blocks and for irreversible pulpitis, others studies show their clinical effectiveness is similar (12, 13). For further discussion of the use of articaine in nerve blocks, see Section 7.10.5 • Safety and efficacy in children <4 years has not been established; therefore it is not recommended in this age group (10)

Table 7.2 (cont.)

Local anaesthetic	Comparative information
Bupivacaine	• Bupivacaine is similar in structure to mepivacaine but is more lipophilic. Its high potency allows it to be formulated in low concentrations of 0.5% • Bupivacaine has greater risk for cardiotoxicity (arrhythmias) compared with lidocaine due to its affinity for binding to cardiac sodium channels, potency and increased lipid solubility (14, 15) • Due to its prolonged anaesthesia of up to 10 hours, it is preferentially used in procedures where prolonged postoperative pain is predicted. Bupivacaine is not recommended for use in children <12 years of age (10)
Lidocaine	• Commonly used in dental practice, lidocaine is available in various formulations, including ointments and gels for topical oral application. It is also available in a topical cream combined with prilocaine as a 'eutectic mixture of local anaesthetics' (EMLA) that can anaesthetise intact skin to a depth of 5mm (4) • Use smallest possible amount of topical lidocaine; orally ingested topical lidocaine has a bioavailability of 30–35%, permitting systemic adverse effects (16)
Mepivacaine	• Mepivacaine is not a potent vasodilator, and so is formulated both with and without a vasoconstrictor • Mepivacaine should not be used in children <3 years (10) • It produces a similar clinical effect to lidocaine but has a shorter half-life (17)

7.4 LA effectiveness in inflammation

The clinical performance of LA is influenced by the presence of inflammation. There are three theories used to explain the decreased effectiveness of LA when injected into an area of infection and inflammation. The first and most commonly quoted relates to the decrease in tissue pH in the presence of infection and inflammation which ranges between pH 5–8 (5). As LAs are weak bases, the equilibrium shifts to produce more ionised forms of LA. The charged forms cannot cross the axonal membrane to access their target binding site. While this explains why LAs given by infiltration can be less effective, it does not explain why LA delivered as a block injection can be less effective when it is given at a site remote from the inflammation.

A second hypothesis is that peripheral inflammation sensitises and increases the excitability of peripheral nerves. This is thought to interfere with the ability of LA to block the action potentials in peripheral sensory nerves (5, 18).

As inflammation leads to increased capillary permeability and vascularity, increased systemic absorption of the LA is seen in the presence of inflammation (5). This third theory supports the use of vasoconstrictors to retain the LA at the local site (5).

7.5 Resistance to local anaesthetic

Many factors are likely to be responsible for the failure of LA, including inadequate technique, insufficient concentration at the intended site of action, loss of LA into the systemic circulation and the presence of inflammation. However, limited recent research demonstrates that idiosyncratic resistance to the effect of LA is another rare but possible reason why patients do not achieve full local anaesthesia (19, 20). Genetic variants have been identified that encode for mutations of the voltage-gated sodium channel which are thought to be the possible cause of LA resistance (20). *In vitro* studies have shown that point mutations in the LA binding site in the sodium channel subtypes have decreased affinity for binding of LA (21). A prospective clinical study demonstrated that a small percentage of the cohort who experienced ineffective regional anaesthesia had hypoesthesia to selective LAs, with some demonstrating hypoesthesia to all tested LAs (22). While LA resistance is established, complete resistance to LAs is rare and further research is required into the incidence and genetic predisposition in this small cohort of patients (19).

7.6 Vasoconstrictors

The addition of a vasoconstrictor to LA formulations has many benefits including reduction of the LA dose required to produce analgesia, prolonged duration of action, slowed loss of LA to the circulation, and reduced systemic absorption and adverse effects. Adrenaline and felypressin are the most commonly used vasoconstrictors in dental cartridges.

7.6.1 Adrenaline

Adrenaline is a naturally occurring sympathomimetic amine produced by the adrenal glands, which exerts its physiological effects via agonism on α-1, α-2, β-1 and β-2 adrenoceptors around the body. Activation of α-1 and α-2 receptors in arterioles is responsible for the vasoconstrictive effects, while activation of β-1 receptors in cardiac muscle and the conducting system are responsible for increased heart rate, contractility and cardiac output if the LA solution is inadvertently injected into a vessel or if systemic effects are seen (23).

When adrenaline is added to LAs with a moderate half-life, such as lidocaine or mepivacaine, their duration of action is extended by approximately 1 hour (19). Use of adrenaline in dental preparations is not contraindicated in patients with stable cardiovascular disease due to their limited local administration in the mouth and use of small doses (e.g. 1–2 cartridges per patient) (24).

Adrenaline itself is unstable and can easily undergo degradation via oxidation if exposed to certain conditions, such as heat, light and alkaline conditions (25). Sodium metabisulfite, an antioxidant, is commonly added to adrenaline-containing products of LA to lower the pH of the formulation, prevent oxidation and prolong its shelf life (25, 26).

7.6.2 Felypressin

Felypressin is another vasoconstrictor used in dental LAs as an alternative to adrenaline. Felypressin is a synthetic analogue of vasopressin (also known as antidiuretic hormone) (27). It can stimulate vascular smooth muscle, has myocardial effects and has been shown to increase diastolic blood pressure in hypertensive patients (28). Use of prilocaine with felypressin is associated with causing an increase in cardiac sympathetic nervous activity and an increase in myocardial contraction force compared to lidocaine with adrenaline (29). The clinical significance of this in dentistry is unknown. Doses used in dentistry are considered safe for patients with pre-existing stable cardiovascular conditions (30). Despite its structural similarity to vasopressin, which has been known to increase uterine contractility, use of felypressin is not contraindicated in pregnancy (30).

7.7 Drug interactions

A number of drug interactions are mentioned in dental LA product information and other resources such as the proposed interactions between LAs and mono-amine oxidase inhibitors and tricyclic antidepressants. However, many of these cited interactions are theoretical at best or only likely to occur with doses much higher than those used for dental procedures.

7.7.1 Dynamic interactions

There are a few significant pharmacodynamic interactions with LA when used in the small doses administered for dental procedures. Dentists are often concerned about potential drug interactions between adrenaline-containing LAs and antihypertensives. However, the low adrenaline doses used for dental procedures, minimal likely systemic exposure, and single occasion of use allows these potential interactions to be considered insignificant.

7.7.2 Kinetic interactions

Some significant pharmacokinetic interactions can occur with dental LAs, mainly in the processes of absorption and metabolism.

- **Absorption:** If a LA is administered into a site with active infection and inflammation, the increased pH of the local tissues promotes the conversion of the weakly basic LA molecules to the ionised form, making them less effective.
- **Metabolism:** Concomitant use of drugs that inhibit or induce CYP1A2 metabolism can slow down or speed up the elimination of drugs that are substrates for these enzymes, including lidocaine and ropivacaine. This will result in higher or systemic levels and prolonged half-life. However, this interaction is largely irrelevant to dental LAs as the quantity that reaches the systemic circulation after local administration is so small. This interaction is therefore only likely to be relevant to LAs administered systemically (i.e. for medical procedures).

7.8 Pregnancy and lactation recommendations

See Table 14.2.

7.9 Allergy to local anaesthetics

Despite many people claiming allergy to LAs, true hypersensitivity reactions are rare and reported to be less than 1% (19, 31). When taking a medication history, dental practitioners should document the adverse effects experienced by the patient and how long ago they occurred in order to distinguish between reactions that are psychogenic, due to inadvertent intravascular injection, or from an overdose resulting in cardiovascular and central nervous system (CNS) effects, or from a true immunologic reaction (31).

Psychogenic effects are the most common adverse effects in dentistry often stemming from needle phobias, anxiety and fear, and can produce a variety of symptoms including tachycardia, hyperventilation, nausea, bronchospasm and vasovagal syncope (31).

Inadvertent intravascular injection of the LA solution can lead to increased systemic absorption of the LA itself, increasing the risk of toxic effects. Tremor and agitation are some initial CNS signs of systemic effects (see Section 7.11). If a LA solution containing adrenaline has been injected into the vascular system, systemic effects of adrenaline are often experienced, including increased heart rate and contractility. However, some of this effect may be attributed to the patient's own adrenaline released in response to anxiety. Since the half-life of adrenaline is short (5–10 minutes after intravenous administration), these effects are generally short-lived and of little or no significance (10).

True allergic reactions (Type 1 or Type 4) can occur to either the LA itself, the preservatives in the solution, or metabolites. Latex allergy associated with the bung of LA cartridges is no longer an issue as latex has been removed from cartridges used in Australia (32).

Type 1 allergic reactions to LAs are rare but real and include anaphylaxis. Type 4 allergic reactions can also occur, presenting as a delayed generalised rash. If a patient is suspected of having a true allergic response, they should be referred to an allergist for appropriate testing, such as skin prick testing and/or drug provocation challenge (31) (see Chapter 3).

Hypersensitivity reactions can also occur to the excipients or preservatives in the solution. Sulphites, such as sodium metabisulfite or potassium metabisulfite, are used in formulations to prevent the oxidation of adrenaline (31). As the meta-bisulphite preservative is only included to preserve the adrenaline, patients with a documented hypersensitivity to sulphites should be given an adrenaline-free LA. Sulphite preservatives are not used in formulations that do not contain a vasoconstrictor.

Hypersensitivity reactions can also be due to metabolites. PABA, a metabolite of ester LAs, is associated with hypersensitivity reactions (31). A cross-reactivity exists between patients allergic to sulphonamide antibiotics and PABA, due to chemical structural similarities. Although articaine has an ester linkage, it is not associated with this cross-reactivity as it does not contain the same chemical structure as PABA (6).

7.10 Local adverse effects

7.10.1 Post-injection pain

The most common adverse effect of LA is pain at the site of injection. This can last up to 5–10 days, but is self-limiting and responds well to anti-inflammatories, such as ibuprofen, if appropriate for the patient (30, 33). Multiple injections into the same site, as well as other predisposing underlying pain conditions, such as fibromyalgia, increase the risk of postoperative pain (30).

7.10.2 Local ischemia of soft tissues

If LA is injected in large volumes or too quickly, local ischemia and necrosis of the soft tissues can occur, usually due to the effect of the vasoconstrictor (6).

7.10.3 Facial nerve paralysis

The facial nerve (cranial nerve VII) traverses through and divides in the parotid gland. Its function is to provide motor innervation to the muscles that control facial movement and expression, as well as taste sensation to the anterior two-thirds of the tongue and innervation of the lacrimal glands. If LA is deposited near or in the parotid gland, it can disrupt the facial nerve, resulting in a temporary paralysis of the muscles and lacrimal glands for the duration of the anaesthetic. The patient will recover when the effect of the LA has worn off. Reassurance for the patient and an eye patch on the affected eye is recommended as paralysis of the periocular muscles will result in the patient being unable to blink and, with diminished lacrimal secretion, creates a risk of corneal abrasion. If worn, the contact lens should also be removed from the affected eye to reduce any damage to the cornea (33). The patient should not drive for the remainder of the day and should be referred if paralysis is still present 12 hours later (30).

7.10.4 Trismus

Trismus is the myospasm and increased tone of the muscles that can develop from a LA injection and can result in limitation of mouth opening. Most commonly it is the mesial pterygoid muscle that is affected with a mandibular nerve block, but the temporalis and masseter may also be involved (33). The muscle can be damaged by the needle piercing the muscle fibres, from the LA itself, or from bleeding into the muscle (33, 34). Following muscle damage, pain develops that causes the muscle to contract resulting in a limitation in range of motion (33). The likelihood of trismus occurring increases if multiple injections are given.

Trismus usually presents clinically on the day of the procedure but can also present a few days later. Infection should be ruled out by ensuring there is no fever, lymphadenopathy or swelling. Anti-inflammatories, such as ibuprofen, can be recommended if the patient is able to tolerate them (see Chapter 5). Treatment includes referral to a physiotherapist who specialises in the jaw joint to increase the range of mouth opening. The aim is to achieve gentle functioning of the jaw early to prevent fibrosis of the muscle. While it takes 2–3 days to show some improvement, normal jaw functioning can take between days to several weeks to recover (34). If no improvement is seen within 2–3 days, referral is recommended for investigation of other pathologies or diagnoses such as haematoma or infection (34).

7.10.5 Neurotoxicity

The definition of neurotoxicity is alteration of normal nervous system activity due to exposure to neurotoxins (35). Prolonged loss of sensation can occur in dentistry due to the use of LA. While rare, it is most commonly seen with the mandibular and lingual nerves, which are both protected by an epineurium and innervated by a fibrous perineurium and endoneurial connective tissue layer. The lingual nerve is most at risk when administering a standard block injection; it is positioned only 3–5mm from the mucosal surface, and when the patient has their mouth open for a block injection the lingual nerve is stretched within the interpterygoid fascia and less able to deflect if the needle is aimed directly at the nerve (36).

The incidence of nerve damage from LA is low, with reported ranges from 1:27,415 to 1:785,000 (36). However, approximately one-third of LA-associated nerve damage manifests as dysaesthaesias, thereby causing significant functional and psychological discomfort for the patient.

The proposed mechanisms of LA-associated neurotoxicity are thought to be (36):

1. **Direct needle injury to the nerve.** Although this is unlikely—as the diameter of the largest needle is <0.5mm, the diameter of the mandibular nerve is around 3mm and lingual nerve is approximately 2mm—often the nerve will deflect (36). Some nerve fibres or individual axons may be affected, but it is unlikely for the needle to traverse the nerve to produce the effects that affect the entire nerve as seen in clinical practice (36). The 'electric-shock' reaction that can be reported by patients during the needle injection is a clinical sign that nerve injury may have occurred

2. **Direct needle injury to the blood supply within the nerve.** This causes a haematoma within the nerve sheath but not injury to the nerve itself. The haematoma then causes compression against the nerve, with nerve damage forming within 30 minutes (36)

3. **Chemical toxicity from the LA.** This causes nerve damage if injected within the nerve (see Section 7.10.6).

7.10.6 LA solution and neurotoxicity

Chemical damage to nerves from the LA solution can lead to inflammation of the nerve fibres with subsequent demyelination and oedema. Formation of oxygen radicals can also be produced that causes cytotoxic injury to nerve fibres (37, 38).

While all LAs are associated with this adverse effect, higher concentration LAs (such as prilocaine 3% and articaine 4%) have been associated with neurotoxicity more commonly than lower concentration LAs (such as lidocaine 2%) when given by mandibular block anaesthesia (36, 39, 40). It is thought that the breakdown of the amide bond around the neuron was responsible for the production of the alcohol derivatives that are thought to be toxic to the nerve. With higher concentration anaesthetics, this results in an increased production of these alcohol by-products (38).

There is no significant difference in the effectiveness of analgesia when comparing articaine with adrenaline and lidocaine with adrenaline after buccal maxillary infiltration (13), and no significant difference between the use of articaine and lidocaine for mandibular block analgesia (41). However, articaine has been shown to be more effective than lidocaine for supplementary anaesthesia as infiltration in the mandible for patients with irreversible pulpitis after mandibular block anaesthesia (41).

There is also no significant difference between articaine with adrenaline and lidocaine with adrenaline regarding pain on injection, although lidocaine is associated with slightly less pain on injection (42). Thus, it is not recommended to use articaine for mandibular block injections.

If neurotoxicity develops, prompt specialist referral is recommended. Most nerve injuries heal spontaneously within 8 weeks (in 85–94% of cases) (37). Healing can take up to 2 years, although if sensation has not returned to normal after 6 months, complete recovery and normal sensation is unlikely (36).

7.11 Systemic adverse effects in overdose

7.11.1 Central nervous system effects

As LAs are absorbed into the blood stream, they also have dose-dependent membrane-stabilising effects in the CNS. In the context of overdose, toxic symptoms occur as central inhibitory tracks are depressed, leaving excitatory tracks to fire uncontrollably (6). Clinically, this presents as restlessness, tremor, and can progress to seizures, confusion and agitation (1). As toxic levels continue to increase, the membrane-inhibitory effect occurs on the excitatory pathways as well, resulting in depression of the CNS, coma, and eventually respiratory and cardiovascular depression (3).

7.11.2 Cardiovascular adverse effects

With increasing LA concentrations, adverse cardiovascular effects tend to be seen after the CNS effects. Depressant cardiac effects generally occur at lower doses, at which they can slow down and normalise cardiac rhythm. For example, lignocaine is used for suppression of ventricular arrhythmias due to its negative inotropic effect and reduction on the automaticity of myocardial tissue (11). As systemic levels increase, LAs also have an affinity for sodium channels in cardiac muscle, causing an inhibition of the sodium current and producing a negative inotropic effect. Ultimately this causes myocardial depression and partial or complete heart block. Concurrently, LAs cause vasodilatation of the vascular smooth muscle, causing a fall in blood pressure. Eventually, as plasma concentrations become toxic, cardiac arrest can occur (1).

Bupivacaine has greater cardiotoxicity compared with other LAs, thought to be due to the increased potency and affinity for cardiac sodium channels (14, 15). This causes an increased recovery time for the neuron to restore the intracellular sodium and potassium concentrations, delaying recovery of the action potential and increasing the likelihood of arrhythmias (6).

7.11.3 Methaemoglobinaemia

Methaemoglobinaemia is a form of functional anaemia characterised by oxidation of the iron on haemoglobin from the ferrous (Fe^{2+}) to the ferric (Fe^{3+}) form to become methaemoglobin. This form of haemoglobin is a poor oxygen carrier and causes overall impairment of oxygen delivery to tissues with varying degrees of hypoxia and cyanosis (30). There are two types of methaemoglobinaemia: congenital and acquired. People with congenital methaemoglobinaemia have life-long cyanosis but are generally asymptomatic (43–45). Acquired is the most common type and is typically caused by ingestion of drugs or other oxidising agents. Methaemoglobinaemia can be acute or chronic and often occurs in the context of drug poisoning/overdose but can also occur with medications in their usual dose (43, 44).

Methaemoglobinaemia has been associated with a range of LAs, most frequently with prilocaine, topically applied benzocaine, and occasionally articaine and lidocaine (30). With prilocaine, this occurs most commonly with doses greater than 600mg (30).

Signs and symptoms of methaemoglobinaemia correlate with an increasing level of methaemoglobin and can occur within a few minutes and up to 1–2 hours after using LAs (46, 47). Early symptoms typically occur when methaemoglobin fractions exceed 10–15%, including sedation, cyanosis and a bluish tinge in lips and fingers (3, 48). Headache, dizziness, tachycardia, dyspnoea and weakness occur at levels around 30–40% (45). Death is associated with methaemoglobin levels greater than 70% (45). It can be a life-threatening condition and requires emergency referral to hospital (30).

Predisposing factors for methaemoglobinaemia include young age (infants <6 months), the condition of the skin to which the drug is applied (inflamed and broken skin absorbs more drug), concomitant use of other methaemoglobinaemia-causing drugs, malnutrition, and the genetic make-up of the patient (altered haemoglobin, G6PD deficiency or methemoglobin reductase enzyme deficiency) (45). LAs should be used in lower doses for these types of patients (45, 49).

The use of topical benzocaine and prilocaine by any route is contraindicated in patients with hereditary methaemoglobinaemia (10).

7.12 Other considerations

7.12.1 Myasthenia gravis

Myasthenia gravis (MG) is an auto-immune condition in which antibodies are made against the patient's own nicotinic acetylcholine receptors (AChRs) at the neuromuscular junction (50). These antibodies attack the AChRs and prevent skeletal muscle contraction (51). Therefore, MG results in skeletal muscle weakness, including facial muscles, soft palate muscles, neck muscles, respiratory muscles and the diaphragm (50).

LAs have some skeletal muscle relaxant properties which occurs as a result of their 'switching off' nerve impulses to the muscles surrounding the site of administration. As a result, there is a theoretical risk that LAs may exacerbate the muscle weakness of MG; however, it is only likely to occur in patients with severe disease.

Because of this, LAs are often included in lists of drugs which can exacerbate MG. However, current evidence suggests that patients with MG are only at risk of complications from LAs when administered intravenously and not when they are given for local infiltration or regional anaesthesia (52).

7.12.2 Patients with cardiovascular disease

While submucosal injections of small amounts of adrenaline may still produce cardiac effects, such as increased heart rate and slightly increased blood pressure, the use of a LA with vasoconstrictors is associated with insignificant changes on ECGs (6, 53). In addition, a single episode of slight elevation in these parameters does not constitute a significant impact on cardiovascular disease. The patient's own endogenous adrenaline from anxiety relating to the procedure may also be contributing to symptoms. Guidelines and reviews have advised that the use of small doses of LAs (e.g. 1–2 cartridges per patient) containing adrenaline are not contraindicated for patients with stable cardiovascular disease (30, 53).

7.12.3 Patients with epilepsy

Neurologic toxicity of LAs most frequently presents as agitation, restlessness, and tremor (54). A study assessing adverse reactions associated with LA use in the US showed that 17 of approximately 180,000 reports included the term 'seizure' (55).

Overall, patients with epilepsy or a history of seizures are more at risk of LA neurological adverse effects.

7.12.4 Topical use in teething

See Section 8.2.1: Teething gels for children.

7.12.5 Use in the elderly

LAs in dentistry are generally well tolerated in the elderly due to the relatively small doses used. However, increased systemic absorption can occur from topical administration, so older patients would be more at risk of side effects and adverse interactions from systemic exposure to these drugs. Therefore, lower LA starting doses should be used and up-titration conducted more slowly in older patients (56, 57).

7.13 Dosing of local anaesthetic

The maximum single doses of LAs are set out in Table 7.3. The maximum doses are rarely required in dentistry provided that the correct technique has been employed and the anatomical landmarks identified. It is also important to note that dental cartridges are available in varying volumes, ranging between 1.8mL to 2.2mL.

Table 7.3 Maximum single doses of commonly used LA formulations in Australia. Adapted from (30).

Local anaesthetic formulation	Maximum single doses (mg/kg)
Articaine 4% with adrenaline 1:100,000	7
Articaine 4% with adrenaline 1:200,000	7
Lidocaine 2% with adrenaline 1:80,000	7
Mepivacaine 2% with adrenaline 1:100,000 Mepivacaine 3%	The maximum volume specified in the product information based on age is: • adult: 6.6mL • 14–17 years: 4.4mL • 6–14 years: 2.7mL • 3–6 years: 1.8mL
Prilocaine 3% with felypressin 0.03 international units/mL	9
Prilocaine 3% with adrenaline 1:300,000	9
Prilocaine 4%	6

Extended dental procedures where the appointment duration can outlast the period of anaesthesia requires consideration (3). As initial serum levels of LA are declining, any additional doses will cause increasing plasma levels (3). It is difficult to predict the serum levels of LA in this situation and the absorption and elimination is influenced by other factors, such as drug interactions, liver and kidney function and pharmacogenomics. The maximum single dose of LA should not be exceeded in total during any single procedure.

7.13.1 Combining local anaesthetics

There is little research on the safety and appropriate dosing regimen when combining different LAs in dentistry, although in clinical practice this is often done. When administering more than one LA, their effects should be considered to be additive, and the lowest total maximum dose not exceeded (30).

7.13.2 Dose calculations

Concentrations of LA are expressed in percentages, which is equivalent to g/100mL.

Thus, lidocaine 2% is equivalent to 2g in 100mL or 20mg/mL.

The units of concentration used for vasoconstrictors are employed as they are for expressing very small concentrations.

Concentrations of adrenaline are expressed as g:mL. Thus, a concentration of adrenaline of 1:100,000 is 1g of adrenaline in 100,000 mL or 10 mcg/mL.

Concentrations of felypressin are expressed in international units per mL. International units are used to measure mass and differ for each substance. A concentration of felypressin at 0.03 IU/mL is equivalent to 0.54 mcg/mL.

See the online resources available at www.cambridge.org/highereducation/isbn/9781009060059/resources for case studies on dose calculations regarding the use of LA in dental practice.

FURTHER READING

Malamed S. *Handbook of Local Anaesthesia.* 7th edition. Elsevier; 2019.

REFERENCES

1. Ritter J, Flower R, Henderson G, Loke YK, MacEwan D, Rang H. *Rang and Dale's Pharmacology.* 9th edition. Elsevier; 2020.
2. Katzung BG, Trevor AJ. *Basic and Clinical Pharmacology.* 15th edition. McGraw Hill; 2020.
3. Becker DE, Reed KL. Essentials of local anesthetic pharmacology. *Anesth Prog.* 2006;53(3):98–108; quiz 9–10.
4. Stevens CW, Brenner GM. *Brenner and Stevens' Pharmacology.* 5th edition. Elsevier; 2018.
5. Lirk P, Picardi S, Hollmann MW. Local anaesthetics: 10 essentials. *Eur J Anaesthesiol.* 2014;31(11):575–585.
6. Becker DE, Reed KL. Local anesthetics: review of pharmacological considerations. *Anesth Prog.* 2012;59(2):90–101; quiz 2–3.
7. Edgcombe H, Hocking G. *Local Anaesthetic Pharmacology.* AnaesthesiaUK; 2006. https://resources.wfsahq.org/atotw/local-anaesthetic-pharmacology/
8. Moore PA, Hersh EV. Local anesthetics: pharmacology and toxicity. *Dent Clin North Am.* 2010;54(4):587–599.

9. Newton DJ, McLeod GA, Khan F, Belch JJ. Mechanisms influencing the vasoactive effects of lidocaine in human skin. *Anaesthesia.* 2007;62(2):146–150.
10. Medical Director AusDI. *Independent Drug Monographs.* Accessed April 3, 2021. https://ausdi .hcn.com.au/browseDocuments.hcn?filter=PRODUCTS_WITH_MONGRAPH
11. Editorial Advisory Committee. *Australian Medicines Handbook.* AMH Pty Ltd; 2020.
12. Nagendrababu V, Duncan HF, Whitworth J et al. Is articaine more effective than lidocaine in patients with irreversible pulpitis? An umbrella review. *Int Endod J.* 2020;53(2):200–213.
13. Kanaa MD, Whitworth JM, Meechan JG. A comparison of the efficacy of 4% articaine with 1:100,000 epinephrine and 2% lidocaine with 1:80,000 epinephrine in achieving pulpal anesthesia in maxillary teeth with irreversible pulpitis. *J Endod.* 2012;38(3):279–282.
14. Casati A, Putzu M. Bupivacaine, levobupivacaine and ropivacaine: are they clinically different? *Best Pract Res Clin Anaesthesiol.* 2005;19(2):247–268.
15. Clarkson CW, Hondeghem LM. Mechanism for bupivacaine depression of cardiac conduction: fast block of sodium channels during the action potential with slow recovery from block during diastole. *Anesthesiology.* 1985;62(4):396–405.
16. Tucker GT, Mather LE. Clinical pharmacokinetics of local anaesthetics. *Clini Pharmacokinet.* 1979;4:241–278. doi:10.2165/00003088-197904040-00001
17. Gao X, Meng K. Comparison of articaine, lidocaine and mepivacaine for buccal infiltration after inferior alveolar nerve block in mandibular posterior teeth with irreversible pulpitis. *Br Dent J.* 2020;228(8):605–608.
18. Rood JP, Pateromichelakis S. Inflammation and peripheral nerve sensitisation. *Br J Oral Surg.* 1981;19(1):67–72.
19. Lirk P, Hollman MW, Strichartz G. *The Science of Local Anesthesia: Basic Research, Clinical Application, and Future Directions.* International Anesthesia Research Society; 2017.
20. Clendenen N, Cannon AD, Porter S, Robards CB, Parker AS, Clendenen SR. Whole-exome sequencing of a family with local anesthetic resistance. *Minerva Anestesiol.* 2016;82(10):1089–1097.
21. Panigel J, Cook SP. A point mutation at F1737 of the human Nav1.7 sodium channel decreases inhibition by local anesthetics. *J Neurogenet.* 2011;25(4):134–139.
22. Trescot AM. Local anesthetic "resistance". *Pain Physician.* 2003;6(3):291–293.
23. Sisk AL. Vasoconstrictors in local anesthesia for dentistry. *Anesth Prog.* 1992;39(6):187–193.
24. Seminario-Amez M, Gonzalez-Navarro B, Ayuso-Montero R, Jane-Salas E, Lopez-Lopez E. Use of local anesthetics with a vasoconstrictor agent during dental treatment in Hypertensive and Coronary disease patients. A systematic review. *Journal of Evidence-Based Dental Practice.* 2021;21(2):101569.
25. Hoellein L, Holzgrabe U. Ficts and facts of epinephrine and norepinephrine stability in injectable solutions. *Int J Pharm.* 2012;434(1–2):468–480.
26. Wennberg E, Haljamae H, Edwall G, Dhuner KG. Effects of commercial (pH approximately 3.5) and freshly prepared (pH approximately 6.5) lidocaine-adrenaline solutions on tissue pH. *Acta Anaesthesiol Scand.* 1982;26(5):524–527.
27. Malamed S. *Handbook of Local Anesthesia.* 6th edition. Mosby; 2013.
28. Bronzo AL, Cardoso CG Jr, Ortega KC, Mion D Jr. Felypressin increases blood pressure during dental procedures in hypertensive patients. *Arq Bras Cardiol.* 2012;99(2):724–731.
29. Yamashita K, Kibe T, Shidou R, Kohjitani A, Nakamura N, Sugimura M. Difference in the Effects of Lidocaine With Epinephrine and Prilocaine With felypressin on the Autonomic Nervous System During Extraction of the Impacted Mandibular Third Molar: A Randomized Controlled Trial. *J Oral Maxillofac Surg.* 2020;78(2):215 e1–e8.
30. Oral and Dental Expert Group. *Therapeutic Guidelines Oral and Dental (Version 3).* Therapeutic Guidelines Pty Ltd; 2019.

31. Speca SJ, Boynes SG, Cuddy MA. Allergic reactions to local anesthetic formulations. *Dent Clin North Am.* 2010;54(4):655–664.

32. Allen G, Chan D, Gue S. Investigation and diagnosis of an immediate allergy to amide local anaesthetic in a paediatric dental patient. *Aust Dent J.* 2017;62(2):241–245.

33. Ogle OE, Mahjoubi G. Local anesthesia: agents, techniques, and complications. *Dent Clin North Am.* 2012;56(1):133–148, ix.

34. Wright M. Medial pterygoid trismus (myospasm) following inferior alveolar nerve block: Case report and literature review. *General Dentistry.* 2011;59(1):64–67.

35. National Institute of Neurological Disorders and Stroke. *Neurotoxicity.* 2019. https://www.ninds.nih.gov/disorders/all-disorders/neurotoxicity-information-page

36. Sambrook PJ, Goss AN. Severe adverse reactions to dental local anaesthetics: prolonged mandibular and lingual nerve anaesthesia. *Aust Dent J.* 2011;56(2):154–159.

37. Smith MH, Lung KE. Nerve injuries after dental injection: a review of the literature. *J Can Dent Assoc.* 2006;72(6):559–564.

38. Hopman AJG, Baart JA, Brand HS. Articaine and neurotoxicity—a review. *Br Dent J.* 2017;223(7):501–506.

39. Hillerup S, Jensen RH, Ersboll BK. Trigeminal nerve injury associated with injection of local anesthetics: needle lesion or neurotoxicity? *J Am Dent Assoc.* 2011;142(5):531–539.

40. Hillerup S, Jensen R. Nerve injury caused by mandibular block analgesia. *Int J Oral Maxillofac Surg.* 2006;35(5):437–443.

41. Kung J, McDonagh M, Sedgley CM. Does Articaine Provide an Advantage over Lidocaine in Patients with Symptomatic Irreversible Pulpitis? A Systematic Review and Meta-analysis. *J Endod.* 2015;41(11):1784–1794.

42. St George G, Morgan A, Meechan J et al. Injectable local anaesthetic agents for dental anaesthesia. *Cochrane Database Syst Rev.* 2018;7:CD006487.

43. Rehman HU. Methaemoglobinaemia. *West J Med.* 2001;175(3):193–196.

44. Prchal J. *Clinical features, diagnosis and treatment of methaemoglobinaemia.* UpToDate; 2023. https://www.uptodate.com/contents/methaemoglobinaemia

45. Tandale S, Dave NM, Garasia M. Methaemoglobinaemia: What the anaesthetist must know. *Indian J Anaesth.* 2013;57(4):427–428.

46. US Food and Drug Administration. *FDA Drug Safety Communication: Reports of a rare, but serious and potentially fatal adverse effect with the use of over-the-counter (OTC) benzocaine gels and liquids applied to the gums or mouth.* 2018. https://www.fda.gov/Drugs/DrugSafety/ucm250024.htm

47. US Food and Drug Administration. *FDA Safety Announcement. Risk of serious and potentially fatal blood disorder prompts FDA action on oral over-the counter benzocaine products used for teething and mouth pain and prescription local anesthetics.* 2018. https://www.fda.gov/drugs/drug-safety-and-availability/risk-serious-and-potentially-fatal-blood-disorder-prompts-fda-action-oral-over-counter-benzocaine

48. Sambrook PJ, Smith W, Elijah J, Goss AN. Severe adverse reactions to dental local anaesthetics: systemic reactions. *Aust Dent J.* 2011;56(2):148–153; quiz 234.

49. Guay J. Methaemoglobinaemia related to local anesthetics: a summary of 242 episodes. *Anesth Analg.* 2009;108(3):837–845.

50. Yarom N, Barnea E, Nissan J, Gorsky M. Dental management of patients with myasthenia gravis: a literature review. *Oral Surg Oral Med Oral Pathol Oral Radiol Endod.* 2005;100(2):158–163.

51. Haroutiunian S, Lecht S, Zur AA, Hoffman A, Davidson E. The challenge of pain management in patients with myasthenia gravis. *J Pain Palliat Care Pharmacother.* 2009;23(3):242–260.

52. Kveraga R, Pawlowski J. Anesthesia for the patient with myasthenia gravis. *UptoDate*; 2023. www.uptodate.com/contents/anesthesia-for-the-patient-with-myasthenia-gravis/print

53. Godzieba A, Smektala T, Jędrzejewski M, Sporniak-Tutak K. Clinical assessment of the safe use local anaesthesia with vasoconstrictor agents in cardiovascular compromised patients: A systematic review. *Med Sci Monit*. 2014:10(20):393–398.

54. Harmatz A. Local anesthetics: uses and toxicities. *Surg Clin North Am*. 2009;89(3):587–598.

55. D'Eramo E M, Bookless SJ, Howard JB. Adverse events with outpatient anesthesia in Massachusetts. *J Oral Maxillofac Surg*. 2003;61(7):793–800; discussion.

56. Semla TP, Beizer JL, Higbee MD. *Geriatric Dosage Handbook: Including clinical recommendations and monitoring guidelines*. 21st edition. Lexicomp; 2016.

57. Moore PA. Adverse drug interactions in dental practice: interactions associated with local anesthetics, sedatives and anxiolytics. Part IV of a series. *J Am Dent Assoc*. 1999;130(4):541–554.

58. Nagelhout J. *Local Anesthetics*. Anathesia Key; 2016. https://aneskey.com/local-anesthetics-2/

8 TOPICAL MEDICATIONS

KEY POINTS

- Dentists commonly recommend and use various topical medications.
- Topical agents for dental caries can be very beneficial, while oral antiseptics should be recommended judiciously.
- Topical antifungal, antiviral and anti-inflammatory agents are extremely effective in specific settings.

8.1 Introduction

Topical medications are those that are administered to the surface of the skin or on mucous membranes in the eye, ear, nose, mouth, vagina, etc. with the intent of containing the drug's pharmacological effect to the superficial epithelial layers of skin or nearby structures (1). Drugs for topical application are usually available as creams, ointments, gels, lotions, sprays, powders, aerosols, mouth rinses and toothpastes.

Topical administration provides a high local concentration of the drug, generally without significant exposure to the systemic circulation. However, absorption does occur and can lead to adverse effects. Absorption can be significant as the digestive processes in the gastrointestinal tract and liver that diminish drug absorption (the first pass effect) are avoided. Sometimes, systemic absorption from topical drug application is utilised for its therapeutic value.

Advantages of topical drug administration include (2):

- maximising drug effects via targeted and accurate drug delivery to a specific site
- minimising drug dose by minimising loss to first pass metabolism and unintended sites
- an avoidance of systemic side effects by limiting drug delivery to tissues that may have been adversely affected
- convenient use and easy application
- easy termination
- it permits use of drugs that have little or no oral bioavailability
- a decreased risk of interaction with systemically administered drugs

Disadvantages of topical drug administration include:

- possible local skin irritation at the site of application from the drug, although this rarely occurs on the oral mucosa
- possible absorption after topical application with potential systemic side effects

8.2 Topical anaesthetics

Topical anaesthetics are used to reduce painful stimuli and diminish the effect of a minor procedure, particularly prior to injecting local anaesthetic (LA). Other procedures, such as the placement of crowns, band removal or suture removal, will also be made more comfortable with the use of topical anaesthetics.

Lidocaine is the most frequently used topical and LA. Classified as an amide (1), lidocaine is commercially available as a 2% gel, 5% and 10% ointments, a 10% spray and 5% pellets and is the most common topical anaesthetic used prior to injecting LA.

For anaesthesia of the skin, the eutectic mixture of lidocaine and prilocaine (EMLA) 5% cream (25mg/g lidocaine, 25mg/g prilocaine) is available. EMLA needs to be applied 1 hour before the procedure to provide surface anaesthesia on the skin and lasts 2–3 hours, so it is useful as an emergency local pain management at home but not practical for clinical procedures (2).

Benzocaine is an ester-type topical anaesthetic that blocks the influx of sodium by selectively binding to sodium channels on the intracellular surface of the axon (1). A 20% gel (Hurricane Gel®) is available in the US and Aotearoa New Zealand; however, its use is discouraged in Australia due to the high risk of allergy and methaemoglobinaemia.

Compounded gels and creams containing various combinations and strengths of tetracaine, prilocaine and lidocaine can be prepared by compounding pharmacies. If these products are used, it is important to be aware that compounded formulations have rarely been subjected to clinical trials, stability and safety testing and do not have government regulatory approval. In addition, state and territory regulations require that compounded products are only ever ordered for individual patients (and not the practice), using an individual prescription for the named patient in order to prevent compounding pharmacies that are not licensed with the Therapeutic Goods Administration (TGA) from manufacturing large quantities of unregulated products. This is because 'manufacturing' is defined by the TGA as making batches of large quantities of a product for unknown users, and manufacturing is legally restricted to TGA-registered manufacturers only (3, 4).

8.2.1 Teething gels for children

Current recommendations for management of teething include giving the child cooled items to gnaw on, such as chilled teething rings, cold washcloths and pacifiers, or massaging the child's gum with a clean finger.

Despite their ready availability, topical agents are not recommended (5). Teething gels containing 0.5–0.66% lidocaine are available in stores and online, and pharmacies can compound products containing up to 2% lidocaine (5). Accurate dosing of teething gels is difficult to achieve, and overenthusiastic application can lead to toxicity (5). It is difficult to ascertain the exact dose of a teething gel in the oral cavity as it quickly becomes mixed with saliva and increases the child's risk of swallowing and ingestion (5). If the child is crying, drooling or salivating, it is even more difficult to determine the actual dose applied and increases the risk of swallowing. Swallowing of the LA can numb the child's mucous membranes, increasing the risk of aspiration. Systemic exposure can also occur as lidocaine has an oral bioavailability of 30–35%, and aspirated lidocaine is absorbed directly through the respiratory tract (5, 6).

The UK's Medicine and Healthcare products Regulatory Agency (MHRA) extensively reviewed the literature to ascertain the effectiveness of lidocaine for teething and concluded that 'there are no robust data providing convincing evidence of efficacy for oral lidocaine products in the treatment of teething in children' (7). Furthermore, the concentrations and specific formulations currently available vary widely and can be different to what was trialled in the published literature for efficacy.

While the literature regarding efficacy is scant and difficult to interpret due to the flawed trial design and varied formulations used, the risk of LA-containing teething gels likely outweighs their benefit as many case reports have identified adverse reactions and toxicity. Lidocaine-based teething gels used in infants and young children have been associated with seizures, respiratory arrest and death (8–11). Topical lidocaine-based gels are not recommended for treatment of teething in infants and children.

Teething gels available in Australia also contain choline salicylate in addition to LAs. These products have little evidence of benefit and case reports exist of salicylate intoxication and Reye's syndrome (12, 13). The MHRA have recommended against the use of salicylate-containing gels in children younger than 16 years (5).

8.3 Topical products for dental caries

8.3.1 Topical fluoride

Topical fluoride products are available in various concentrations as gels, foams, and varnish (for professional use only), as well as in toothpastes and mouthwashes for patients to use at home. Fluoride has also been combined with casein phosphopeptide-amorphous calcium phosphate (CPP-ACP) to augment the effect of CPP-ACP (see Section 8.3.2). See the *Therapeutic Guidelines Oral and Dental* (*Version 3*) for recommendations on when to use specific formulations and concentrations of fluoride formulations (14).

The use of fluoride has been a key factor in prevention of dental caries, mostly through community water fluoridation and widespread use of fluoridated toothpaste (15). When present in low concentrations in oral fluids, fluoride is incorporated into the surface of apatite crystals where it forms fluoride-containing apatites, fluorhydroxyapatite and fluorapatite, which are less soluble and more resistant to acid challenges than hydroxyapatite (16).

In Australia, community water fluoridation began in 1953 in the city of Beaconsfield, Tasmania, and now the majority of Australians have access to a fluoridated public water supply. The benefit of water fluoridation has been established through extensive population oral health research, which has demonstrated a reduction in prevalence and severity of tooth decay in children and adults. National guidelines for fluoride use in Australia have been developed since 2005 and were last updated in 2019 (17). The National Health and Medical Research Council (NHMRC) established that water fluoridation at the current levels is safe and not associated with any other adverse health outcomes, such as lowered IQ or cancer (15). In addition, when considering all sources of fluoride—including diet, water and fluoridated toothpaste—levels of fluoride ingestion for infants and children up to 8 years old in Australia and Aotearoa New Zealand were found to be less than the upper level of intake for the nutrient reference values. Fluoride ingestion above the upper level is associated with an increased risk of adverse effects (15).

Dental fluorosis can occur due to the excessive exposure to fluoride during odontogenesis, where the fluoride causes subsurface porosities and mottling of enamel (15). The Australian National Child Oral Health Study found just less than 1% of children had definitive dental fluorosis (18). In Australia, the prevalence of fluorosis is mild or very mild, and is not found to be of aesthetic concern or to have long-term negative impacts (15).

As fluorosis is associated with excess ingestion of fluoride, systemically administered fluoride supplements such as drops and tablets are no longer recommended. It is also recommended to spit out excess toothpaste after cleaning, although the mouth should not be rinsed after brushing to retain the remaining toothpaste in the saliva to aid with remineralisation of the enamel (14).

8.3.2 Casein phosphopeptide-amorphous calcium phosphate

Topically applied CPP-ACP has anticariogenic activity. CPP-ACP is derived from the milk protein casein and can stabilise a supersaturated solution of calcium and phosphate, preventing their precipitation. The calcium and phosphate ions are thus bioavailable to enhance remineralisation, and CPP-ACP has been shown to be efficacious in remineralising white spot lesions (19), slowing the progression of coronal caries, and promoting the regression of caries lesions (20). CPP-ACP is also used to prevent caries in patients with moderate to high caries risk in combination with other measures, such as fluoride (21). It must not be used in patients with documented allergy to milk proteins such as casein.

CPP-ACP is currently available in various formulations, including chewing gum, mousse, paste and varnish. Some of these products also contain fluoride. The addition of fluoride to CPP-ACP has shown to improve remineralisation in both permanent and primary teeth compared to CPP-ACP alone (22, 23).

8.3.3 Silver compounds

Topically applied silver compounds, specifically 38% silver diamine fluoride (SDF), has been shown to prevent and arrest caries in both the primary and permanent dentition. However, there is risk of black tooth discolouration and pulp irritation (24). It is thought that this compound's mode of action is exerted by inhibition of demineralisation as well as by an antibacterial effect exerted via inhibition of bacterial DNA replication, interfering in both cytoplasmic enzymes and cell membranes (24). A recent systematic review (25) of SDF's prevention caries in the primary dentition concluded that, when applied to carious lesions in primary teeth and compared with no treatment, placebo or fluoride varnish, SDF appears to effectively prevent dental caries in the entire dentition (25). Furthermore, in 2016 the American Academy of Pediatric Dentistry published evidence-based recommendations for the use of SDF for arresting cavitated caries lesions in primary teeth as part of a comprehensive caries management program (26). It was recommended that 'SDF therapy for caries arrest is indicated for cavitated lesions on coronal or root surfaces that are not suspected to have pulpal involvement, are not symptomatic, and are cleansable. Ideally, these conditions should be verified by radiographic evaluation' (27).

The use of 38% SDF in elderly patients for preventing and arresting root caries has been clearly demonstrated in recent systematic reviews (28, 29) demonstrating a significant decrease in new active lesions post intervention. The likelihood of a lesion arresting with treatment in one case series was shown to be from 82.9–91.6% (30) and there is now well-established recommendations for its use (31).

8.4 Oral antiseptics

Oral antiseptics used as mouthwash and oral rinses have been thought to be much more effective that systemic antibiotics to diminish oral biofilm causing disease. Oral antiseptics have also been used to not only improve gingival and oral health but also to aid in diminishing ventilator-associated pneumonia (VAP) in vulnerable patients (32, 33).

However, recent evidence has questioned this dogma with evidence suggesting that the oral microbial ecosystem, or oral 'microbiome', should be considered an integral part of both oral and systemic health. Indeed, genetic sequencing of the oral microbiome has demonstrated that antiseptic mouthwash, particularly chlorhexidine (CHX), which has been extensively used, adversely effects the oral microbial ecosystem resulting in less bacterial diversity, with less 'good' bacteria for oral and systemic health (34). Although this research is new and our understanding of the effects of oral dysbiosis caused by oral antiseptics is incomplete, good oral hygiene practices should not rely on the use of oral antiseptics alone and their long-term use is now discouraged.

8.4.1 Chlorhexidine

CHX, a bis-biguanide antiseptic with broad spectrum antimicrobial activity, has been used extensively in dentistry and medicine. It was used initially in dentistry, particularly in endodontics for the pre-surgical disinfection of the mouth (35). CHX exerts broad activity against fungi, bacteria and viruses (36, 83). The antimicrobial effect of CHX is dose dependent. At high concentrations (>0.12%) it is bactericidal, while at lower concentrations it has (0.02–0.06%) bacteriostatic activity (37). Brown discoloration of the teeth and tongue, as well as temporary taste alterations, are common adverse reactions (36). As such, CHX is recommended for a maximum of 2 weeks of consecutive use to minimise the development of these side effects (14). Although allergic reactions are very rare, they may cause significant severe reactions particularly when surgical equipment has been soaked in high concentrations of chlorhexidine preoperatively (38). A case of anaphylaxis following the use of CHX mouthwash to irrigate a dry socket has been reported; a problem that is potentially under-reported (39).

Very robust evidence has confirmed the antiplaque and antigingivitis effects of CHX (40). Oral hygiene care, including CHX mouthwash or gel, has been shown to reduce ventilator-associated pneumonia risk in critically ill patients; however, this did not influence mortality, duration of ventilation, or length of intensive care unit stay (33, 83).

Nevertheless, there are concerns about emerging resistance to CHX (41), potentially associated with resistance to other antibiotics resulting in multi-drug resistant organisms in oral plaque (42). It is recommended to limit the use of CHX in dentistry to short-term use for surgical sites to improve wound healing (34).

8.4.2 Povidone iodine

Povidone iodine (PI) exerts a bactericidal, fungicidal, and virucidal effect by releasing iodine that destabilises lipid membranes and lyses proteins as well as degenerating nucleoproteins and scavenging free radicles. Frequently used in hospitals for skin and mucous membrane disinfection before surgery and wound cleansing in both aqueous and alcohol solutions, PI is also employed as a dental antiseptic (35). Commercially available most commonly as a 10% solution, PI products have been shown to be effective at killing most oral bacteria including periodontal fungi, mycobacteria, pathogens, protozoa and viruses (43) with no cytotoxic effects on human cells (44, 83). However, PI can cause allergic reactions in patients with a history of allergy to iodine or shellfish (83). Prolonged intake should be avoided in patients with thyroid dysfunction due to the risk of systemic absorption of excessive iodine (35), although this is not a concern for patients without pre-existing thyroid disease (45) and if the mouthwash is spat out after rinsing. For many years, PI mouth rinse has also been recommended for decontamination of periodontal sites before invasive procedures to reduce the risk of bacteraemia (46).

8.4.3 Hydrogen peroxide

Hydrogen peroxide (HP) is a bleach with strong oxidising action that works by liberating oxygen free radicals, disrupting lipid structures of microbial cell walls to kill obligate anaerobes and to loosen debris present in infection. At concentrations of approximately 0.5%, HP has been shown to be virucidal to enveloped viruses, including coronavirus (47). At concentrations greater than 5% it may cause caustic tissue damage, so lower concentrations between 1–3% have been shown to be acceptable as a mouthwash without adverse effects (48). These HP mouthwashes are broad spectrum antimicrobials shown to reduce gingivitis and staining (49). HP mouthwash can also reduce gingival inflammation for patients with a physical or intellectual impairment, which limits oral hygiene. It can also be used for stain removal and as a soaking solution for dentures (50).

8.4.4 Essential oils

Mouthwashes that contain essential oils, such as thymol, eucalyptol, menthol and methyl salicylate, in solutions of up to 26% alcohol are purported to kill microorganisms through penetration of the plaque biofilm. These mouthwashes have been shown to have broad spectrum antimicrobial activity, preventing aggregation of bacteria and decreasing plaque mass (51). Clinical short-term studies have demonstrated that these mouthwashes reduce plaque, gingivitis and halitosis (51).

The use of mouthwashes that contain essential oils has been recommended as an adjunct to mechanical oral hygiene for those whose oral hygiene is impaired, as well as for the support of gingival health around dental implants. However, patients whose mouth or experiencing oral mucosal ulceration often report essential oil mouth rinses worsen oral dryness and mucosal pain. Finally, the accidental ingestion of high doses of alcohol make these mouthwashes unsuitable for children (50).

8.4.5 Pre-procedural mouthwash and SARS-CoV-2

The use of a CHX mouthwash (0.12%) for 30 seconds twice daily by COVID-19 infected patients eliminates the virus in 62% of cases, and the use of an additional oropharyngeal CHX spray reduces this further to 86% (52). Such evidence resulted in the recommendation for CHX mouthwash to be used prior to dental procedures in patients infected with COVID-19 to diminish risk of transmission (53).

Despite extremely small sample sizes, imperfect study designs and inconclusive results, a recent review found that a 30-second pre-procedural 0.5% PI mouthwash was an effective risk mitigation strategy to diminish the oropharyngeal load of SARS-CoV-2 in patients infected with COVID-19 (53). A recent systematic review concluded that PI at concentrations of 1% (without dilution) and 7% (diluted at 1:30) for 15 seconds appeared to be the most effective mouthwash for reducing salivary viral load of COVID-19 (54).

The European guidelines on infection control during the COVID-19 pandemic reported that the WHO recommendation of pre-procedural mouthwash was followed by 24 of 30 European countries, all of which recommended the use of HP mouthwash (55). However, a very recent thorough systematic review of the current literature concluded that guidelines for the use of HP is based on insufficient scientific evidence to support its recommendation (54). There is a need for further studies, both *in vitro* and clinical, on virus load and risk of transmission during dental treatment. However, currently with the limited and vague scientific evidence it is difficult to justify the benefit of pre-procedural mouthwash use (55).

The Australian Dental Association 'Risk Management Principles for Dentistry: During the COVID-19 pandemic', published in 2021, suggested that 'there is some evidence that ... commercially available mouth rinses when used before dental treatment reduce the viral load in saliva' (84). This recommendation is endorsed by the Dental Board of Australia and Infection Control Expert Group of the Australian Government. Further evidence will undoubtably influence future guidelines, but until then current recommendations should be adhered to.

8.4.6 Alcohol in mouthwash

Alcohol (ethanol) in mouthwashes has been used as a preservative, solvent, and antiseptic. High alcohol concentrations alone will have activity against most microbes due to protein denaturation and lipid dissolution. Further, high levels of alcohol can cause keratosis, mucosal ulceration, petechiae and pain (50). A recent investigation demonstrated that exposure to 20% alcohol causes marked cytotoxicity to oral mucosal cells even after 20 hours of recovery (56).

Farah et al. state that 'there is increasing evidence that there may be a direct relationship between the alcohol content of mouthwashes and the development of oral cancer' (50). The risk of acquiring oral cancer increases 6.4 fold in those who drink alcohol heavily and 2.1 fold for smokers (57). A previous review of the literature 'suggested that it would be inadvisable to recommend the long-term use of alcohol-containing mouthwashes' (50, 58). Recently, there have been a number of systematic reviews and meta-analyses (59–61)—some of which attracted methodological criticism (62)—but all concluding that, using epidemiological data alone, it is currently impossible to establish a clear causal relationship between alcohol in mouthwash and the development of oral cancer. The most recent meta-analysis found that there was a statistically significant correlation between frequent mouthwash usage (more than once per day) and an increased risk for upper aerodigestive tract cancer, with a risk increase for oral cancer compared to laryngeal cancer, potentially implying a connection between regular direct contact of the mouthwash constituents (most plausibly alcohol) with the oral mucosa (60).

Given the trend in the literature associating alcohol-content in mouthwash with oral cancer, it would appear to be inadvisable to recommend the long-term use of this product.

8.5 Topical antifungals

The main topical preparations used in dentistry to treat oral fungal infections are the azoles and polyene drugs.

Oral candidosis is by far the most common mycosis in the mouths of healthy and immunocompromised people. The transition from a harmless commensal to a pathogen is facilitated by both systemic as well as local factors, contributed by candida virulence factors (63). Oral candidosis results from host defences and fungal virulence factors becoming imbalanced (63, 64). The clinical features of fungal disease vary from when the condition is acute to chronic, and may cause asymptomatic lesions, but may also cause pain and discomfort and limit nutritional intake in elderly or hospitalised patients (65).

Before commencing patients on antifungal therapy, the dentist should take a thorough medical history with detailed information on the patient's current medication due to the chance of complex drug interactions. Furthermore, underlying patient factors that might contribute to susceptibility such as immunocompromise, hematinic deficiencies and diabetes need to be identified. Patients should be reminded to remove their dentures/dental prosthesis before taking the medication to ensure distribution of medication at the site of infection. Topical agents are usually preferred for treatment of oral fungal infections, not only because direct topical application is very effective but also to avoid systemic side effects and drug interactions. However, systemic agents are indicated for disseminated systemic infections and, in cases of immunocompromised patients, may be indicated for oropharyngeal candidosis, candidosis refractory to topical agents, and when topical agents are not tolerated (64).

Ergosterol biosynthesis is specific for fungi and required for cell membrane function, and as such most antifungals have either a direct or indirect action on this biosynthetic pathway, causing cell death by the loss of cytoplasmic components and altered cell wall permeability (63). However, some *Candida* species, such as *C. krusei* and *C. glabrata,* have shown to have azole-resistance and as such it is recommended to use the polyenes as a first line of treatment (63, 85).

8.5.1 Azoles

The main azole antifungals used in dentistry are clotrimazole, miconazole, and fluconazole. Azole antifungals inhibit CYP450 -14α demethylation which inhibits ergosterol in the fungal cell membrane. This CYP inhibition also occurs in humans. It can affect vitamin D and cholesterol metabolism and the metabolism of many other drugs such as oral anticoagulants (warfarin), hypoglycaemics, and benzodiazepines. It is also important in cell differentiation during organogenesis and is thought to explain why azole antifungals are teratogenic.

Clotrimazole is an imidazole that is available as cream, mouth rinse, lotion and vaginal formulations with negligible topical absorption. It can be used to treat erythematous and pseudomembranous candidiasis and angular cheilitis.

Miconazole is available in topical and parenteral forms. For oral use, the 2% miconazole gel is very effective; however, it is well absorbed via mucous membranes and the risk of systemic effect and drug interactions must be considered. Fluconazole is administered systemically for treatment of oropharyngeal and oesophageal candidiasis, but its use is restricted to specialist prescribers only due to the risk of adverse effects and serious drug interactions.

All azole antifungals carry a significant risk of drug interactions due to their inhibition of CYP enzyme-mediated drug metabolism. Due to clotrimazole's very poor transdermal absorption, drug interactions are not considered significant. However, miconazole is more significantly absorbed, especially through inflamed mucosa, and can cause clinically significant interactions. The interactions are caused by inhibition of the enzymes CYP2C9, CYP3A4 and to a lesser extent CYP2D6 (63). In the presence of miconazole, the metabolism of other drugs via these enzymes may be impaired, which will cause their intracellular and serum levels to rise, increasing their risk of side effects and toxicity (see Section 4.16.4).

8.5.1.1 Pregnancy and lactation

See Table 14.2.

8.5.2 Polyenes

Nystatin and amphotericin B are polyene antifungals derived from the *Streptomyces* species. These drugs bind to ergosterol in the fungal cell membrane and alter cell membrane permeability by causing formation of aqueous pores or channels that leak cellular components and cause fungal cell death.

Amphotericin B is formulated for topical use in lozenges used four times a day to treat oral candidiasis (66). It has a very broad spectrum of activity against almost all yeasts and filamentous fungi. Resistance to amphotericin B is rare and the new lipid forms (for intravenous use only) are associated with fewer side effects (67). As amphotericin is not absorbed systemically from topical application or oral ingestion, its use is not associated with drug interactions or systemic adverse effects (see Section 4.16.4).

Nystatin is available as oral drops which are swirled around the mouth four times a day. The drops contain a high concentration of sucrose and may promote dental caries in susceptible individuals. The dose is 100,000 units of nystatin, given 4 times daily for 7–14 days, and treatment needs to be extended for several days after lesions disappear to minimise the risk of the recurrence of candidiasis. Nystatin is also not absorbed systemically and therefore not associated with systemic side effects or drug interactions (67) (see Section 4.16.4; for doses, see Section 4.16.5).

8.5.2.1 Pregnancy and lactation

See Table 14.2.

8.6 Topical antivirals

Topical antivirals used in dentistry include aciclovir and penciclovir. Secondary herpes simplex 1 (HSV-1) infection of the mouth typically affects the vermillion of the lip termed 'herpes labialis' (commonly known as 'cold sores') but can also arise on the perioral and perinasal skin (83). Herpes labialis has a characteristic pattern in its presentation, initially with some patients reporting slight paraesthesia, subsequent redness, vesicle formation, pustulation and ulceration of the superficial mucosa that eventually heals over about a 7-day period (68).

A 5% aciclovir cream is effective against recurrent herpes labialis if applied in the prodromal stage of the infection, 5 times a day for 5 days. It lessens the size of lesions and the duration of lesions and pain. Aciclovir is a synthetic acyclic analogue of 2'-deoxyguanosine that has inhibitory activity against HSV-1. Aciclovir affects HSV DNA polymerase and prevents synthesis of viral DNA; it is therefore selective to virally infected cells and has minimal toxicity in other tissues.

Penciclovir is applied topically as a 1% cream every 2 hours (minimum of 6 times daily) during waking hours for 4 days in the treatment of herpes labialis. It has antiviral activity similar to that of aciclovir HSV-1 and 2 and against varicella zoster virus. This activity is due to intracellular conversion by virus-induced thymidine kinase into penciclovir triphosphate, which inhibits replication of viral DNA and persists in infected cells for more than 12 hours (80). This conversion and activation of thymidine kinase is very specific against virally infected cells and as such penciclovir is effective against recurrent herpes infection. For doses, see Section 4.13.5.

8.7 Topical anti-inflammatories

8.7.1 Corticosteroids

Topical corticosteroid preparations used in dentistry include triamcinolone acetonide 0.1%, hydrocortisone acetate 1% ointment, and betamethasone dipropionate 0.05% ointment. Glucocorticoids (GCs) have both anti-inflammatory and immunosuppressive effects and their use in dentistry is mainly for the management of immunologically mediated oral mucosal diseases like oral lichen planus (OLP), pemphigus vulgaris (PV), and benign mucous membrane pemphigoid (BMMP) and for minimising disease severity in conditions like recurrent aphthous stomatitis (RAS) (69). The action of corticosteroids is via receptor-binding within the cytoplasm, multiple gene transcription modulation leading to the production of diminished inflammatory substances, such as leukotrienes and prostaglandins, and the inhibition of the recruitment of inflammatory cells (69).

There is considerable variation in both the strength and vehicles for topical corticosteroids such that their efficacy, absorption and potency is dependent not only on the active compound, but also on the concentration and vehicle, which ultimately affects their potency, absorption and efficacy. This is particularly important for topical use of betamethasone dipropionate 0.05% which, when it is present in a cream, has moderate potency; its potency increases when present in an ointment. When it is delivered in an optimised vehicle (OV), it becomes very potent.

The *Australian Medicines Handbook* classes topical steroids as mild, moderate, potent and very potent (70); however, this potency often manifests differently on oral mucosa compared with other types of skin. In the general dental practice setting, only mild or moderate potency corticosteroid creams or ointments should be used. Potent or very potent creams or ointments, or other formulations of topical corticosteroids, should not be started without specialist advice.

Ointments consist predominantly of water suspended in oil. By occluding the skin, enhancing hydration and absorption, ointments tend to improve a drug's penetration although they also can be greasy and difficult to spread, resulting in potentially poor patient compliance. Creams tend to be less greasy and easier to spread as they are semi-solid emulsions of oil in 20–50% water and can be washed off (71).

The principal adverse reactions of topical corticosteroids include secondary candidiasis, refractory response, mucosal atrophy, striae, and delayed healing. There is the potential for systemic absorption if incorrectly or excessively used (69, 86). There is always some absorption of small amounts through the oral mucosa, although clinical experience and laboratory studies have shown this not to be clinically significant. Exceptions are when multiple corticosteroids are used in conjunction and a cumulative dose may cause side effects, such as glaucoma and cataracts. Finally, diabetic patients and those using corticosteroids to cover extensive areas, or who use it excessively without monitoring, may develop adverse reactions (69).

Almost all currently available topical corticosteroid products are not legally registered for use in the oral cavity, and therefore prescription for this purpose is off-label. In addition, these products are often labelled 'For external use only' which can alarm the dispensing pharmacist and patient. Therefore, dentists prescribing topical corticosteroids for use inside the mouth should anticipate this concern and reassure the patient and pharmacist that these products are safe to be used on oral mucosa and are safe even if a small amount is swallowed (14).

8.7.2 Calcineurin inhibitors

The main calcineurin inhibitor used topically in the oral cavity is pimecrolimus, a 1% cream applied twice a day. Calcineurin inhibitors are immunosuppressive agents used mainly in transplant patients and in patients with immune-mediated disease that bind to T-lymphocytes cytoplasmic proteins and inhibit inflammatory cytokine production. Binding results in T-cells failing to release their cytokines, diminishing inflammation, redness and itching (72). Calcineurin inhibitors can be considered for management of chronic inflammatory mucosal disorders when topical corticosteroids fail, particularly OLP (72). They are minimally absorbed through the oral mucosa with few clinically significant adverse side effects, and there is little evidence that the long-term use of calcineurin inhibitors increase the risk of oral malignancy (72). Thus, topical tacrolimus has been suggested as an effective therapy for erosive or ulcerative OLP (73). A recent systematic review and meta-analysis also concluded that these are alternative approaches when OLP does not respond to the standard protocols (74). A Cochrane Review on the treatment of OLP concluded that there was very low-certainty evidence suggesting that calcineurin inhibitors may be more effective at resolving pain than corticosteroids (75, 87). However, a recent meta-analysis found a significantly higher risk of adverse effects concluding that topical corticosteroids were still the most effective drug class for treating OLP (76, 87).

8.8 Botulinum toxin therapy

Botulinum toxin (BT) is the exotoxin produced by the gram-negative anaerobic bacterium *Clostridium botulinum*, and there are eight subtypes (A, B, C1, C2, D, E, F and G). Botulinum toxin A (BT-A), also known as onabotulinumtoxin A, is marketed as Botox, Dysport and Xeomin, and has been used in the treatment of muscular temporomandibular disorders (TMDs); Botulinum B is mostly used in neurology (77).

In myofascial pain, there can be excessive acetylcholine release from motor and autonomic nerves, causing contraction of muscle fibres (78). BT-A causes inhibition of the presynaptic release of acetylcholine, thereby inhibiting muscle innervation at the neuromuscular junction and thus inhibiting skeletal muscle contraction (79). In addition, BT inhibits the release of pain mediators in peripheral nerve endings and neurons in the spinal cord, thus modulating pain transmissions pathways to reduce central and peripheral sensitisation (79). After injection, its onset of action takes 2–3 days after which it causes paresis and atrophy of the muscle, and the duration of action depends on regeneration of the skeletal muscle, usually around 2–4 months (77). The paresis level is dose dependent. Adverse effects usually arise from diffusion of BT-A into adjacent tissues to the target site. Necrosis or fibrotic changes do not occur from BT-A into the muscle (77). However, at high doses, widespread systemic weakness, dysphagia and shortness of breath can occur from the effects of BT-A on other skeletal muscle (77).

The use of BT-A for the treatment of patients with TMDs has been studied. An early prospective randomised double-blind placebo-controlled study of patients reported improvement when compared with those injected with saline after 28 days (80). Although reported to be a safe and effective treatment (81), an extensive randomised, placebo-controlled, cross-over multi-centre study comparing BT-A and saline for persistent masticatory myofascial pain showed that BT-A reduced pain intensity by 33% and saline by 40% at 1 month, yet at 3 months this was 30% for BT-A and 33% for saline with no significant difference in pain reduction between both (82). Although BT-A may be a safe treatment, its benefits are unclear for chronic masticatory myofascial pain.

FURTHER READING

Cochrane NJ, Reynolds EC. Calcium phosphopeptides—mechanisms of action and evidence for clinical efficacy. *Adv Dent Res.* 2012;24(2):41–47.

Do LG. Guidelines for use of fluorides in Australia: update 2019. *Aust Dent J.* 2020;65(1):30–38.

Farah CS, McIntosh L, McCullough MJ. Mouthwashes. *Aust Prescr.* 2009;32:162–164.

Manfredi M, Polonelli L, Aguirre-Urizar J, Carrozzo M, McCullough M. Urban legends series: oral candidosis. *Oral diseases.* 2013;19(3):245–261.

REFERENCES

1. Mundiya J, Woodbine E. Updates on Topical and Local Anesthesia Agents. *Oral Maxillofac Surg Clin North Am.* 2022;34(1):147–155.

2. Pharmapproach. *Topical Route of Drug Administration: Advantages and Disadvantages.* 22 November 2020. https://www.pharmapproach.com/ topical-route-of-drug-administration-advantages-and-disadvantages

3. Boyce RA, Kirpalani T, Mohan N. Updates of Topical and Local Anesthesia Agents. *Dent Clin North Am.* 2016;60(2):445–471.

4. Pharmacy Board of Australia. *Guidelines on Compounding of Medicines.* Pharmacy Board of Australia; 2015.

5. Teoh L, Moses GM. Are teething gels safe or even necessary for our children? A review of the safety, efficacy and use of topical lidocaine teething gels. *J Paediatr Child Health.* 2020;56(4):502–505.

6. Curtis LA, Dolan TS, Seibert HE. Are one or two dangerous? Lidocaine and topical anesthetic exposures in children. *J Emerg Med.* 2009;37(1):32–39.

7. Medical and Healthcare Products Regulatory Authority. *Oral lidocaine products: risk minimisation measures for use in teething.* MHRA UK Public Assessment Report; 2018.

8. Balit CR, Lynch AM, Gilmore SP et al. Lignocaine and chlorhexidine toxicity in children resulting from mouth paint ingestion: a bottling problem. *J Paediatr Child Health.* 2006;42(6):350–353.

9. Giard MJ, Uden DL, Whitlock DJ, Watson DM. Seizures induced by oral viscous lidocaine. *Clin Pharm.* 1983;2(2):110.

10. Gonzalez del Rey J, Wason S, Druckenbrod RW. Lidocaine overdose: another preventable case? *Pediatr Emerg Care.* 1994;10(6):344–346.

11. Rothstein P, Dornbusch J, Shaywitz BA. Prolonged seizures associated with the use of viscous lidocaine. *J Pediatr.* 1982;101(3):461–463.

12. Nguyen T, Cranswick N, Rosenbaum J, Gelbart B, Tosif S. Chronic use of teething gel causing salicylate toxicity. *J Paediatr Child Health.* 2018;54(5):576–578.

13. Williams GD, Kirk EP, Wilson CJ et al. Salicylate intoxication from teething gel in infancy. *Med J Aust.* 2011;194(3):146–148.

14. Oral and Dental Expert Group. *Therapeutic Guidelines Oral and Dental (Version 3).* Therapeutic Guidelines Ltd; 2019.

15. Do LG. Guidelines for use of fluorides in Australia: update 2019. *Aust Dent J.* 2020;65(1):30–38.

16. Buzalaf MAR, Pessan JP, Honório HM, Ten Cate JM. Mechanisms of action of fluoride for caries control. *Monogr Oral Sci.* 2011;22:97–114.

17. Do LG. Guidelines for use of fluorides in Australia: update 2019. *Aust Dent J.* 2020 Mar;65(1):30–38.

18. Ha DH, Roberts-Thomson KF, Arrow P, Peres KG, Do LG. Children's oral health status in Australia, 2012–14. In Do LG, Spencer AJ (eds). *Oral health of Australian children: the National Child Oral Health Study 2012–14*. University of Adelaide Press; 2016.

19. Ma X, Lin X, Zhong T, Xie F. Evaluation of the efficacy of casein phosphopeptide-amorphous calcium phosphate on remineralization of white spot lesions in vitro and clinical research: a systematic review and meta-analysis. *BMC Oral Health*. 2019;19(1):295. doi:10.1186/s12903-019-0977-0

20. Reynolds EC. Calcium phosphate-based remineralization systems: scientific evidence? *Aust Dent J*. 2008;53(3):268–273.

21. Cochrane NJ, Reynolds EC. Calcium phosphopeptides—mechanisms of action and evidence for clinical efficacy. *Adv Dent Res*. 2012;24(2):41–47.

22. Salman NR, ElTekeya M, Bakry N et al. Comparison of remineralization by fluoride varnishes with and without casein phosphopeptide amorphous calcium phosphate in primary teeth. *Acta Odontol Scand*. 2019;77(1):9–14.

23. Duraisamy V, Xavier A, Nayak UA et al. An in vitro evaluation of the demineralization inhibitory effect of F(-) varnish and casein phosphopeptide-amorphous calcium phosphate on enamel in young permanent teeth. *J Pharm Bioallied Sci*. 2015;7(Suppl 2):S513– S517.

24. Young DA, Quock RL, Horst J et al. Clinical Instructions for Using Silver Diamine Fluoride (SDF) in Dental Caries Management. *Compend Contin Educ Dent*. 2021;42(6):e5-e9.

25. Oliveira BH, Rajendra A, Veitz-Keenan A et al. The Effect of Silver Diamine Fluoride in Preventing Caries in the Primary Dentition: A Systematic Review and Meta-Analysis. *Caries Res*. 2019;53(1):24–32.

26. Crystal YO, Marghlani AA, Ureles SD et al. Use of Silver Diamine Fluoride for Dental Caries Management in Children and Adolescents, Including Those with Special Health Care Needs. *Pediatr Dent*. 2018;40(6):152–161.

27. Crystal YO, Niederman R. Evidence-Based Dentistry Update on Silver Diamine Fluoride. *Dent Clin North Am*. 2019;63(1):45–68.

28. Castelo R, Attik N, Catirse A, Pradelle-Plasse N, Tirapelli C, Grosgogeat B. Is there a preferable management for root caries in middle-aged and older adults? A systematic review. *Br Dent J*. 2021. doi:10.1038/s41415-021-3003-2

29. Grandjean ML, Maccarone NR, McKenna G, Müller F, Srinivasan M. Silver Diamine Fluoride (SDF) in the management of root caries in elders: a systematic review and meta-analysis. *Swiss Dent J*. 2021;131(5):417–424.

30. Mitchell C, Gross AJ, Milgrom P, Mancl L, Prince DB. Silver diamine fluoride treatment of active root caries lesions in older adults: A case series. *J Dent*. 2021;105:103561.

31. Seifo N, Robertson M, MacLean J et al. The use of silver diamine fluoride (SDF) in dental practice. *Br Dent J*. 2020;228(2):75–81.

32. Bellissimo-Rodrigues WT, Menegueti MG et al. Effectiveness of a dental care intervention in the prevention of lower respiratory tract nosocomial infections among intensive care patients: a randomized clinical trial. *Infect Control Hosp Epidemiol*. 2014;35(11):1342–1348.

33. Hua F, Xie H, Worthington HV, Furness S, Zhang Q, Li C. Oral hygiene care for critically ill patients to prevent ventilator-associated pneumonia. *Cochrane Database Syst Rev*. 2016;10(10):Cd008367.

34. Brookes ZLS, Belfield LA, Ashworth A et al. Effects of Chlorhexidine mouthwash on the oral microbiome. *J Dent*. 2021;113:103768. doi:10.1016/j.jdent.2021.103768

35. Slots J. Low-cost periodontal therapy. *Periodontol 2000*. 2012;60(1):110–137.

36. Karpiński TM, Szkaradkiewicz AK. Chlorhexidine—pharmaco-biological activity and application. *Eur Rev Med Pharmacol Sci*. 2015;19(7):1321–1326.

37. Jenkins S, Addy M, Wade W. The mechanism of action of chlorhexidine. A study of plaque growth on enamel inserts in vivo. *J Clin Periodontol.* 1988;15(7):415–424.

38. Krishna MT, York M, Chin T et al. Multi-centre retrospective analysis of anaphylaxis during general anaesthesia in the United Kingdom: aetiology and diagnostic performance of acute serum tryptase. *Clin Exp Immunol.* 2014;178(2):399–404.

39. Pemberton MN. Allergy to Chlorhexidine. *Dent Update.* 2016;43(3):272–274.

40. James P, Worthington HV, Parnell C et al. Chlorhexidine mouthrinse as an adjunctive treatment for gingival health. *Cochrane Database Syst Rev.* 2017;3(3):Cd008676.

41. Kampf, G Acquired resistance to chlorhexidine—is it time to establish an 'antiseptic stewardship' initiative? *J Hosp Infect.* 2016;94(3):213–227.

42. Saleem HGM, Seers CA, Sabri AN, Reynolds AC. Dental plaque bacteria with reduced susceptibility to chlorhexidine are multidrug resistant. *BMC Microbiol.* 2016 Sep 15:16:214.

43. Schreier H, Erdos G, Reimer K et al. Molecular effects of povidone-iodine on relevant microorganisms: an electron-microscopic and biochemical study. *Dermatology.* 1997;195(Suppl 2):111–6.

44. Niedner R. Cytotoxicity and sensitization of povidone-iodine and other frequently used anti-infective agents. *Dermatology.* 1997;195(Suppl 2):89–92.

45. Adamietz IA, Rahn R, Böttcher HD, Schäfer V, Reimer K, Fleischer W. Prophylaxis with povidone-iodine against induction of oral mucositis by radiochemotherapy. *Support Care Cancer.* 1998;6(4):373–377.

46. Dajani AS, Taubert KA, Wilson W et al. Prevention of bacterial endocarditis: recommendations by the American Heart Association. *Clin Infect Dis.* 1997;25(6):1448–1458.

47. O'Donnell VB, Thomas D, Stanton R et al. Potential Role of Oral Rinses Targeting the Viral Lipid Envelope in SARS-CoV-2 Infection. *Function (Oxf).* 2020;1(1):zqaa002.

48. Reis INR, do Amaral G, Mendoza AAH et al. Can preprocedural mouthrinses reduce SARS-CoV-2 load in dental aerosols? *Med Hypotheses.* 2021;146:110436.

49. Hasturk H, Nunn M, Warbington M et al. Efficacy of a fluoridated hydrogen peroxide-based mouthrinse for the treatment of gingivitis: a randomized clinical trial. *J Periodontol.* 2004;75(1):57–65.

50. Farah CS, McIntosh L, McCullough MJ. Mouthwashes. *Aust Prescr.* 2009;32:162–164.

51. Fine DH, Furgang D, Sinatra K et al. In vivo antimicrobial effectiveness of an essential oil-containing mouth rinse 12 h after a single use and 14 days' use. *J Clin Periodontol.* 2005;32(4):335–340.

52. Huang YH, Huang JT. Use of chlorhexidine to eradicate oropharyngeal SARS-CoV-2 in COVID-19 patients. *J Med Virol.* 2021;93(7):4370–4373.

53. Chen MH, Chang PC. The effectiveness of mouthwash against SARS-CoV-2 infection: A review of scientific and clinical evidence. *J Formos Med Assoc.* 2022;121(5):879–885.

54. Cavalcante-Leão BL, de Araujo CM, Basso IB et al. Is there scientific evidence of the mouthwashes effectiveness in reducing viral load in Covid-19? A systematic review. *J Clin Exp Dent.* 2021;13(2):e179–e189.

55. Becker K, Gurzawska-Comis K, Brunello G, Klinge B. Summary of European guidelines on infection control and prevention during COVID-19 pandemic. *Clin Oral Implants Res.* 2021;32(Suppl 21):353–381.

56. Calderón-Montaño JM, Jiménez-Alonso JJ, Guillén-Mancina E et al. A 30-s exposure to ethanol 20% is cytotoxic to human keratinocytes: possible mechanistic link between alcohol-containing mouthwashes and oral cancer. *Clin Oral Investig.* 2018;22(8):2943–2946.

57. Maasland DH, van den Brandt PA, Kremer B et al. Alcohol consumption, cigarette smoking and the risk of subtypes of head-neck cancer: results from the Netherlands Cohort Study. *BMC Cancer.* 2014;14:187.

58. McCullough MJ, Farah CS. The role of alcohol in oral carcinogenesis with particular reference to alcohol-containing mouthwashes. *Australian Dental Journal*. 2008;53(4):302–305.

59. Aceves Argemí R, González Navarro B, Ochoa García-Seisdedos P, Estrugo Devesa A, López-López J. Mouthwash With Alcohol and Oral Carcinogenesis: Systematic Review and Meta-analysis. *J Evid Based Dent Pract*. 2020;20(2):101407.

60. Hostiuc S, Ionescu IV, Drima E. Mouthwash Use and the Risk of Oral, Pharyngeal, and Laryngeal Cancer. A Meta-Analysis. *Int J Environ Res Public Health*. 2021;18(15):8215.

61. Ustrell-Borràs M, Traboulsi-Garet B, Gay-Escoda C. Alcohol-based mouthwash as a risk factor of oral cancer: A systematic review. *Med Oral Patol Oral Cir Bucal*. 2020;25(1):e1–e12.

62. Brignardello-Petersen R. Uncertainty about association between mouthrinses and oral and pharyngeal cancer owing to serious limitations in systematic review addressing this question. *J Am Dent Assoc*. 2020;151(11):e104.

63. Manfredi M, Polonelli L, Aguirre-Urizar JM et al. Urban legends series: oral candidosis. *Oral Diseases*. 2013;19(3):245–261.

64. Samaranayake LP, Keung Leung W, Jin L. Oral mucosal fungal infections. *Periodontol 2000*. 2009;49:39–59.

65. Manfredi M, Polonelli L, Aguirre-Urizar J, Carrozzo M, McCullough M. Urban legends series: oral candidosis. *Oral diseases*. 2013;19(3):245–261.

66. MIMS. *Data Version*. MIMS Australia; August 2021.

67. Telles DR, Karki N, Marshall MW. Oral Fungal Infections: Diagnosis and Management. *Dent Clin North Am*. 2017;61(2):319–349.

68. Porter S, Leao JC, Gueiros LA. Oral and Maxillofacial Viral Infections. In Farah CBR, McCullough M (eds.) *Contemporary Oral Medicine: A Comprehensive Approach to Clinical Practice*. Springer Nature; 2019.

69. Savage NW, McCullough MJ. Topical corticosteroids in dental practice. *Australian Dental Journal*. 2005;50(4):S40–S44.

70. Rossi S (ed). *Australian Medicines Handbook*. Australian Medicines Handbook Pty Ltd; 2021.

71. Carlos G, Uribe P, Férnandez-Peñas P. Rational use of topical corticosteroids. *Aust Prescr*. 2013;36:5–6

72. Al Johani KA, Hegarty AM, Porter SR, Fedele S. Calcineurin inhibitors in oral medicine. *J Am Acad Dermatol*. 2009;61(5):829–840.

73. Kaliakatsou F, Hodgson TA, Lewsey JD et al. Management of recalcitrant ulcerative oral lichen planus with topical tacrolimus. *J Am Acad Dermatol*. 2002;46(1):35–41.

74. Sun SL, Liu JJ, Zhong B et al. Topical calcineurin inhibitors in the treatment of oral lichen planus: a systematic review and meta-analysis. *Br J Dermatol*. 2019;181(6):1166–1176.

75. Lodi G, Manfredi M, Mercadante V et al. Interventions for treating oral lichen planus: corticosteroid therapies. *Cochrane Database Syst Rev*. 2020;2(2):Cd001168.

76. Sridharan K, Sivaramakrishnan G. Interventions for oral lichen planus: a systematic review and network meta-analysis of randomized clinical trials. *Aust Dent J*. 2021;66(3):295–303.

77. Sipahi Calis A, Colakoglu Z, Gunbay S. The use of botulinum toxin-a in the treatment of muscular temporomandibular joint disorders. *J Stomatol Oral Maxillofac Surg*. 2019;120(4):322–325.

78. Chaurand J, Pacheco-Ruíz L, Orozco-Saldívar H et al. Efficacy of botulinum toxin therapy in treatment of myofascial pain. *J Oral Sci*. 2017;59(3):351–356.

79. Park J, Park HJ. Botulinum toxin for the treatment of neuropathic pain. *Toxins (Basel)*. 2017;9(9):260.

80. Kurtoglu C, Gur OH, Kurkcu M et al. Effect of botulinum toxin-A in myofascial pain patients with or without functional disc displacement. *J Oral Maxillofac Surg*. 2008;66(8):1644–1651.

81. Baker JS, Nolan PJ. Effectiveness of botulinum toxin type A for the treatment of chronic masticatory myofascial pain: a case series. *J Am Dent Assoc*. 2017;148(1):33–39.

82. Ernberg M, Hedenberg-Magnusson B, List T et al. Efficacy of botulinum toxin type A for treatment of persistent myofascial TMD pain: a randomized, controlled, double-blind multicenter study. *Pain*. 2011;152(9):1988–1996.

83. Goncalves S, Dionne RA, Moses G, Carrozzo M. Pharmacotherapeutic Approaches in Oral Medicine. In Farah C, Balasubramaniam R, McCullough M (eds.) *Contemporary Oral Medicine*. Springer Cham; 2019.

84. Australian Dental Association. *Risk Management Principles for Dentistry: During the COVID-19 pandemic*. 22 October 2021. https://www.ada.org.au/getdoc/d3eecaba-d0aa-4803-a7ea-89facae6f274/Risk-Management-Principles-for-Dentistry-(1).aspx

85. Epstein JB, Polsky B. Oropharyngeal candidiasis: a review of its clinical spectrum and current therapies. *Clinical Therapeutics*. 1998;20(1):40–57.

86. Pramick M, Whitmore E. Cushing's syndrome caused by mucosal corticosteroid therapy. *International Journal of Dermatology*. 2009;40:100–101.

87. Ezzat O, Helmy IM. Topical pimecrolimus versus betamethasone for oral lichen planus: a randomized clinical trial. *Clinical Oral Investigations*. 2019;23(8):947–956.

DRUGS ASSOCIATED WITH INCREASED BLEEDING RISK

9

KEY POINTS

- Dentists are responsible for a patient's adverse bleeding event in two main ways: first, by performing an invasive dental procedure with inadequate preoperative assessment of the patient's bleeding risk; or second, by prescribing medicines which cause bleeding as a side effect.
- Many drugs contribute to bleeding risk, including antiplatelet agents, anticoagulants, non-selective NSAIDs, serotonergic antidepressants, drugs that can cause thrombocytopenia and some complementary medicines.
- In order to assess bleeding risk from medications accurately, the dentist must take an up-to-date medication history including all prescription, non-prescription and complementary medicines.
- To calculate a patient's overall bleeding risk, dentists should assess the cumulative effect of patient-, drug- and procedure-related factors.

9.1 Introduction

Antithrombotic drugs are those used to slow down blood clot formation, including antiplatelet agents and anticoagulants. Dentists commonly encounter patients who are on antithrombotic drugs, as these drugs are used to manage common conditions. For example, direct oral anticoagulant (DOACs) drugs are drugs frequently prescribed for management of atrial fibrillation, which affects approximately 5% of the Australian population aged 55 and over (1). As a result, DOACs were among the top 100 drugs dispensed on the PBS in 2018 (2). Increased risk of oral bleeding is thus a complication dentists may have to manage. The risk of post-extraction bleeding is increased three-fold in patients taking anticoagulants compared with those not taking these drugs (3, 4). Understanding the principles of haemostasis, how to balance the risk of bleeding against the risk of clotting, and how to manage these patients is an integral part of dentistry.

9.2 General principles of haemostasis

Haemostasis is a physiological process defined as the arrest of blood loss from a damaged blood vessel (5). It consists of blood vessel constriction, platelet activation and aggregation, and stimulation of the coagulation process (2, 6).

Under normal circumstances in the blood stream a fine balance is maintained between pro- and anticoagulant factors. Historically, coagulation was divided into extrinsic and intrinsic pathways, but now it is accepted that the cell-based model of coagulation involves one pathway that occurs in three sequential steps: initiation, amplification and propagation (6, 7).

9.2.1 Coagulation process

For coagulation to take place, a series of circulating inactive coagulation factors are activated in sequence that interact with platelets and lead to the formation of fibrin that is incorporated into the platelet plug (see Figures 9.1 and 9.2).

Initiation:

- Upon rupture of the blood vessel, subendothelial cells are exposed and express tissue factor (TF) which binds to Factor VII and activates it forming TF-VIIa complex (6).
- This complex triggers the coagulation process involving conversion of Factor IX and X to Factor IXa and Xa respectively (6).
- Factor Xa catalyses the activation of prothrombin to thrombin.

Amplification:

- The small amount of thrombin produced in the initiation phase is used to amplify the thrombin generated from platelets and serine proteases (6, 8).
- Several positive feedback loops are generated that increase coagulation of proteins on the surface of platelets, reinforcing platelet activation and thrombin generation (8).
- Thrombin increases the production of Factors Va, VIIIa, IXa and Xa that are also involved in the positive feedback system (6).

Propagation:

- This final step involves a large amount of thrombin being generated on activated platelets.
- Thrombin catalyses the conversion of fibrinogen to fibrin that binds to the GP IIb/IIIa receptors on platelets.
- Factor XIII (fibrin-stabilising factor) is generated that covalently links the fibrin strands and stabilises the fibrin meshwork (7).

9.2.2 Negative feedback on coagulation

Blood vessel endothelium produces vitamin K-dependent proteins C and S that, when activated, are involved in inhibiting coagulation by inactivating Factors Va and VIIIa (6, 9). Antithrombin (formerly known as antithrombin III) is an endogenous glycoprotein that inhibits the effect of thrombin and other coagulation factors, including Factors Xa and IXa (6).

9.2.3 Platelet plug formation

Upon initial rupture of a blood vessel, the endothelium (inner lining of blood vessels) changes from being non-thrombogenic to thrombogenic by expression of tissue factor. Circulating platelets are exposed to this thrombogenic endothelium and adhere to damaged

Figure 9.1 Coagulation cascade (7).

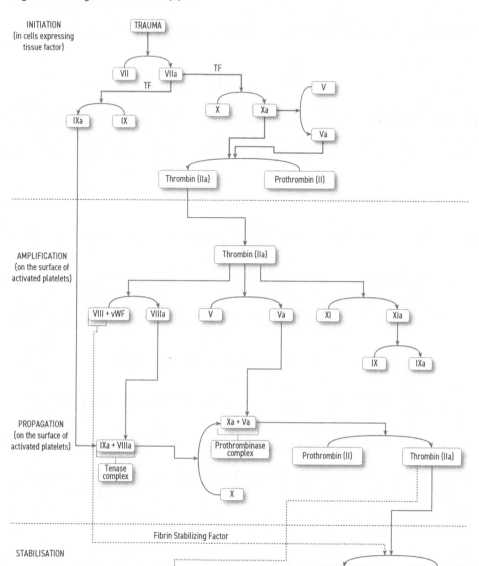

areas by the action of von Willebrand factor. Platelets subsequently undergo a shape change, secrete granules containing adenosine diphosphate (ADP), serotonin and other factors such as thromboxane A2 (TXA2) via the enzyme COX-1 that promotes platelet aggregation (5).

Agonists generated by the platelet activation and coagulation processes, such as ADP and thrombin, cause platelets to express glycoprotein (GP) IIb/IIIa receptors on their surface to amplify the platelet response. GP IIb/IIIa receptors are targeted by fibrinogen, which is then converted to fibrin to form the stabilised platelet plug (5).

Finally, ADP binds to $P2Y_1$ and $P2Y_{12}$ receptors on the platelet for activation of the GP IIb/IIIa receptor. The $P2Y_{12}$ receptor binding by ADP is mostly responsible for TXA2 production and enhancing platelet activation and aggregation (10).

9.2.4 Fibrinolysis

When thrombosis occurs, the fibrinolytic system (to dissolve the clot) is also activated. Several endogenous factors that activate plasminogen are triggered, including tissue plasminogen activator (5). Plasminogen is a circulating, inactive precursor of plasmin; plasmin is a proteolytic enzyme that breaks down fibrin, as well as fibrinogen, Factors II, V and VIII to dissolve the blood clot (5, 11).

Figure 9.2 The process of formation of an arterial thrombus (5).

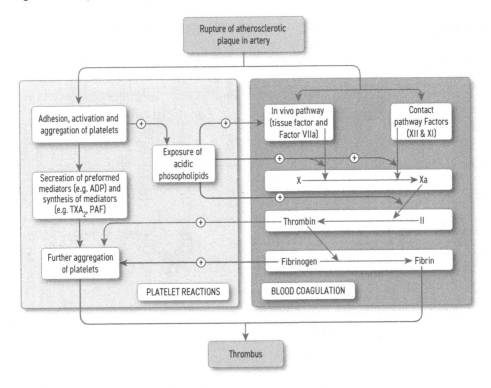

9.3 Antithrombotic effects of drugs

Drugs can affect coagulation and haemostasis by acting on:

- the coagulation pathway
- platelet aggregation
- fibrinolysis

Some of the most common types of drugs encountered in clinical practice are those with antithrombotic effects. The increased risk of bleeding associated with these drugs should be carefully considered when determining perioperative patient management. Table 9.1 presents an overview of the drugs with antithrombotic effects.

Table 9.1 Antithrombotic drugs relevant to dental practice.

Antithrombotic	Drug class	Drug	Mode of administration
Antiplatelet drugs	Salicylate	Aspirin	Oral
	Phosphodiesterase inhibitor	Dipyridamole	Oral
	P2Y$_{12}$ inhibitors	Clopidogrel	Oral
		Ticagrelor	Oral
	GP IIb/IIIa inhibitors	Eptifibatide	IV
		Tirofiban	IV
Anticoagulants	Heparins	Low molecular weight heparins: dalteparin, danaparoid, enoxaparin, nadroparin	SC
		Heparin	IV or SC
	Synthetic heparin	Fondaparinux	IV
	Vitamin K antagonists	Warfarin	Oral
	Direct thrombin inhibitors	Dabigatran	Oral
	Factor Xa inhibitors	Apixaban	Oral
		Rivaroxaban	Oral
Non-selective NSAIDs: see Section 9.4.2			Oral
Antidepressants with a relevant serotonin inhibition: see Section 9.6.1			Oral
Medications that are associated with thrombocytopenia (e.g. cytotoxics, immunomodulators): see Section 9.6.2			Oral or parenteral
Complementary medicines with antithrombotic effects: see Section 9.6.3			Oral

9.4 Antiplatelet drugs

9.4.1 Aspirin

9.4.1.1 Drug class

Salicylate.

9.4.1.2 Pharmacodynamics

Aspirin (acetylsalicylic acid) is a COX-1 selective non-steroidal anti-inflammatory drug (NSAID) that has antiplatelet, antipyretic and analgesic properties. Its antiplatelet effect is exerted by acetylation and irreversible inhibition of COX-1 on the surface of platelets, leading to a reduction in TXA2 and inhibition of platelet aggregation (12). As aspirin's inactivation of platelet activity is permanent, it lasts for the remaining lifetime of the platelet which is 7–10 days.

9.4.1.3 Indications

Aspirin is commonly used for acute coronary syndrome, prevention of ischaemic stroke and transient ischaemic attack, and prevention of pre-eclampsia in women at moderate–high risk (2, 12).

Practice points

- The duration of aspirin's antiplatelet effect is related to its permanent inactivation of platelet function (7–10 days) rather than its half-life, which is 20 minutes (13). Recovery of the patient's platelet function occurs once sufficient new platelets are formed after the drug is discontinued—generally a further 10 days (14).
- Aspirin is no longer recommended for primary prevention of cardiovascular (CV) disease, even in elderly or diabetic patients. This is because clinical trials have shown that the benefit of aspirin for primary prevention of CV events is outweighed by the risk of bleeding (15–17). Thus, in clinical practice, aspirin is now most commonly used in secondary prevention of CV disease where its benefits still outweigh the risk, and in combination with other antithrombotics for prevention of stroke and myocardial infarction (MI) post-PCI (e.g. stenting or valve replacement) (12).

9.4.2 Non-selective non-steroidal anti-inflammatory drugs (NSAIDs)

9.4.2.1 Drugs

The NSAIDs most frequently used in clinical practice are:

- diclofenac
- ibuprofen
- indomethacin
- ketoprofen
- ketorolac
- mefenamic acid
- naproxen
- piroxicam

9.4.2.2 Pharmacodynamics

Non-selective NSAIDs inhibit COX-1 on platelets, causing inhibition of TXA2 production and platelet aggregation, which can lead to increased bleeding risk (12). Unlike aspirin that binds irreversibly to platelets, NSAIDs bind reversibly. The duration of effect therefore depends on the half-life of the respective NSAID and not on the lifetime of the platelet (2). Nonetheless, when taken continuously for a period of time, the effect of NSAIDs on platelet function can contribute to increased risk of bleeding. Although NSAID-associated bleeding can occur anywhere in the body, the most likely location is in the GI tract due to the negative impact of NSAIDs on prostaglandin production in the gut. Fortunately, use of NSAIDs with a short half-life such as ibuprofen for management of postoperative pain does not produce a clinically significant risk of postoperative bleeding (18).

Practice points

- Continuous use of non-selective NSAIDs prior to a procedure can contribute to increased risk of intra- and postoperative bleeding, especially in patients with other bleeding risk factors.
- Short half-life NSAIDs such as ibuprofen contribute little or no postoperative bleeding risk on their own.
- For more information on prescribing NSAIDs in dental practice see Section 5.7.1.

9.4.3 Dipyridamole

9.4.3.1 Pharmacodynamics

Dipyridamole reversibly inhibits cyclic guanine monophosphate phosphodiesterase and adenosine uptake on erythrocytes and on endothelial cells, allowing for increased adenosine binding on platelets, resulting in an increased blood flow and reduced platelet aggregation (12, 19). It also has coronary vasodilating properties (14).

9.4.3.2 Indications

Dipyridamole is used for prevention of recurrent ischaemic stroke and transient ischaemic attack (12).

Practice points

- Dipyridamole is used as a fixed-dose combination with aspirin to confer an additive antiplatelet effect (20).
- Dipyridamole alone has a weak, reversible antiplatelet effect that is lost after about 24 hours following cessation (14, 19).

9.4.4 P2Y$_{12}$ inhibitors

9.4.4.1 Clopidogrel

Pharmacodynamics

Clopidogrel is a pro-drug metabolised by six liver enzymes, but principally by CYP2C19 to its active metabolite (10). The latter irreversibly inhibits the P2Y$_{12}$ receptor on the platelets, preventing binding of ADP and subsequent activation of the GP IIb/IIIa complex, thus inhibiting platelet aggregation.

Indications

Clopidogrel is used as monotherapy for prevention of vascular ischaemia in patients with history of symptomatic atherosclerosis. Together with aspirin, clopidogrel is used for prevention of acute coronary syndrome-related thrombosis (myocardial infarction and stroke) (12).

Practice point

Clopidogrel is most frequently used in combination with aspirin, so the cumulative effect of the two drugs combined on bleeding must be considered.

9.4.4.2 Ticagrelor

Pharmacodynamics

Ticagrelor works by reversible inhibition of the $P2Y_{12}$ receptor on platelets, preventing binding of ADP and subsequent activation of the GP IIb/IIIa complex, thus inhibiting platelet aggregation (2).

Indications

Ticagrelor is used with aspirin for prevention of acute coronary syndrome and for patients who have percutaneous coronary interventions such as stenting or coronary artery bypass grafting (12, 20).

Practice points

- Ticagrelor has a synergistic antiplatelet effect when administered in combination with aspirin (12). The combination increases the potential benefit, but also increases the bleeding risk.
- Ticagrelor is more effective than clopidogrel in prevention of major coronary events (myocardial infarction and stroke) without an increase in the rate of major bleeding, as demonstrated in the landmark Platelet Inhibition and Patient Outcomes (PLATO) study (21).

9.4.5 GP IIb/IIIa Inhibitors

9.4.5.1 Drugs

- eptifibatide
- tirofiban

9.4.5.2 Pharmacodynamics

These drugs work by blocking GP IIb/IIIa receptor on platelets, inhibiting the final step of platelet aggregation by preventing fibrinogen and other adhesive ligands from binding to the platelet (12).

9.4.5.3 Indications

These drugs are used for prevention of thrombosis in patients who have undergone percutaneous coronary interventions, intracoronary stenting or who have been diagnosed with unstable angina (12).

Practice point

These potent inhibitors of platelet function are mostly used short term in settings where monitoring of prothrombin time (PT), activated partial thromboplastin time (aPTT), CrCl, platelet count, haemoglobin and haemotocrit is provided (12).

Table 9.2 summarises the key features of antiplatelet drugs currently used in clinical practice.

Table 9.2 Summary of the pharmacokinetic, pharmacodynamic and pharmacotherapeutic features of commonly used antiplatelet agents. Based on (2, 12, 14, 20, 22).

Drug	Aspirin	Dipyridamole	Clopidogrel	Ticagrelor
Some commercial names	Spren Cardiprin Cartia Astrix	Persantin Asasantin SR (Dipyridamole + aspirin)	Clovix Iscover Piax Plavix CoPlavix (Clopidogrel + aspirin)	Brilinta
Mechanism of action	Irreversible inhibitor of platelet COX-1	Inhibits cGMP phosphodiesterase and adenosine uptake	Pro-drug, irreversible $P2Y_{12}$ antagonist	Reversible $P2Y_{12}$ antagonist
Onset and maximum effect	Maximum effect: 30–60 minutes	Time to peak plasma levels: 2–3 hours (SR formulation)	Onset 1–2 hours. Time to maximum effect depends on dose: 2–3 hours after 600mg; 4–5 hours after 300mg; 7 days after 75mg	After loading dose: Onset: 30 minutes. Maximum effect: 2–4 hours
Half-life	20 minutes	30–60 minutes (SR formulation)	Clopidogrel: 6 hours Active metabolite: 30 minutes	Ticagrelor: 7 hours Active metabolite: 8.6 hours
Pro-drug	No	No	Yes	No
Bioavailability	50%	70% (SR formulation)	Active metabolite: >50%	36%
Practice points	No longer used as primary prevention; used in combination with other antithrombotics for secondary prevention	Synergistic effect with aspirin; commonly used in combination	15–40% of the population will have a reduced response to clopidogrel due to pharmacogenomic variability	Synergistic effect with aspirin; commonly used in combination

Note: cGMP: guanosine 3'5'-cyclic monophosphate

9.5 Anticoagulants

9.5.1 Heparin, low molecular weight heparins and fondaparinux

9.5.1.1 Pharmacodynamics

Heparin comprises a family of mucopolysaccharides naturally present in mast cells. Low molecular weight heparins (LMWH) are fragments of heparin. Fondaparinux is a synthetic analogue of heparin.

While heparin, LMWHs and fondaparinux have no intrinsic anticoagulant activity, they work by binding to and activating antithrombin III, an endogenous anticoagulant, leading to inhibition of clotting Factors IIa (thrombin), Xa and some serine proteases (5, 12, 14, 23). While LMWH activates antithrombin III, it predominately inhibits Factor IIa only (5). Heparin also prevents the activation of fibrin stabilising factor, thus preventing a stable clot forming. Fondaparinux primarily works by activating antithrombin III to target Factor Xa (24).

9.5.1.2 Indications

Heparin, LMWH, and fondaparinux are often used for initial treatment of venous thrombosis and pulmonary embolism because of their rapid onset of action (54). They are also used for prevention of venous thromboembolism during and after surgery, and in acute coronary syndromes such as peripheral arterial occlusion (12).

9.5.1.3 Administration

These drugs are large molecules with poor oral bioavailability, so must be administered parenterally. Heparin is administered as continuous intravenous infusion, usually in a hospital setting with the dose individualised based on the aPTT. LMWH and fondaparinux are administered once or twice daily by subcutaneous injection which can be self-administered by patients from pre-filled syringes. Dose is based on body weight and monitoring of their anticoagulant effect is not usually required (23).

9.5.1.4 Monitoring

Anti-factor Xa and aPTT can be used to monitor and individualise the dose of heparin.

9.5.1.5 Antidote

Protamine sulfate is used to reverse the effects of heparin.

Practice points

- The rapid onset and offset of heparin are useful for patients who require anticoagulation during and after surgery.
- Administration is parenteral, which limits their clinical use.
- LMWHs and fondaparinux have relatively predictable pharmacokinetics with reduced need for monitoring and reduced risk of adverse effects, such as heparin-induced thrombocytopenia (2, 8).
- These drugs are used in the outpatient setting and may be used by patients attending their dentist.

9.5.2 Warfarin

9.5.2.1 Pharmacodynamics

Warfarin works by competitively inhibiting the enzyme vitamin K epoxide reductase component 1 (VKORC1) in the liver. This action inhibits conversion of vitamin K from the oxidised form to the reduced form, thus impairing the hepatic synthesis of vitamin K-dependent clotting Factors II, VII, IX and X (see Figure 9.3). Warfarin also prevents the synthesis of the vitamin K-dependent Protein C and co-factor Protein S, which are involved in the coagulation pathway (5).

Figure 9.3 Mechanism of action of warfarin (5).

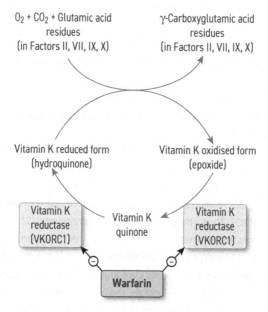

9.5.2.2 Indications

Warfarin is used for atrial fibrillation, prevention of stroke, and prevention and treatment of venous thromboembolism (VTE) in patients with risk factors such as prosthetic heart valves (12).

9.5.2.3 Pharmacokinetics

While peak plasma concentrations of warfarin are achieved within one hour of oral administration, it takes 2–3 days before warfarin-induced depletion of clotting factors in the liver produces a significant reduction in coagulation time (5). This is also dependent on the half-lives of the affected clotting factors, which vary considerably. For example, Factor VII has a half-life of 6 hours, but Factor II has a half-life of 60 hours. Therefore, a single dose of warfarin may not exert clinically useful effects for up to 4–5 days, which accounts for its long duration of action (5).

Warfarin itself also has a long half-life of 20–60 hours (which can vary depending on pharmacogenomic variation in the enzymes: see Practice points below), as well as being highly protein bound (99% to albumin) (12, 20, 25). Dose alterations also take 2–3 days before clinical changes are detected.

9.5.2.4 Doses and monitoring

Doses are individualised and adjusted regularly by measuring the PT, which is then standardised to the International Normalised Ratio (INR).

9.5.2.5 Antidote

Vitamin K (phytomenadione).

Practice points

- Use of warfarin is declining in the community due to preference for the newer DOACs, which act more quickly and more predictably and do not require regular monitoring of anticoagulation.
- Warfarin has a narrow therapeutic index and, due to genetic, drug and dietary interactions, works slightly differently in every person. Therefore, regular monitoring is required by measuring PT, which is standardised to the INR.
- For most indications, such as prevention of VTE or stroke, warfarin is usually prescribed in a dose to reach an INR between 2 and 3.5.
- Warfarin is formulated as a racemic mixture of R- and S-warfarin, and each isomer is metabolised by different enzymes. R-warfarin is a substrate for CYP1A2, CYP3A4, CYP2C19; S-warfarin is a substrate for CYP2C9. Thus, there are many drug interactions (2).
- S-warfarin is four times more potent than R-warfarin. This is important to understanding the stereoselective nature of how drugs interact with the different isomers of warfarin (26).
- Foods, drinks and nutritional supplements containing significant concentrations of vitamin K, including leafy green vegetables, can oppose the effect of warfarin. Patients do not need to avoid these substances completely but consume similar amounts each day so their INR can stabilise.
- Pharmacogenomic variation in the enzymes CYP2C9 and VKORC also affect the clinical response to warfarin and duration of action and offset.

9.5.2.6 Warfarin and the INR

It is well established that there is no need for most patients to cease their warfarin prior to dental procedures, as long as the dentist has ready access to local haemostatic measures including topical tranexamic acid. However, the patient's INR should be checked immediately prior to the procedure (within 24 hours) and protocols generally advise that dentoalveolar procedures conducted with an INR <4 are unlikely to result in significant intra- or postoperative bleeding (27, 28).

However, INR should not be used alone as an assessment of the patient's bleeding risk (29). Other factors should also be considered, including other drugs, underlying medical conditions, and the procedure itself. The INR will only indicate the prolonged bleeding time due to warfarin. An INR does not reflect changes in platelet function, so if the patient is on antiplatelet agents these drugs will also elevate the patient's bleeding risk without increasing the INR (see Chapter 11).

9.5.3 Direct oral anticoagulants

DOACs have many advantages over warfarin, such as more predictable pharmacokinetics, faster onset and offset, less need for regular monitoring and fewer drug interactions. As the DOACs work directly in the blood stream at the site of clot formation, they start working within 12–16 hours of the first dose (14). This rapid onset is also associated with rapid offset, which allows for significant reduction of effect if the drug is temporarily stopped prior to surgery.

The more predictable pharmacokinetics of DOACs confers less interindividual variation in the anticoagulant effect. Because of this, regular monitoring is not required, which is attractive to doctors and patients and enhances adherence. However, DOACs are not without adverse effects, as all are subject to many drug interactions with similar risks of major and minor bleeding. A drawback to the use of DOACs is that only one, dabigatran, currently has a specific antidote (see Table 9.3) although others are in the pipeline. As antidotes are only required prior to major surgery or in overdose, antidote availability is not relevant to dental practice.

9.5.3.1 Dabigatran

Drug class

Direct thrombin inhibitor.

Pharmacodynamics

Dabigatran is a reversible competitive inhibitor of free and fibrin-bound thrombin, as well as thrombin-induced platelet aggregation (14).

Indications

Dabigatran is used for prevention and treatment of VTE after total hip or knee replacement and prevention of stroke in patients with non-valvular atrial fibrillation (2, 12).

Pharmacokinetics

Dabigatran etexilate is the pro-drug presented in the medication, which has no pharmacological activity and poor oral bioavailability (3–7%) so relatively high doses are given to ensure adequate efficacy. After oral administration and absorption, it undergoes transformation in the liver and plasma to dabigatran, which is the active form and confers the anticoagulant effect (14). Dabigatran etexilate is a substrate of p-glycoprotein transporter, so other drugs that are substrates or inhibitors of p-glycoprotein can affect its gastrointestinal absorption and plasma concentrations (14).

Peak dabigatran concentrations and its onset of action occurs within 30 minutes, and with a half-life of 12–14 hours, it produces a more predictable and much faster clinical effect than warfarin. Approximately 80% of a dabigatran dose is renally excreted, so patients with impaired renal function require a lower dose, and dabigatran is contraindicated in patients with severe renal impairment (Cr/Cl <30mL/minute) (14).

Table 9.3 Summary of the pharmacokinetic, pharmacodynamic and pharmacotherapeutic features of anticoagulants commonly seen in dental practice. Based on (2, 12, 14, 31).

	Heparin and low molecular weight heparin	Warfarin	Dabigatran	Apixaban	Rivaroxaban
Commercial names	Heparin: heparin sodium LMWH: Clexane, Fragmin	Coumadin Marevan	Pradaxa	Eliquis	Xarelto
Mechanism of action	Heparin: enhances antithrombin III Low MW heparin: inhibits Factor Xa	Vitamin K antagonist	Direct thrombin inhibitor	Factor Xa inhibitor	Factor Xa inhibitor
Onset of action	Heparin IV: immediate subcutaneous: 20–60 minutes LMWH: 3 hours	36–72 hours	30 minutes	30 minutes	30 minutes
Half-life	Heparin: half-life depends on dose and route LMWH (dalteparin, enoxaparin): 3–6 hours LMWH (danaparoid): 25 hours	20–60 hours	Elderly: 12–14 hours Young adults: 7–9 hours (half-life is prolonged in impaired renal function)	12 hours	Elderly: 11–13 hours Young adults: 5–9 hours
Pro-drug	No	No	Yes	No	No
Oral bioavailability (%)†	–	100	7	50	>80 (when administered with food; bioavailability reduces when fasting)

Metabolism/ transport	–	CYP1A2, CYP3A4, CYP2C19, CYP2C9	P-glycoprotein	P-glycoprotein, CYP3A4, CYP3A5	P-glycoprotein, CYP3A4, CYP3A5
Renal excretion (%)	–	0	80	27	36
Antidote	Protamine sulfate	Vitamin K	Idaricuzumab	Andexanet alfa*	Andexanet alfa*
Practice points	LMWH is more convenient and produces more predictable anticoagulation than heparin; no need for monitoring LMWH	Effect reduced by high intake of dietary vitamin K. Narrow therapeutic index. Pharmacogenomic variability via CYP2C9 and VKORC status. Many drug interactions; penicillin antibiotics can increase the INR	More predictable pharmacokinetics compared with warfarin; no need for regular monitoring. Levels reduce to trough 12–24 hours after cessation	More predictable pharmacokinetics compared with warfarin; no need for regular monitoring. Levels reduce to trough 12–24 hours after cessation	More predictable pharmacokinetics compared with warfarin; no need for regular monitoring. Levels reduce to trough 12–24 hours after cessation

Notes:

† Values in young, healthy individuals.

* Not available in Australia.

LMWH: [low molecular weight heparin]; VKORC: [vitamin K epoxide reductase component]; INR: [international normalised ratio].

Antidote

Idarucizumab is a humanised monoclonal antibody specifically manufactured as the antidote to dabigatran. It can be administered as an IV infusion or bolus IV injection. It binds to dabigatran in the blood stream, reversing the effect of dabigatran within 5 minutes. It is generally used prior to emergency surgery to reduce the risk of major intraoperative bleeding.

9.5.3.2 Apixaban

Drug class

Factor Xa inhibitor.

Pharmacodynamics

Apixaban selectively inhibits Factor Xa, preventing the conversion of prothrombin to thrombin as well as inhibition of prothrombinase, thus preventing thrombus development (7, 14). Factor Xa inhibitors are effective anticoagulants as they prevent the formation of thrombin (rather than blocking the effect of thrombin), and work at the amplification site of the coagulation process (2, 6). As they inhibit both free Factor Xa as well as Factor Xa interacting with platelets, they are called 'direct' oral anticoagulants (6).

Indications

Apixaban is used for prevention and treatment of VTE and prevention of stroke in patients with atrial fibrillation (12).

Pharmacokinetics

After oral absorption (50% bioavailability), peak plasma concentrations are achieved 3–4 hours later but the onset of action begins within 30 minutes (14). Apixaban is a substrate for p-glycoprotein and is metabolised by CYP3A4 and CYP3A5 so is susceptible to many drug interactions.

Renal excretion accounts for the elimination of approximately 27% of apixaban and it is contraindicated in individuals with severe hepatic or renal impairment (CrCl <15mL/ minute) (14). The elimination half-life is approximately 12 hours, allowing for reasonably rapid trough levels to be achieved by the next day of drug cessation if necessary (14).

Antidote

Andexanet alfa is a specific reversal agent that neutralises the anticoagulant effects of Factor Xa inhibitors such as apixaban (30). Although marketed in the US and Europe, at time of writing andexanet is not yet available in Australia.

9.5.3.3 Rivaroxaban

Drug class

Factor Xa inhibitor.

Pharmacodynamics

Factor Xa inhibitors selectively inhibit Factor Xa, preventing the conversion of prothrombin to thrombin in the prothrombinase complex and preventing thrombus development

(7, 14). Factor Xa inhibitors are effective anticoagulants as they prevent the formation of thrombin (rather than blocking the effect of thrombin) and work at the amplification site of the coagulation process (2, 6). Factor Xa inhibitors inhibit both free Factor Xa as well as Factor Xa interacting with platelets in the blood stream so are called 'direct' oral anticoagulants (6).

Indications

Rivaroxaban is used for 'prevention and treatment of VTE, and prevention of stroke in patients with atrial fibrillation' (2, 12).

Pharmacokinetics

After oral absorption (>80% bioavailability), peak rivaroxaban plasma concentrations are achieved 2–4 hours later, but its onset of action starts within 30 minutes (14). Rivaroxaban is a substrate for p-glycoprotein in the gut wall, and around two-thirds undergoes hepatic metabolism by several CYP enzymes (including CYP3A4, CYP2J2 and others); hence, it is subject to many drug interactions (2). Rivaroxaban is contraindicated in individuals with moderate and severe hepatic impairment. Renal excretion accounts for the elimination of the remaining one-third (14). The elimination half-lives are 5–9 hours in young people and 11–13 hours in older people, allowing for reasonably rapid trough levels to be achieved by the next day of drug cessation if necessary (2, 7, 14).

Antidote

Andexanet alfa is a specific reversal agent that neutralises the anticoagulant effects of Factor Xa inhibitors such as rivaroxaban (30). Although available in the US and Europe, at time of writing, andexanet alfa is not yet available in Australia.

9.6 Other medications associated with increased bleeding

9.6.1 Serotonergic antidepressants

9.6.1.1 Pharmacodynamics of bleeding risk

Antidepressants which inhibit serotonin reuptake can impair platelet aggregation by inhibiting the reuptake of serotonin on platelets. Serotonin is a factor involved in platelet aggregation; however, platelets are unable to make their own serotonin so they acquire it from the blood stream. It is thought that serotonergic antidepressants impair clotting function by further depleting platelet serotonin (32).

The main bleeding risk associated with selective serotonin reuptake inhibitors (SSRIs) is gastrointestinal (GI) bleeding. Studies suggest that the estimated risk of GI bleeding is between 1.55 and 3.6 times greater than the risk for matched controls (2, 33–35). Venlafaxine and its active metabolite desvenlafaxine, both of which are selective serotonin and noradrenaline reuptake inhibitors (SNRIs), have also been shown to increase bleeding risk (20, 36, 37).

The combination of an SSRI and NSAID increases the risk of bleeding between 4.25 and 12.2 times (2, 33–35). Since antidepressants cannot be abruptly ceased prior to surgery, their additional bleeding risk should be considered when contemplating use of NSAIDs for postoperative pain management in people taking SSRIs.

9.6.1.2 Indications

Serotonergic antidepressants are used to treat a wide variety of conditions from depression, anxiety, post-traumatic stress disorder, and bulimia nervosa to non-registered indications such as migraine prophylaxis and menopausal hot flushes (12, 38).

Practice points

- SSRIs and SNRIs alone carry a low risk of bleeding when no other drug- or patient-related bleeding risk factors are present (32).
- In combination with other antithrombotics or other patient-related risk factors, SSRIs and SNRIs can significantly increase bleeding risk and should be carefully assessed prior to invasive procedures (39).
- As antidepressants must be ceased gradually over several weeks, they should not be stopped prior to dental procedures, unless there was a very high risk of bleeding with potential catastrophic consequences. Medical advice needs to be sought for these cases.
- Table 9.4 lists all the antidepressants with a relevant serotonin inhibition and their common uses.

Table 9.4 Common uses and brand names of antidepressants that contribute to bleeding risk in dentistry (2). Based on (12, 40).

Generic name	Some commercial names	Drug class	Registered uses
Citalopram	Cipramil Citalo Celapram	Selective serotonin reuptake inhibitor	Major depression
Escitalopram	Lexapro Esipram Escicor	Selective serotonin reuptake inhibitor	Major depression Generalised anxiety disorder Social phobia Obsessive-compulsive disorder
Fluoxetine	Lovan Prozac Auscap Zactin	Selective serotonin reuptake inhibitor	Major depression Obsessive-compulsive disorder Premenstrual dysphoric disorder
Fluvoxamine	Faverin Luvox Movox Voxam	Selective serotonin reuptake inhibitor	Major depression Obsessive-compulsive disorder
Paroxetine	Aropax Extine Paxtine	Selective serotonin reuptake inhibitor	Major depression Obsessive-compulsive disorder Panic disorder Generalised anxiety disorder Post-traumatic stress disorder Social phobia

Table 9.4 (cont.)

Generic name	Some commercial names	Drug class	Registered uses
Sertraline	Sertra Eleva Xydep Zoloft	Selective serotonin reuptake inhibitor	Major depression Obsessive-compulsive disorder Panic disorder Social phobia Premenstrual dysphoric disorder
Venlafaxine	Efexor Efexor-XR	Serotonin and noradrenaline reuptake inhibitor	Major depression Generalised anxiety disorder Panic disorder Social phobia

Antidepressants are rarely ceased prior to surgery due to high risk of withdrawal syndrome. If an antidepressant is no longer clinically necessary and requires cessation, withdrawal should only be conducted under close medical supervision with gradual dose tapering over 2–4 weeks as outlined in *Therapeutic Guidelines Psychotropic* (*Version 7*) (40).

9.6.2 Cytotoxics and other drugs that can cause thrombocytopenia

9.6.2.1 What is thrombocytopenia?

Thrombocytopenia is a reduced platelet count, which is typically defined as a platelet count of $<150 \times 10^9$/L (usual reference range is 150–450 $\times 10^9$/L) (41).

9.6.2.2 How do drugs cause thrombocytopenia?

Drug-induced thrombocytopenia (DITP) is an adverse effect associated with over 300 different drugs (42). Several mechanisms can be responsible for this adverse effect including inhibition of platelet production in the bone marrow and/or increased destruction or elimination from the blood stream via the spleen (43).

Many conventional antineoplastic agents are associated with causing myelosuppression, thereby causing depletion of all blood cell lines. However, some cytotoxic drugs specifically affect megakaryocytopoiesis (the development of megakaryocytes: cells in the bone marrow that develop into platelets), thereby specifically inhibiting platelet production (43).

Several drugs can also cause DITP by destroying circulating platelets through an immunological mechanism by the formation of drug-induced platelet antibodies. Several types of antibodies have been described in this pathogenesis.

9.6.2.3 What are the signs of drug-induced thrombocytopenia?

DITP can be associated with severe bleeding. Signs to be aware of are purpura-type bleeding and mucocutaneous signs (petechiae, ecchymosis, easy bruising) (43).

Severe thrombocytopenia ($<20 \times 10^9$/L) can be associated with major bleeding (43).

DITP usually occurs around 5–10 days after starting the offending drug, but some can induce thrombocytopenia hours after administration (e.g. GP IIa/IIIb inhibitors) (42).

9.6.2.4 What drugs are associated with thrombocytopenia?

Heparin is the drug most commonly associated with thrombocytopenia, but is managed differently as it is also associated with a prothrombotic state.

The drugs typically associated with thrombocytopenia are the conventional cytotoxic drugs, antineoplastic agents and targeted therapies. However, many other drugs, such as quinine, GP IIb/IIIa inhibitors, some cephalosporins, and anticonvulsants are also associated with rarely causing thrombocytopenia (42, 43).

9.6.2.5 Why is this relevant for dental practice?

Dentists need to be aware that many drugs are associated with thrombocytopenia, which means that the patient can be at increased risk of severe bleeding after invasive dentoalveolar procedures. For patients taking drugs associated with thrombocytopenia, their most recent blood test should be assessed prior to invasive dental procedures via portals such as My Health Record or via consultation with a member of the patient's medical or oncology team. If the platelet count is outside the standard range ($<150 \times 10^9$/L), consider delaying procedures until it has improved. Depending on the urgency of the procedure and the patient's co-morbidities, seek medical advice about how to proceed.

9.6.3 Complementary medicines with antithrombotic properties

9.6.3.1 What are complementary medicines?

Complementary medicines (CM) are non-prescription products used with conventional treatments to treat health conditions. Examples of CMs include vitamins, minerals, herbal remedies, aromatherapy and homeopathic products (44). They can also be called 'traditional' medicines if their use is supported by traditional health practices from a particular ethnic culture. Natural health products are called 'alternative medicines' if they are used instead of conventional medicines (44).

9.6.3.2 How prevalent is CM use?

CM are used regularly by approximately two-thirds of the Australian population, with CMs often used to treat chronic unrelenting disease such as rheumatoid arthritis, osteoporosis, osteoarthritis, asthma, cardiovascular disease, diabetes and mental health conditions (45, 46). Pregnancy, menopause and cancer are also popular reasons for CM use (46).

9.6.3.3 What are the difficulties with determining the safety and efficacy of CMs?

Regulation of CMs in Australia is governed to some extent by the Therapeutic Goods Administration (TGA) in terms of registration of products and establishment of manufacturing standards (44). By mandating that all therapeutic products must be listed in the Australian Register of Therapeutic Goods, there is some assurance that products are made by reputable manufacturers and their manufacturing facility has been inspected by the TGA (44). However, CMs in Australia are not required to prove they are effective in order to receive marketing authorisation. In addition, CMs in Australia are not required to be subjected to safety assessment. It is assumed that if the manufacturers states that the products contains only unscheduled (non-prescription) substances, then the products are safe enough for general sale. Health professionals should understand these limitations on the safety and efficacy of CMs and be alert to potential adverse events as they would with any other medicine.

CMs are often obtained online through channels outside Australian regulation. Therefore, these products may be completely unregulated, and the dose, potency and formulation unknown (46).

Most adverse effects of CMs are unreported to the TGA, and products do not usually carry warnings about adverse effects, including bleeding risk (2). In addition, patients do not necessarily advise their dental professional they are taking CMs, as they are often seen as being separate to conventional healthcare (47). However, dentists should document exactly which CMs their patients are taking in case they impact on their oral health or on procedures.

9.6.3.4 Which complementary medicines contribute to bleeding risk?

Table 9.5 shows CMs known to cause a potential increase in bleeding risk, with effects on blood clotting and interactions with antithrombotic medicines (2, 47). It is important to consider that there are other CMs that may also increase bleeding risk that are not listed, and many have not had appropriate studies to determine if they contribute towards bleeding risk.

Table 9.5 Selected complementary medicines with potential to increase bleeding risk (2). Based on (47).

Herbal supplements	Effects on blood clotting	Potential interactions with antithrombotic medications	Time to cease before surgery
Dong quai	Coumarins and ferulic acid have anticoagulant and antiplatelet effects respectively; ferulic acid increases bleeding by inhibiting release of serotonin and ADP	Increased risk of bleeding with warfarin, and also possibly with aspirin and other NSAIDs	All complementary medicines that are not clinically necessary and increase risk of bleeding should be ceased wherever possible prior to surgery. Duration required is 10–14 days to allow time for platelet function to be restored (48)
Evening primrose	Constituents associated with reduction of TXA2, decreased platelet aggregation and increased bleeding time	Increased risk of bleeding with aspirin, warfarin and some NSAIDs	

Table 9.5 (cont.)

Herbal supplements	Effects on blood clotting	Potential interactions with antithrombotic medications	Time to cease before surgery
Fish oil	Associated with reduction of TXA2, decreased platelet aggregation and increased bleeding time (48)	Doses 3g or higher have antiplatelet effect (48)	
Garlic	Certain constituents inhibit platelet aggregation and induce bleeding under different conditions by inhibiting production/release of various mediators including TXA2, ADP, PAF and adenosine	Augments the antithrombotic effects of aspirin, NSAIDs and warfarin	
Ginger	Certain constituents reduce platelet aggregation by inhibiting synthesis of TXA2, with the potential to increase bleeding risk	Increased bleeding reported with warfarin	
Ginkgo	Certain components, particularly ginkgolides, inhibit platelet aggregation and cause bleeding by inhibiting PAF formation	Increased bleeding risk reported with antiplatelet drugs and warfarin	
Ginseng	Some components have antiplatelet effects with the risk of causing increased bleeding via inhibition of TXA2	No reports of interactions with antiplatelet medications; potential interaction with warfarin	
Glucosamine	Glucosamine is associated with inhibition of platelet function by inhibition of the ADP receptor $P2Y_1$	Several case reports associate glucosamine alone with an increased INR with patients who are taking warfarin	
Turmeric	Curcuminoids inhibit platelet aggregation by inhibiting arachidonic acid metabolism and TXA2 synthesis	Curcuminoids can inhibit CYP3A4 which metabolizes all oral anticoagulants to some extent, and may block p-glycoprotein transport. Outcome is increased serum levels of anticoagulants.	

Notes: ADP: adenosine diphosphate; PAF: platelet activating factor.

9.6.3.5 How is the bleeding risk by CMs managed in dentistry?

Dental professionals should always ask patients specifically what CMs they are taking to ensure these are captured in the patient's medication history. The brand name of the product should be specified so that the exact ingredients of the product can be determined and assessed, not just the main or most well-known ingredient.

All CMs that are known to promote bleeding and are not clinically necessary should be ceased prior to dentoalveolar surgical procedures, wherever possible. As platelets take up to two weeks to regenerate, the CMs should be stopped 10–14 days prior to the procedure (2).

9.7 Tranexamic acid

The antifibrinolytic, tranexamic acid (TXA), is a pro-thrombotic agent used to manage bleeding in patients on warfarin. TXA is a synthetic derivative of lysine and works by preventing lysine from binding to plasminogen, thus inhibiting the activation of plasmin by plasminogen. Plasmin breaks down the fibrin polymers in the blood clot; hence, TXA works as an antifibrinolytic (12, 49).

When applied topically for oral surgery, TXA has low systemic absorption. It has been shown to be effective as a local haemostatic measure that does not increase CV events when applied as surgical site irrigation or used as a mouthwash by the patient for up to a week after dental extractions for patients taking vitamin K antagonists (e.g. warfarin) (49, 50). TXA has not been shown to be effective in reducing bleeding in patients on other antithrombotics, including DOACs (4, 49, 50). Australian guidelines recommend TXA to be used at a concentration of 4.8% to be applied topically at the surgical site, followed by use as a mouthwash for 2 days after the extractions as an adjunctive measure for patients taking warfarin (29). Refer to the most recent edition of the *Therapeutic Guidelines Oral and Dental* for the protocol when managing patients taking warfarin (29).

9.8 Assessment of bleeding risk in dental practice

Appropriate assessment of dental patients' bleeding risk relies on a good understanding of why the medications have been prescribed, especially when used for CV disease. Antiplatelet and anticoagulant drugs are generally used to prevent major adverse CV events (i.e. heart attack and stroke) so temporary cessation to reduce bleeding risk can have life-threatening consequences. The risk of bleeding from a dentoalveolar procedure and the ability to manage it with local measures needs to be weighed against the risk of an adverse coronary event if the medications were stopped (2).

In the vast majority of cases, the medications do not need to be stopped and the risk of the patient developing a clot and subsequent coronary event is much higher than the risk of prolonged bleeding. For a simple extraction, several studies show that local haemostatic measures are sufficient to manage the post-extraction bleeding (51–53). However, each case needs to be assessed individually, taking into account all the factors that contribute towards bleeding risk: individual patient factors, the degree of tissue trauma caused by the procedure itself, as well as all the drugs that contribute towards bleeding risk (2). If the dentist is unsure or thinks the medication regimen needs to be altered, consultation needs to be undertaken with the prescribing medical practitioner and adjustment of the patient's medication regimen undertaken with their supervision. Dentists should never undertake alteration of the medication regimen themselves as this can lead to the patient being at risk of an acute coronary event.

9.9 Perioperative bleeding risk management of patients prior to dental procedures

This assessment is based on the patient-, procedure-related risk factors, and all the drugs and any complementary medicines that can contribute to increased bleeding risk. For perioperative management of the risk factors, see Section 11.2.

FURTHER READING

Abebe W. Review of herbal medications with the potential to cause bleeding: dental implications, and risk prediction and prevention avenues. *EPMA J.* 2019;10(1):51–64.

Scottish Dental Clinical Effectiveness Programme. *Management of Dental Patients taking Anticoagulant or Antiplatelet Drugs.* Dental Clinical Guidance; 2015.

Teoh L, Moses G, McCullough MJ. A review of drugs that contribute to bleeding risk in general dental practice. *Aust Dent J.* 2020;65(2):118–130.

Vayne C, Guery EA, Rollin J, Baglo T, Petermann R, Gruel Y. Pathophysiology and Diagnosis of Drug-Induced Immune Thrombocytopenia. *J Clin Med.* 2020;9(7).

REFERENCES

1. Australian Institute of Health and Welfare. *Atrial fibrillation in Australia.* 2022. https://www.aihw.gov.au/reports/heart-stroke-vascular-diseases/atrial-fibrillation-in-australia/contents/how-many-australians-have-atrial-fibrillation

2. Teoh L, Moses G, McCullough MJ. A review of drugs that contribute to bleeding risk in general dental practice. *Aust Dent J.* 2020;65(2):118–130.

3. Bensi C, Belli S, Paradiso D, Lomurno G. Postoperative bleeding risk of direct oral anticoagulants after oral surgery procedures: a systematic review and meta-analysis. *Int J Oral Maxillofac Surg.* 2018;47(7):923–932.

4. Ockerman A, Miclotte I, Vanhaverbeke M et al. Tranexamic acid and bleeding in patients treated with non-vitamin K oral anticoagulants undergoing dental extraction: The EXTRACT-NOAC randomized clinical trial. *PLoS Med.* 2021;18(5):e1003601.

5. Ritter J, Flower R, Henderson G, Loke YK, MacEwan D, Rang H. *Rang and Dale's Pharmacology.* 9th edition. Elsevier; 2020.

6. Thean D, Alberghini M. Anticoagulant therapy and its impact on dental patients: a review. *Aust Dent J.* 2016;61(2):149–156.

7. Fortier K, Shroff D, Reebye UN. Review: An overview and analysis of novel oral anticoagulants and their dental implications. *Gerodontology.* 2018;35(2):78–86.

8. Toschi V, Lettino M. Inhibitors of propagation of coagulation: factors V and X. *Br J Clin Pharmacol.* 2011;72(4):563–580.

9. Esmon CT, Vigano-D'Angelo S, D'Angelo A, Comp PC. Anticoagulation proteins C and S. *Adv Exp Med Biol.* 1987;214:47–54.

10. Wallentin L. P2Y(12) inhibitors: differences in properties and mechanisms of action and potential consequences for clinical use. *Eur Heart J.* 2009;30(16):1964–1977.

11. Castellino FJ. Plasmin. *Handbook of Proteolytic Enzymes*. ScienceDirect; 2013. https://www
    .sciencedirect.com/topics/immunology-and-microbiology/plasmin

12. Editorial Advisory Committee. *Australian Medicines Handbook*. AMH Pty Ltd; 2022.

13. Awtry EH, Loscalzo J. Aspirin. *Circulation*. 2000;101(10):1206–1218.

14. eMIMS. 2021. www.emims.com.au [Subscription only]

15. McNeil JJ, Nelson MR, Woods RL et al. Effect of Aspirin on All-Cause Mortality in the
    Healthy Elderly. *N Engl J Med*. 2018;379(16):1519–1528.

16. McNeil JJ, Wolfe R, Woods RL et al. Effect of Aspirin on Cardiovascular Events and
    Bleeding in the Healthy Elderly. *N Engl J Med*. 2018;379(16):1509–1518.

17. McNeil JJ, Woods RL, Nelson MR et al. Effect of Aspirin on Disability-free Survival in the
    Healthy Elderly. *N Engl J Med*. 2018;379(16):1499–1508.

18. Kelley BP, Bennett KG, Chung KC, Kozlow JH. Ibuprofen May Not Increase Bleeding
    Risk in Plastic Surgery: A Systematic Review and Meta-Analysis. *Plast Reconstr Surg*.
    2016;137(4):1309–1316.

19. Pototski M, Amenabar JM. Dental management of patients receiving anticoagulation or
    antiplatelet treatment. *J Oral Sci*. 2007;49(4):253–258.

20. AusDI. *Independent Drug Monographs*. 2021. https://ausdi.hcn.com.au/browseDocuments
    .hcn?filter=PRODUCTS_WITH_MONGRAPH

21. Wallentin L, Becker RC, Budaj A et al. Ticagrelor versus clopidogrel in patients with acute
    coronary syndromes. *N Engl J Med*. 2009;361(11):1045–1057.

22. Rocca B, Petrucci G. Variability in the responsiveness to low-dose aspirin: pharmacological
    and disease-related mechanisms. *Thrombosis*. 2012;2012:376721. doi:10.1155/2012/376721

23. Brunton L, Knollman BC, Chabner B. *Goodman & Gilman's The Pharmacological Basis of
    Therapeutics*. 12th edition. McGraw Hill Medical; 2011.

24. Zhang Y, Zhang M, Tan L, Pan N, Zhang L. The clinical use of Fondaparinux: A synthetic
    heparin pentasaccharide. *Prog Mol Biol Transl Sci*. 2019;163:41–53.

25. Salam S, Yusuf H, Milosevic A. Bleeding after dental extractions in patients taking warfarin.
    Br J Oral Maxillofac Surg. 2007;45(6):463–466.

26. Katzung BG, Trevor AJ. *Basic and Clinical Pharmacology*. 15th edition. McGraw Hill; 2020.

27. Carter G, Goss AN, Lloyd J, Tocchetti R. Current concepts of the management of dental
    extractions for patients taking warfarin. *Aust Dent J*. 2003;48(2):89–96; quiz 138.

28. Lu SY, Lin LH, Hsue SS. Management of dental extractions in patients on warfarin and
    antiplatelet therapy. *J Formos Med Assoc*. 2018;117(11):979–986.

29. Oral and Dental Expert Group. *Therapeutic Guidelines Oral and Dental* (*Version 3*).
    Therapeutic Guidelines Ltd; 2019.

30. Carpenter E, Singh D, Dietrich E, Gums J. Andexanet alfa for reversal of factor Xa inhibitor-
    associated anticoagulation. *Ther Adv Drug Saf*. 2019;10:2042098619888133.

31. Chin P. Long-term prescribing of new oral anticoagulants. *Aust Prescr*. 2016;39(6):200–204.

32. Napenas JJ, Hong CH, Kempter E et al. Selective serotonin reuptake inhibitors and oral
    bleeding complications after invasive dental treatment. *Oral Surg Oral Med Oral Pathol Oral
    Radiol Endod*. 2011;112(4):463–467.

33. Dalton SO, Johansen C, Mellemkjaer L et al. Use of selective serotonin reuptake inhibitors
    and risk of upper gastrointestinal tract bleeding: a population-based cohort study. *Arch
    Intern Med*. 2003;163(1):59–64.

34. Jiang HY, Chen HZ, Hu XJ et al. Use of selective serotonin reuptake inhibitors and risk of
    upper gastrointestinal bleeding: a systematic review and meta-analysis. *Clin Gastroenterol
    Hepatol*. 2015;13(1):42–50 e3.

35. Weinrieb RM, Auriacombe M, Lynch KG, Lewis JD. Selective serotonin re-uptake inhibitors
    and the risk of bleeding. *Expert Opin Drug Saf*. 2005;4(2):337–344.

36. Sarma A, Horne MK. Venlafaxine-induced ecchymoses and impaired platelet aggregation. *Eur J Haematol.* 2006;77(6):533–537.

37. de Abajo FJ, Rodriguez LA, Montero D. Association between selective serotonin reuptake inhibitors and upper gastrointestinal bleeding: population based case-control study. *BMJ.* 1999;319(7217):1106–1109.

38. Skanland SS, Cieslar-Pobuda A. Off-label uses of drugs for depression. *Eur J Pharmacol.* 2019;865:172732.

39. Scottish Dental Clinical Effectiveness Program. *Management of Dental Patients taking Anticoagulant or Antiplatelet Drugs.* Dental Clinical Guidance; 2015.

40. Psychotropic Expert Group. *Therapeutic Guidelines Psychotropic (Version 7).* Therapeutic Guidelines Pty Ltd; 2013.

41. Nagrebetsky A, Al-Samkari H, Davis NM et al. Perioperative thrombocytopenia: evidence, evaluation, and emerging therapies. *Br J Anaesth.* 2019;122(1):19–31.

42. Bakchoul T, Marini I. Drug-associated thrombocytopenia. *Hematology Am Soc Hematol Educ Program.* 2018;2018(1):576–583.

43. Vayne C, Guery EA, Rollin J, Baglo T, Petermann R, Gruel Y. Pathophysiology and Diagnosis of Drug-Induced Immune Thrombocytopenia. *J Clin Med.* 2020;9(7).

44. Therapeutic Goods Administration Department of Health. *Complementary Medicines.* 2020. https://www.tga.gov.au/complementary-medicines

45. von Conrady DM, Bonney A. Patterns of complementary and alternative medicine use and health literacy in general practice patients in urban and regional Australia. *Aust Fam Physician.* 2017;46(5):316–320.

46. Reid R, Steel A, Wardle J, Trubody A, Adams J. Complementary medicine use by the Australian population: a critical mixed studies systematic review of utilisation, perceptions and factors associated with use. *BMC Complement Altern Med.* 2016;16:176.

47. Abebe W. Review of herbal medications with the potential to cause bleeding: dental implications, and risk prediction and prevention avenues. *EPMA J.* 2019;10(1):51–64.

48. NatMed. *NatMed Pro.* 2023. https://naturalmedicines.therapeuticresearch.com/

49. de Vasconcellos SJ, de Santana Santos T, Reinheimer DM et al. Topical application of tranexamic acid in anticoagulated patients undergoing minor oral surgery: A systematic review and meta-analysis of randomized clinical trials. *J Craniomaxillofac Surg.* 2017;45(1):20–26.

50. Engelen ET, Schutgens RE, Mauser-Bunschoten EP et al. Antifibrinolytic therapy for preventing oral bleeding in people on anticoagulants undergoing minor oral surgery or dental extractions. *Cochrane Database Syst Rev.* 2018;7:CD012293.

51. Lanau N, Mareque J, Giner L, Zabalza M. Direct oral anticoagulants and its implications in dentistry. A review of literature. *J Clin Exp Dent.* 2017;9(11):e1346–e1354.

52. Doganay O, Atalay B, Karadag E et al. Bleeding frequency of patients taking ticagrelor, aspirin, clopidogrel, and dual antiplatelet therapy after tooth extraction and minor oral surgery. *Journal of the American Dental Association* (1939). 2018;149(2):132–138.

53. Olmos-Carrasco O, Pastor-Ramos V, Espinilla-Blanco R et al. Hemorrhagic complications of dental extractions in 181 patients undergoing double antiplatelet therapy. *J Oral Maxillofac Surg.* 2015;73(2):203–210.

54. Weitz JI. Blood Coagulation and Anticoagulant, Fibrinolytic, and Antiplatelet Drugs. In Brunton L, Chabner BA, Knollmann BC (eds). *Goodman & Gilman's: The Pharmacological Basis of Therapeutics.* 12th edition. McGraw Hill; 2021.

DRUGS ASSOCIATED WITH MEDICATION-RELATED OSTEONECROSIS OF THE JAW

10

KEY POINTS

- Medication-related osteonecrosis of the jaw (MRONJ) is a debilitating condition, characterised by non-healing bone, pain and morbidity occurring mostly in patients taking medications affecting bone turnover following a dental extraction.
- Risk of MRONJ depends on patient-, medication-, dental- and procedure-related risk factors.
- The degree of risk conferred by medications increases with their dose and duration of use, combined with non-pharmacological risk factors.
- Although bisphosphonates and RANKL inhibitors such as denosumab are most well known for predisposing to osteonecrosis of the jaw (ONJ), many other drugs also carry this risk.
- The most common dental trigger of MRONJ is tooth extraction, although ill-fitting dentures, implant placement and periodontal surgery have also been implicated.
- The presence of infection and inflammation, including periapical abscess and periodontitis, also increases risk of MRONJ.

10.1 Introduction

Medication-related osteonecrosis of the jaw (MRONJ) is a debilitating condition, characterised by non-healing bone, with subsequent chronic infection, pain and morbidity. While osteonecrosis of the jaw can occur spontaneously in healthy patients, it most commonly occurs in patients taking medications that affect bone turnover and is precipitated by an invasive procedure such as a dental extraction.

Medications that increase MRONJ risk are commonly used in the Australian population, therefore awareness of their association with MRONJ is critical in dental practice.

In 2015, approximately 470,000 Australians were dispensed a medication for osteoporosis on the PBS (1). Other bone diseases that require medical treatments include Paget's disease and cancers that metastasise to bone such as multiple myeloma, breast, and prostate cancer. Corticosteroids contribute to MRONJ risk and are frequently used in the Australian population for acute and chronic disease. Anti-angiogenic drugs are increasingly in use not just for treatment of malignancy, but also post-transplant and for autoimmune disease.

10.2 Definition

MRONJ is diagnosed when all three of the following criteria are met as stated in the 2022 American Association of Oral and Maxillofacial Surgeons' (AAOMS) *Position Paper on MRONJ* (2):

1. Current or previous treatment with antiresorptive or antiangiogenic agents.
2. Exposed bone or bone that can be probed through an intraoral or extraoral fistula in the maxillofacial region that has persisted for longer than 8 weeks.
3. No history of radiation therapy to the jaws or obvious metastatic disease to the jaws (2).

10.3 Pathophysiology

The pathophysiology of MRONJ has been widely studied but is still uncertain. Current thought is centred around five main mechanisms: inhibition of bone remodelling and turnover; increased infection and inflammation; reduced innate or acquired immune response; suppression of soft tissue healing; and inhibition of angiogenesis (2–5).

10.4 Incidence of MRONJ

The incidence of MRONJ has only been closely studied in patients on antiresorptive agents. In these populations, MRONJ frequency varies directly with the drug dose and the setting in which it is used. The latter is most relevant because the indication determines the dose and, due to their possible exposure to chemotherapy and radiation, cancer patients are likely to have been exposed to more osteonecrosis of the jaw (ONJ) risk factors than just antiresorptive drugs. See Table 10.1.

Table 10.1 Incidence of MRONJ. Based on (4).

Indication for use	Incidence		
	Oral BPs	IV BPs	Denosumab (subcut.)
Osteoporosis (low dose, few ONJ risk factors)	1.04-69/100,000 patient-years	Up to 90/100,000 patient-years	Up to 30 per 100,000 patient-years
Oncology (high dose, multiple ONJ risk factors)	–	Up to 12,222/100,000 patient-years	Up to 2,316/100,000 patient-years

In patients on bisphosphonates (BPs) or denosumab for osteoporosis, the frequency of MRONJ is estimated to range between 0.001–0.01%, and in patients on higher doses in the setting of cancer treatment, MRONJ frequency is much higher at 1–15% (3).

10.5 Patient risk factors

In general, people with multiple co-morbidities and polypharmacy are at increased risk of MRONJ (6, 7). Specific co-morbidities that predispose to ONJ risk are those associated with impairing wound healing, including autoimmune disease, diabetes mellitus, cardiovascular (CV) disease, chronic kidney disease and tobacco use (3, 6).

Certain genetic factors have been associated with MRONJ, predisposing some to increased risk. These include genes involved in collagen formation, bone turnover or angiogenesis (such as drug and bone metabolism single nucleotide polymorphisms) genes involved with VEFG polymorphisms, or polymorphisms with farnesyl diphosphate synthase (which is the enzyme targeted by BPs) (2, 6, 8). Collectively, these suggest there may be genetic predisposition to increased ONJ risk (2, 8).

Cancer and chemotherapy place patients at risk if antiresorptive and anti-angiogenic drugs are used. Antiresorptives are used in higher doses and of more frequent administration for bone cancers or skeletal metastases compared to osteoporosis. The most common cancers associated with MRONJ are multiple myeloma, breast cancer, prostate cancer and renal cancer because these malignancies have a greater tendency to metastasise to bone (6).

10.6 Medications associated with MRONJ

The first peer-reviewed publication associating medications with MRONJ was by Marx in 2003 that described ONJ cases occurring in association with BPs (9). Since 2003, an increasing number of drugs have been associated with MRONJ, mostly BPs and denosumab, but also many other drugs that affect angiogenesis or bone turnover. While the literature is still scant and risk is considered low, these other agents include TNF-α inhibitors, methotrexate, corticosteroids and drugs that affect angiogenesis (2, 5, 8). See Table 10.2 for medications associated with osteonecrosis of the jaw.

10.6.1 Common medication doses

MRONJ is dependent on dose and duration. Table 10.3 shows the various doses used for different conditions in clinical practice (11).

10.6.2 Bisphosphonates

Clinical uses of BPs include osteoporosis, Paget's disease, prevention and treatment of cancer metastases in bone, and hypercalcaemia of malignancy (12). Doses and regimens vary widely, depending on the medical condition being treated.

10.6.2.1 Chemistry

Bisphosphonates are structurally similar to inorganic pyrophosphate, which is a naturally occurring compound in bone (12). *Bis* refers to 'two' in Latin, as BPs are comprised of two phosphonate groups linked by an ester bond, with the substitutions at the R1 and R2 groups (see Figure 10.1). It was determined in the 1960s that pyrophosphate could bind to hydroxyapatite crystals in bone matrix and, as such, BPs were developed and similarly have a high affinity for hydroxyapatite crystals in bone (12).

Table 10.2 Medications associated with osteonecrosis of the jaw. Based on (10).

Drug class	Medication	Common brand names	Common indications	Route of administration
Bisphosphonates	Alendronate	Fonat Fosamax	Osteoporosis Paget's disease	Oral
	Ibandronic acid	Bondronat	Bone metastases Hypercalcaemia of malignancy Osteoporosis	Oral
	Pamidronate	Pamisol	Bone metastases Paget's disease Hypercalcaemia of malignancy	IV
	Risedronate	Actonel	Osteoporosis Paget's disease	Oral
	Zoledronic acid	Aclasta Osteovan Zometa	Osteoporosis Paget's disease Bone metastases Hypercalcaemia of malignancy	IV
RANKL inhibitor	Denosumab	Prolia (60mg) Xgeva (120mg)	Osteoporosis Bone tumours Bone metastases Hypercalcaemia of malignancy	SC
Antiangiogenic drugs				
VEGF inhibitor	Bevacizumab	Mvasi	Various cancers (e.g. colorectal, breast, renal cell, cervical)	Infusion
Tyrosine kinase inhibitors	Sorafenib	Nexavar	Various cancers (e.g. hepatocellular, renal cell, thyroid)	Oral
	Sunitinib	Sutent	Various cancers (e.g. renal cell, GI stromal tumour)	Oral
mTOR inhibitors	Sirolimus	Rapamune	Prevention of kidney transplant rejection	Oral
	Everolimus	Afinitor	Prevention of transplant rejection Breast and renal cancer	Oral

Other medications

			Route
TNF-α inhibitors	Adalimumab	Amgevita Hadlima Humira Hyrimoz Idacio	Autoimmune conditions (e.g. rheumatoid arthritis, psoriatic arthritis, ankylosing spondylitis)	SC
Corticosteroids	Betamethasone	Celestone	Wide range of conditions for immunosuppressant, anti-inflammatory and anti-emetic properties	Intra-articular Intra-dermal
	Dexamethasone	Dexmethasone		Intra-articular IM IV Oral
	Methylprednisolone	Depo-Medrol Depo-Nisolone Solu-Medrol		Intra-articular IM IV
	Prednisone/ Prednisolone	Prednisone: Panafcort Predsone Sone Prednisolone: Panafcortelone Predsolone Solone		Oral
Folic acid antagonist	Methotrexate	Methoblastin	High doses for various cancers (e.g. breast, SCC of the head/neck, lymphomas) Lower doses for autoimmune conditions (e.g. rheumatoid arthritis, psoriasis)	IM IV Oral SC
Sclerostin inhibitor	Romosozumab	Evenity	Osteoporosis	SC

Notes: IV: intravenous; IM: intramuscularly; SC: subcutaneously; VEGF: vascular endothelial growth factor.

Table 10.3 Common doses of bisphosphonates and denosumab used in clinical practice [11].

| Agent | Low dose | | | | | | High dose | |
| | Osteoporosis | | | Paget's disease of bone | Cancer treatment-induced bone loss | Tumour-induced hypercalcemia | Prevention of SREs in patients with bone malignancies | Giant cell tumour of bone |
	Post-menopausal women	Men	Glucocorticoid-induced					
Alendronate	70mg PO once weekly or 10mg PO once daily	10mg PO once daily	10mg PO once daily					
Ibandronic acid	150mg PO once monthly or 3mg IV once every 3 months					Single dose of 4mg IV (severe) or 2mg IV (moderate)	6mg IV once every 3–4 weeks or 50mg PO daily in patients with breast cancer	
Pamidronate				180–210mg in either 3- or 6-unit doses		15–90 mg (depending on plasma calcium level) as a single dose or over 2–4 infusions	90mg every 4 weeks	
Risedronate	5mg PO once daily or 35mg PO once weekly	35mg PO once weekly	5mg PO once daily	30mg PO once daily for 2 months				
Zoledronic acid	5mg IV once yearly	5mg IV once yearly	5mg IV once yearly	Single dose of 5mg IV		Single dose of 4mg IV	4mg IV once every 3–4 weeks	
Denosumab	60mg SC once every 6 months	60mg SC once every 6 months			60mg SC once every 6 months		120mg SC once every 4 weeks	120mg SC once every 4 weeks plus additional 120mg SC doses on days 8 and 15 during the first month

Notes: IV: intravenous; PO: per orally; SC: subcutaneous; SRE: skeletal-related event.

Figure 10.1 Differences in mechanisms of action between bisphosphonates and denosumab (22).

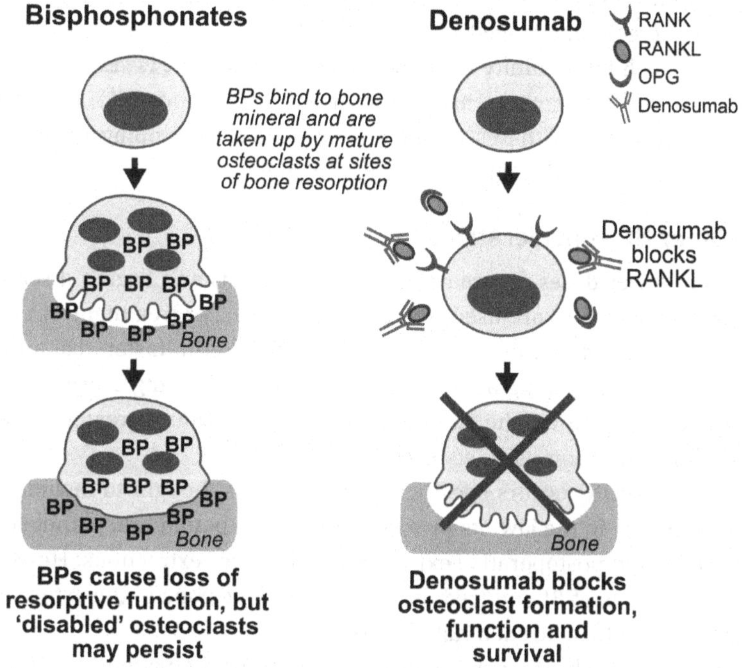

Bisphosphonates

BPs bind to bone mineral and are taken up by mature osteoclasts at sites of bone resorption

BPs cause loss of resorptive function, but 'disabled' osteoclasts may persist

Denosumab

RANK
RANKL
OPG
Denosumab

Denosumab blocks RANKL

Denosumab blocks osteoclast formation, function and survival

10.6.2.2 Pharmacodynamics

BPs preferentially bind to hydroxyapatite in areas of active bone remodelling, particularly at the 'calcification front' in osteoid (12, 13). During bone resorption, BPs are taken up into osteoclasts by the process of endocytosis (13). Intracellularly, they bind to farnesyl pyrophosphate synthase, an enzyme involved in the production of cholesterol and other sterols. This leads to inhibition of osteoclast cellular activities, resulting in osteoclast apoptosis, loss of function and inhibition of bone resorption (10, 12). Recently, BPs have been shown to prevent osteoblast and osteocyte apoptosis, thereby preserving the anabolic actions of osteoblasts to lay down bone matrix (14).

The exact pathophysiology of association with MRONJ is unknown, with proposed theories including altered bone remodelling, inhibition of osteoclast differentiation and inhibition of angiogenesis (2).

10.6.2.3 Pharmacokinetics

Oral BPs have low bioavailability and a very acidic pH. Their absorption is further reduced in the presence of food—in particular, magnesium- or calcium-containing foods, drinks or supplements (12). As a result, orally administered BPs must be taken on an empty stomach, at least 30 minutes prior to any food or drink. Patients must also remain upright after BP ingestion, to ensure the medication does not burn the oesophageal wall causing erosions or ulceration. BP use also frequently causes gastritis and duodenitis (10). Some

BPs are so acidic they cannot be administered orally, such as pamidronate and zoledronic acid, so are administered intravenously. The fraction of drug that is not absorbed into bone is renally excreted unchanged.

As BPs have such high affinity for bone, their bone half-life is very long (months to years); alendronate, for example, has a 10-year half-life in bone (15). This is the main reason why drug holidays with BPs are not recommended, as skipping a few days' dosing will make no difference to the concentration of BP in bone.

10.6.2.4 Other BP considerations

BPs are used in lower doses for treatment of osteoporosis and Paget's disease. Higher doses and more potent BPs are used in the context of cancer treatment. An example is the use of zoledronic acid for osteoporosis: it is generally administered at an IV dose of 5mg once a year; for managing bone metastases, a dose of 3–4mg every 3 to 4 weeks is usually employed (10). Thus, the risk of MRONJ is significantly greater in patients on higher doses for cancer compared to osteoporosis.

Reasons why MRONJ occurs specifically in the jaw is thought to include increased rate of bone turnover in the jaw, its proximity to surface bound oral pathogens, vulnerability to trauma, and postoperative exposure of bone after extractions. However, there have also been reports of BP-induced osteonecrosis of the bone in the external auditory canal, which is not subject to such risk factors (16, 17).

Due to their long half-life in bone, even BPs used in the patient's distant past can contribute to the patient's current MRONJ risk. In addition, the longer the treatment duration (current or past treatment), the higher the risk. Use for four years or more most significantly increases the patient's risk of MRONJ (18).

10.6.3 Denosumab

Clinical uses of denosumab include post-menopausal osteoporosis, increasing bone mineral density in men with prostate cancer or osteoporosis, bone tumours, prevention of skeletal complications due to bone metastases, and hypercalcaemia of malignancy.

The Phase III FREEDOM trial demonstrated that denosumab was effective in increasing bone mineral density and prevented the risk of hip, vertebral and non-vertebral fractures (19). An extension of the FREEDOM trial demonstrated a sustained reduction in bone mineral density and reduced fracture risk (20).

A systematic review and meta-analysis have shown that denosumab is associated with MRONJ (21). Longer treatment durations and increased dosages of denosumab are correlated with increased risk of MRONJ (2, 8). The doses of denosumab for osteoporosis are 60mg every 6 months; for bone cancers, up to 120mg every 4 weeks (10). Thus, patients using denosumab for cancers, coupled with the effect of the medical condition itself and associated immune compromise, are at much higher risk of MRONJ.

10.6.3.1 Pharmacodynamics

Denosumab is a fully humanised monoclonal antibody that blocks the receptor activator of nuclear factor kappa B ligand (RANKL), which is responsible for differentiation and activation of osteoclasts (19). By binding to the RANK receptor on both the precursor and mature osteoclasts, the ligand promotes formation, activity and survival of osteoclasts (15).

By binding to RANKL, denosumab prevents RANKL from binding to and activating its RANK receptor on the osteoclast. Thus, denosumab inhibits osteoclast function, survival and formation, resulting in decreased bone resorption and increased bone density and strength (22). Denosumab works at an earlier step of osteoclast activation than BPs, as it works on the immature osteoclast away from the bone surface (15). In contrast, BPs work by being taken up into the mature osteoclast in cortical bone at sites of bone remodelling (see Figure 10.1).

10.6.3.2 Pharmacokinetics

Unlike BPs, denosumab is comparatively short acting, primarily circulating in extracellular fluid and blood stream and does not take up residence in bone. With a half-life of 26 days (on average; ranging between 6–52 days) (15), systemic exposure to denosumab reaches trough levels after approximately 6 months.

10.6.3.3 Delay or suspension of denosumab treatment for dental procedures

After several treatment doses, cessation of denosumab has been shown to lead to rapid reversal of its therapeutic effect, increase in vertebral fractures, and loss of bone mineral density (23, 24). This occurs progressively, but bone density can deteriorate to baseline measures, and in some cases the bone loss can be greater than the gain achieved while on denosumab therapy (23). This rebound increase in fracture risk is only significant for those who have had more than one dose, as it takes several weeks to reach a significant impact and peaks around 16 weeks after stopping denosumab (24). As discontinuation of denosumab therapy is sometimes clinically necessary, some recommendations include substitution of BPs to transition patients off denosumab and to reduce fracture risk (23, 25). However, due to the increased risk of fractures and negligible benefit to healing and ONJ risk, discontinuation of denosumab is not recommended in dentistry prior to extractions or other invasive procedures.

10.6.4 Other medications associated with MRONJ

10.6.4.1 Anti-angiogenic medicines

Drugs with anti-angiogenic properties are associated with MRONJ, as documented in the 2022 Position Paper from the American Association of Oral and Maxillofacial Surgeons (AAOMS) (2). These drugs include: the antivascular endothelial growth factor monoclonal antibody, bevacizumab; the vascular endothelial growth factor (VEGF) receptor tyrosine kinase inhibitors, sorafenib and sunitinib; as well as the mammalian target of rapamycin inhibitors, everolimus and sirolimus (61). While the use of anti-angiogenic drugs increases a patient's risk of MRONJ in combination with antiresorptives (26), they also are an independent risk factor with many case reports occurring in antiresorptive-naive patients (11, 26, 27). These drugs are mainly used in oncology to target tumour-related angiogenesis. They are currently used for cancers such as breast cancer, colorectal cancer, non-small-cell lung cancer and renal cell cancer (10, 26).

When tumours are small, they are limited in their growth as they can only obtain nutrients and oxygen by diffusion. The tumours then develop collateral blood vessels by the process of angiogenesis in order to obtain nutrients from the blood stream. In this process, pro-angiogenic factors, such VEGF, are released and stimulate endothelial cell development and activity and consequent increased vascularisation of the tumour, enabling growth (28). VEGFs are a family of major angiogenic growth factors that bind to specific tyrosine kinase receptors causing endothelial cells to proliferate, migrate and increase vascular permeability in both normal and pathological conditions (29, 30).

These anti-angiogenic drugs can disrupt the angiogenesis-signalling process and formation of new blood vessels by either directly targeting VEGF (e.g. bevacizumab) or blocking the VEGF receptors downstream by action of the tyrosine kinase inhibitors (e.g. sunitinib, sorafenib) (26). Bevacizumab can also be given by intra-ocular injection to treat age-related macular degeneration. However, there is no current evidence that the risk of MRONJ is increased when it is administered by this route.

The mammalian target of rapamycin (mTOR) inhibitors, such as everolimus and sirolimus, target the production of VEGF and platelet-derived growth factors thereby inhibiting the process of angiogenesis (26). Everolimus has had several case reports implicating it with MRONJ, both alone and in combination with immunosuppressants and antiresorptives (5, 31–34). Other tyrosine kinase inhibitors, including lenvatinib and cabozantinib, have also been reported to be associated with MRONJ, without a concomitant antiresorptive drug (35, 36). It is postulated that the inhibition of angiogenesis after procedures such as extractions may be the pathophysiological process contributing to MRONJ development (2).

10.6.4.2 Adalimumab

Adalimumab, an inhibitor of the cytokine tumour necrosis factor (TNF) α, is a potent anti-inflammatory drug used to treat many different autoimmune diseases such as psoriasis, rheumatoid arthritis and ankylosing spondylitis (10). Adalimumab has been associated with several published case reports of MRONJ (5, 37, 38). This drug may be implicated because TNF-α can cause osteoclast-mediated bone damage in joints by inducing the differentiation of osteoclasts, as well as stimulating RANKL production and increasing osteoclast proliferation (39). TNF-α inhibitors have been reported to positively affect systemic bone loss in patients with rheumatoid arthritis when assessed using bone mineral density (39). It is thought that TNF-α inhibitors could affect bone turnover by a reduction of RANKL or inducing apoptosis of monocytes leading to an impaired immune response after jaw necrosis (37).

10.6.4.3 Corticosteroids

Corticosteroids are steroid hormones produced and released by the adrenal cortex that have both glucocorticoid and mineralocorticoid effects. The term 'corticosteroids' is generally used to refer to glucocorticoids, which include hydrocortisone, dexamethasone, methylprednisolone, prednisone and prednisolone. These drugs have a wide range of pharmacological actions and adverse effects on every part of the body, varying in impact with dose and duration of use. Long-term use can be particularly problematic with some adverse effects shown in Table 10.4.

Table 10.4 Long-term adverse effects of glucocorticoids. Adapted from (40).

Body system	Adverse effects
Musculoskeletal	Osteoporosis, avascular necrosis of the bone
Endocrine	Hyperlipidaemia, diabetes mellitus, dyslipidaemia, growth suppression, adrenal suppression
Gastrointestinal	Gastritis, peptic ulcer, gastrointestinal bleeding, pancreatitis
Cardiovascular	Hypertension, coronary heart disease
Dermatologic	Skin atrophy, ecchymosis, delayed wound healing, purpura, hair loss, hirsutism
Psychiatric	Mood changes, depression, euphoria, cognitive impairment, delirium, anxiety
Ophthamologic	Cataract, glaucoma, ptosis, myadriasis
Immunologic	Increased infection risk, immune system suppression

Corticosteroids have been shown to be associated with the development of MRONJ, as documented in the 2022 AAOMS position paper and the 2015 paper from the International Taskforce on ONJ (2, 3). In a 2018 systematic review of MRONJ risk factors, use of corticosteroids was among the most frequently reported contributors (6). A retrospective cohort study found patients taking corticosteroids, immunosuppressants and biological agents had an association with delayed wound healing and ONJ (5, 41).

The association between corticosteroid use and MRONJ is thought to be due to their well-documented adverse effects on bone, skin structure, blood vessel integrity and wound healing (5). Corticosteroids inhibit bone formation by decreasing osteoblast proliferation differentiation and activity (42, 43), as well as affecting various osteoblast genes, including those for type I collagen in bone and osteocalcin, resulting in reduced osteoblast numbers and bone formation (43). Increased risk of infection due to immunosuppression and elevated blood sugar levels from corticosteroids may also contribute to MRONJ risk.

While systemic corticosteroids have been associated with increased risk of MRONJ, immune compromise is not the main mechanism for this since haematological evidence of reduced white cell count has demonstrated no increased risk of MRONJ (5, 7). Chronic use of systemic corticosteroids is more likely to contribute to MRONJ risk by impairing and delaying wound healing via fibroblast dysfunction, reduced collagen synthesis, decreased angiogenesis, impaired re-epithelialization, as well as increased risk of infection (44).

10.6.4.4 Methotrexate

Methotrexate is a folic acid antagonist and several case reports have suggested an association between methotrexate use and MRONJ, including one case on the TGA's Database of Adverse Event Notifications where it was the sole suspected medicine (5, 45–47). Methotrexate is a folic acid antagonist and inhibits DNA synthesis and cell replication and in higher doses is used for neoplastic conditions. It also has immunomodulatory effects causing a reduction in inflammation and is used in low doses to treat autimmune conditions such as rheumatoid arthritis (10).

Methotrexate is thought to increase MRONJ risk via its potential to inhibit osteoclast formation, suppress bone marrow function, and reduce white blood cell synthesis resulting in immunosuppression (48). Methotrexate also affects bone healing by inhibiting the proliferation of osteoblasts. There are several possible ways it may increase a person's MRONJ risk (49).

10.6.4.5 Leflunomide

Leflunomide is a pro-drug which requires metabolism to its active metabolite, teriflunomide, to exert anti-inflammatory, immunosuppressive, immunomodulating and antiproliferative effects. Its mechanism of action is via inhibition of dihydro-orotate dehydrogenase which impairs pyrimidine synthesis in leucocytes and other rapidly dividing cells involved in inflammation. Leflunomide's mechanism is similar to methotrexate, except that it works on the pyrimidine synthesis pathway as opposed to purine synthesis. For this reason, leflunomide is often used in clinical practice to replace methotrexate if the latter is not tolerated or is inadequately effective. Sometimes the two drugs are used together; however, this can result in profound immunosuppression (10, 50).

To date there have only been a few published case reports of leflunomide-associated MRONJ, several where it is used with other predisposing drugs, and there are two cases of suspected MRONJ on the TGA's Database of Adverse Event Notifications (5). However, it is possible that more cases have simply not been published or reported due to a lack of awareness of leflunomide's potential to contribute to MRONJ risk. Given the similarity of leflunomide to methotrexate, it would be wise to consider it as a risk factor for MRONJ, especially when used in the context of other already recognised predisposing factors (51).

10.6.4.6 Romosozumab

Romosozumab is a monoclonal antibody marketed for treatment of post-menopausal osteoporosis and osteoporosis in men with a high fracture risk (10). Romosozumab binds and inhibits the bone hormone sclerostin, a negative regulator of bone formation, predominantly secreted by mature osteocytes. Sclerostin is a protein produced by osteoclasts that plays a role in promoting bone resorption by blocking the Wnt (pronounced 'Wint') signalling bone formation pathway. The Wnt pathway promotes differentiation, maturation and proliferation of osteoblasts, prevents osteoblast and osteocyte apoptosis, and reduces bone resorption (52). Blocking sclerostin with romosozumab thus leads to an increase in bone density through activation of anabolic signalling, increasing bone formation by osteoblasts and decreasing resorption by osteoclasts (52–54).

While this is a relatively new drug with anabolic activity, two cases of ONJ have already been reported in the literature (53). Therefore, it is important for dentists to be aware that this drug may contribute to MRONJ risk, especially in patients who have been on other osteoporosis drugs prior to treatment with romosozumab.

10.7 Dental risk factors

The most common trigger for MRONJ is dental extractions, although other oral trauma and invasive procedures including ill-fitting dentures, implant placement and periodontal surgery are also implicated (2, 8). An Australian study assessing the frequency of MRONJ associated with bisphosphonate use showed that tooth extractions were the trigger in 73% of cases (55).

Other risk factors relating to infection burden, including periodontitis and periapical abscesses, are also associated with an increased risk of MRONJ. It should be noted that MRONJ can occur without any known precipitating trigger. Filleul et al. found that up to 26% of cases of MRONJ with people taking BPs occurred without any predisposing factors (56). Thus, optimising oral health by treating infections and reducing inflammation is critical in these patients so as to reduce the future need for invasive dental procedures (6).

10.7.1 Assessing risk of MRONJ

Considerations of the risk of MRONJ should be made on an individual basis, taking the following four factors into account (2, 18, 57):

1. **Medication risk**
   - dose of antiresorptive drug used
   - duration of treatment (i.e. >4 years of BP use increases risk)
   - frequency of use (e.g. 120mg/month denosumab versus 60mg/6 months denosumab)
   - all other medications that contribute to risk (e.g. corticosteroids, other anti-angiogenic drugs)
2. **Patient risk factors**
   - advanced age
   - poor oral hygiene
   - smoking
   - medical conditions that can contribute to risk (e.g. cancer where antiresorptive and/or anti-angiogenic drugs are used, osteoporosis, poorly controlled diabetes mellitus, chronic kidney disease, autoimmune disease such as rheumatoid arthritis)
3. **Dental risk factors**
   - periapical abscesses, active periodontitis
4. **Procedure and operator skill and difficulty of the procedure.**

Based on these factors, algorithms have been devised such as those detailed in the *Therapeutic Guidelines Oral and Dental (Version 3)* that can be used to assess individual patient risk and guide management (18).

10.7.2 Role of C-terminal telopeptide test

C-terminal telopeptide (CTX) is a breakdown product of bone resorption from Type 1 collagen and an indicator of bone turnover. As BPs suppress bone turnover, there is a correlation between serum CTX levels and the use of these drugs. Some research has shown that a minimum level of CTX of >150pg/mL is associated with reduced risk of developing ONJ (58, 59).

However, systematic reviews and recent research have shown that an individual's CTX level in isolation is not a reliable indicator of ONJ risk, as CTX is affected by many variables, not only the use of antiresorptive medication. These variables include age, alcohol consumption, smoking, sex, exercise, circadian rhythms, and other medications such as corticosteroids (58, 60).

Furthermore, using CTX as an indicator of ONJ risk has only been validated in patients taking BPs and, as such, it is not yet applicable to patients on other medications (58). Indeed, CTX levels vary widely between patients even with the same BP dose, therefore the value of 150pg/mL is not an accurate predictor of risk which is why it is not currently recommended as a predictor of MRONJ risk (18, 59).

FURTHER READING

Nicolatou-Galitis O, Schiodt M, Mendes RA et al. Medication-related osteonecrosis of the jaw: definition and best practice for prevention, diagnosis, and treatment. *Oral Surg Oral Med Oral Pathol Oral Radiol.* 2019;127(2):117–135.

Pimolbutr K, Porter S, Fedele S. Osteonecrosis of the Jaw Associated with Antiangiogenics in Antiresorptive-Naive Patient: A Comprehensive Review of the Literature. *Biomed Res Int.* 2018;8071579. doi:10.1155/2018/8071579

Ruggiero SL, Dodson TB, Aghaloo T et al. American Association of Oral and Maxillofacial Surgeons: position paper on Medication-Related Osteonecrosis of the Jaw—2022 Update. Position Paper. *J Oral Maxillofac Surg.* 2022;80(5):920–943.

REFERENCES

1. Australian Government Department of Health. *Osteoporosis medicines.* 2017. https://www.pbs.gov.au/pbs/industry/listing/participants/public-release-docs/2016-09/medicines-osteoporosis-2016-09

2. Ruggiero SL, Dodson TB, Aghaloo T et al. American Association of Oral and Maxillofacial Surgeons: Position Paper on Medication-Related Osteonecrosis of the Jaw—2022 Update. *J Oral Maxillofac Surg.* 2022;80(5):920–943.

3. Khan AA, Morrison A, Hanley DA et al. Diagnosis and management of osteonecrosis of the jaw: a systematic review and international consensus. *J Bone Miner Res.* 2015;30(1):3–23.

4. Lombard T, Neirinckx V, Rogister B et al. Medication-Related Osteonecrosis of the Jaw: New Insights into Molecular Mechanisms and Cellular Therapeutic Approaches. *Stem Cells Int.* 2016;2016:8768162.

5. Teoh L, Moses G, Nguyen AP, McCullough MJ. Medication-related osteonecrosis of the jaw: Analysing the range of implicated drugs from the Australian database of adverse event notifications. *Br J Clin Pharmacol.* 2021;87(7):2767–2776.

6. McGowan K, McGowan T, Ivanovski S. Risk factors for medication-related osteonecrosis of the jaws: A systematic review. *Oral Dis.* 2018;24(4):527–536.

7. McGowan K, Acton C, Ivanovski S, Johnson NW, Ware RS. Systemic comorbidities are associated with medication-related osteonecrosis of the jaws: Case-control study. *Oral Dis.* 2019;25(4):1107–1115.

8. Ruggiero SL, Dodson TB, Fantasia J et al. American Association of Oral and Maxillofacial Surgeons: Position Paper on Medication-related Osteonecrosis of the Jaw—2014 update. *J Oral Maxillofac Surg.* 2014;72(10):1938–1956.

9. Marx RE. Pamidronate (Aredia) and zoledronate (Zometa) induced avascular necrosis of the jaws: a growing epidemic. *J Oral Maxillofac Surg.* 2003;61(9):1115–1117.

10. Editorial Advisory Committee. *Australian Medicines Handbook.* AMH Pty Ltd; 2020.

11. Nicolatou-Galitis O, Schiodt M, Mendes RA et al. Medication-related osteonecrosis of the jaw: Definition and best practice for prevention, diagnosis, and treatment. *Oral Surg Oral Med Oral Pathol Oral Radiol.* 2019;127(2):117–135.

12. Drake MT, Clarke BL, Khosla S. Bisphosphonates: Mechanism of action and role in clinical practice. *Mayo Clin Proc.* 2008;83(9):1032–1045.

13. Cremers S, Drake MT, Ebetino FH et al. Pharmacology of bisphosphonates. *Br J Clin Pharmacol.* 2019;85(6):1052–1062.

14. Bellido T, Plotkin LI. Novel actions of bisphosphonates in bone: preservation of osteoblast and osteocyte viability. *Bone.* 2011;49(1):50–55.

15. AusDI. *Independent Drug Monographs.* https://ausdi.hcn.com.au/browseDocuments .hcn?filter=PRODUCTS_WITH_MONGRAPH.

16. Wickham N, Crawford A, Carney AS, Goss AN. Bisphosphonate-associated osteonecrosis of the external auditory canal. *J Laryngol Otol.* 2013;127 Suppl 2:S51–S53.

17. Thorsteinsson AL, Vestergaard P, Eiken P. External auditory canal and middle ear cholesteatoma and osteonecrosis in bisphosphonate-treated osteoporosis patients: A Danish national register-based cohort study and literature review. *Osteoporos Int.* 2014;25(7):1937–1944.

18. Oral and Dental Expert Group. *Therapeutic Guidelines Oral and Dental (Version 3).* Therapeutic Guidelines Pty Ltd; 2019.

19. Cummings SR, San Martin J, McClung MR et al. Denosumab for prevention of fractures in postmenopausal women with osteoporosis. *N Engl J Med.* 2009;361(8):756–765.

20. Brown JP, Reid IR, Wagman RB et al. Effects of up to 5 years of denosumab treatment on bone histology and histomorphometry: the FREEDOM study extension. *J Bone Miner Res.* 2014;29(9):2051–2056.

21. Boquete-Castro A, Gomez-Moreno G, Calvo-Guirado JL et al. Denosumab and osteonecrosis of the jaw: A systematic analysis of events reported in clinical trials. *Clin Oral Implants Res.* 2016;27(3):367–375.

22. Baron R, Ferrari S, Russell RG. Denosumab and bisphosphonates: Different mechanisms of action and effects. *Bone.* 2011;48(4):677–692.

23. Lamy O, Stoll D, Aubry-Rozier B, Rodriguez EG. Stopping Denosumab. *Curr Osteoporos Rep.* 2019;17(1):8–15.

24. Lyu H, Yoshida K, Zhao SS et al. Delayed Denosumab Injections and Fracture Risk Among Patients With Osteoporosis: A Population-Based Cohort Study. *Ann Intern Med.* 2020;173(7):516–526.

25. Pang KL, Low NY, Chin KY. A Review on the Role of Denosumab in Fracture Prevention. *Drug Des Devel Ther.* 2020;14:4029–4051.

26. Pimolbutr K, Porter S, Fedele S. Osteonecrosis of the Jaw Associated with Antiangiogenics in Antiresorptive-Naive Patient: A Comprehensive Review of the Literature. *Biomed Res Int.* 2018; 2018:8071579.

27. Abel Mahedi Mohamed H, Nielsen CEN, Schiodt M. Medication related osteonecrosis of the jaws associated with targeted therapy as monotherapy and in combination with antiresorptive: A report of 7 cases from the Copenhagen Cohort. *Oral Surg Oral Med Oral Pathol Oral Radiol.* 2018;125(2):157–163.

28. Clarke SJ, Sharma R. Angiogenesis inhibitors in cancer—mechanisms of action. *Aust Prescr.* 2006;29:9–12.

29. Maniscalco WM, D'Angio CT. Vascular Endothelial Growth Factor. In *Encyclopedia of Respiratory Medicine.* ScienceDirect; 2006. https://www.sciencedirect.com/referencework/9780123708793/encyclopedia-of-respiratory-medicine

30. Sherbet GV. Vascular Endothelial Growth Factor. In *Growth Factors and Their Receptors in Cell Differentiation, Cancer and Cancer Therapy.* ScienceDirect; 2011. https://www.sciencedirect.com/book/9780123878199/growth-factors-and-their-receptors-in-cell-differentiation-cancer-and-cancer-therapy

31. Mian M, Sreedharan S, Kumar R. Osteonecrosis of the jaws associated with protein kinase inhibitors: a systematic review. *Oral Maxillofac Surg.* 2021;25(2):149–158.

32. Martini V, Bonacina R, Mariani U. Osteonecrosis of the jaw in a patient treated with zoledronic acid and everolimus: A case report. *Ann Stomatol.* 2014;5(2 Suppl):26.

33. Kim DW, Jung YS, Park HS, Jung HD. Osteonecrosis of the jaw related to everolimus: A case report. *Br J Oral Maxillofac Surg.* 2013;51(8):e302–e304.

34. Akkach S, Shukla L, Morgan D. Everolimus-induced osteonecrosis of the jaw in the absence of bisphosphonates: A case report. *Br J Oral Maxillofac Surg.* 2019;57(7):688–690.

35. Lu W, Guo Q, Ma Z et al. Lenvatinib and osteonecrosis of the jaw: A pharmacovigilance study. *Eur J Cancer.* 2021;150:211–213.

36. Marino R, Orlandi F, Arecco F et al. Osteonecrosis of the jaw in a patient receiving cabozantinib. *Aust Dent J.* 2015;60(4):528–531.

37. Cassoni A, Romeo U, Terenzi V et al. Adalimumab: Another Medication Related to Osteonecrosis of the Jaws? *Case Rep Dent.* 2016;2016:2856926.

38. Preidl RH, Ebker T, Raithel M et al. Osteonecrosis of the jaw in a Crohn's disease patient following a course of Bisphosphonate and Adalimumab therapy: A case report. *BMC Gastroenterol.* 2014;14:6.

39. Manara M, Sinigaglia L. Bone and TNF in rheumatoid arthritis: Clinical implications. *RMD Open.* 2015;1(Suppl 1):e00065.

40. Oray M, Abu Samra K, Ebrahimiadib N et al. Long-term side effects of glucocorticoids. *Expert Opin Drug Saf.* 2016;15(4):457–465.

41. Hayashi M, Morimoto Y, Iida T et al. Risk of Delayed Healing of Tooth Extraction Wounds and Osteonecrosis of the Jaw among Patients Treated with Potential Immunosuppressive Drugs: A Retrospective Cohort Study. *Tohoku J Exp Med.* 2018;246(4):257–264.

42. Ritter J, Flower R, Henderson G, Loke YK, MacEwan D, Rang H. *Rang and Dale's Pharmacology.* 9th edition. Elsevier; 2020.

43. Reid IR. Glucocorticoid effects on bone. *J Clin Endocrinol Metab.* 1998;83(6):1860–1862.

44. Levine JM. The Effect of Oral Medication on Wound Healing. *Adv Skin Wound Care.* 2017;30(3):137–142.

45. Henien M, Carey B, Hullah E, Sproat C, Patel V. Methotrexate-associated osteonecrosis of the jaw: A report of two cases. *Oral Surg Oral Med Oral Pathol Oral Radiol.* 2017;124(6):e283–e287.

46. Furudate K, Satake A, Narita N, Kobayashi W. Methotrexate-Related Lymphoproliferative Disorder in Patients With Osteonecrosis of the Jaw: A 3-Case Report and Literature Review. *J Oral Maxillofac Surg.* 2018;76(1):97–111.

47. Furukawa S, Oobu K, Moriyama M et al. Oral Methotrexate-related Lymphoproliferative Disease Presenting with Severe Osteonecrosis of the Jaw: A Case Report and Literature Review. *Intern Med.* 2018;57(4):575–581.
48. Mathai PC, Andrade NN, Aggarwal N et al. Low-dose methotrexate in rheumatoid arthritis: a potential risk factor for bisphosphonate-induced osteonecrosis of the jaw. *Oral Maxillofac Surg.* 2018;22(2):235–240.
49. Annussek T, Kleinheinz J, Thomas S et al. Short time administration of antirheumatic drugs—methotrexate as a strong inhibitor of osteoblast's proliferation in vitro. *Head Face Med.* 2012;8:26.
50. Shankaranarayana S, Barret C, Kubler P. The Safety of Leflunomide. *Aust Prescr.* 2013;36:28–32.
51. Patel D, Patel V. Pharmacology: MRONJ risk factor. *Br Dent J.* 2018;224(4):198.
52. Bandeira L, Lewiecki EM, Bilezikian JP. Romosozumab for the treatment of osteoporosis. *Expert Opin Biol Ther.* 2017;17(2):255–263.
53. Cosman F, Crittenden DB, Adachi JD et al. Romosozumab Treatment in Postmenopausal Women with Osteoporosis. *N Engl J Med.* 2016;375(16):1532–1543.
54. NPSMedicineWise. Romosozumab for osteoporosis. *Aust Prescr.* 2021;44:109–110.
55. Mavrokokki T, Cheng A, Stein B, Goss A. Nature and frequency of bisphosphonate-associated osteonecrosis of the jaws in Australia. *J Oral Maxillofac Surg.* 2007;65(3):415–423.
56. Filleul O, Crompot E, Saussez S. Bisphosphonate-induced osteonecrosis of the jaw: A review of 2,400 patient cases. *J Cancer Res Clin Oncol.* 2010;136(8):1117–1124.
57. Engelbrecht H. ONJ Medication-related osteonecrosis of the jaws. *ADA News Bulletin.* 2021(October).
58. Enciso R, Keaton J, Saleh N et al. Assessing the utility of serum C-telopeptide cross-link of type 1 collagen as a predictor of bisphosphonate-related osteonecrosis of the jaw: A systematic review and meta-analysis. *J Am Dent Assoc.* 2016;147(7):551–560 e11.
59. Awad ME, Sun C, Jernigan J, Elsalanty M. Serum C-terminal cross-linking telopeptide level as a predictive biomarker of osteonecrosis after dentoalveolar surgery in patients receiving bisphosphonate therapy: Systematic review and meta-analysis. *J Am Dent Assoc.* 2019;150(8):664–675 e8.
60. Hannon R, Eastell R. Preanalytical variability of biochemical markers of bone turnover. *Osteoporos Int.* 2000;11(Suppl 6):S30–S44.
61. Bracarda S, Hutson TE, Porta C et al. Everolimus in metastatic renal cell carcinoma patients intolerant to previous VEGFr-TKI therapy: a RECORD-1 subgroup analysis. *British Journal of Cancer.* 2012;106:1475–1480.

11 PERIPROCEDURAL MEDICINES MANAGEMENT

KEY POINTS

- Perioperative medicine is a sub-specialty branch of healthcare aimed at comprehensively caring for patients before, during and after surgery to promote positive outcomes and minimise adverse events.
- An integral part of perioperative patient care is perioperative medication management.
- The principles of perioperative medicines management apply as much to the conduct of dental procedures as they do to any other type of invasive procedure or surgery.

11.1 Introduction

Many commonly used medicines can adversely impact patient outcomes of dental procedures. This awareness means it is important for dentists to ensure medications are appropriately managed perioperatively.

Managing medicines taken by patients before and after their dental procedures is a common and sometimes confusing clinical problem. Traditionally, the responsibility for perioperative medication management has been deferred to the patient's prescribing doctor. However, doctors are often unfamiliar with the physiological impacts of dental procedures and few have access to oral and dental prescribing guidelines. The prescriber can still be consulted, but dentists are encouraged to take a more active role in the clinical decision-making regarding medication management, especially since the dentist is responsible for the procedure itself.

Medication management is also becoming more important due to the ever-growing list of medicines that can adversely impact dental procedures. Medication-related risks include increased chance of perioperative bleeding, infection, impaired wound healing, diabetic ketoacidosis, and medication-related osteonecrosis of the jaw (MRONJ).

11.1.1 What is perioperative medicine?

Perioperative medicine is a relatively new sub-speciality of healthcare that 'emphasises the importance of an integrated, planned, and personalised approach to patient care before, during, and after any surgical procedure' (1). Perioperative medication management is an integral part of perioperative medicine.

Figure 11.1 The ANZCA perioperative medicine care model (1).

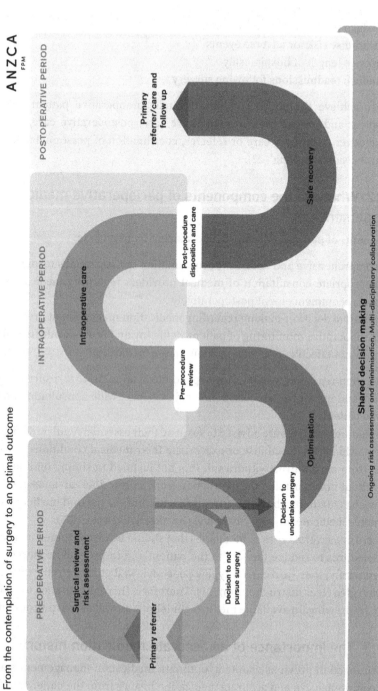

The Perioperative Care Framework
From the contemplation of surgery to an optimal outcome

PREOPERATIVE PERIOD

INTRAOPERATIVE PERIOD

POSTOPERATIVE PERIOD

Surgical review and risk assessment

Intraoperative care

Primary referrer/care and follow up

Primary referrer

Decision to not pursue surgery

Pre-procedure review

Post-procedure disposition and care

Decision to undertake surgery

Optimisation

Safe recovery

Shared decision making
Ongoing risk assessment and minimisation, Multi-disciplinary collaboration

ANZCA

FPM

© October 2021

ANZCA acknowledges the work of the POM Care Working group in the development of this framework.

The goals of the perioperative medicine care model (see Figure 11.1) are to:

- improve the patient experience
- reduce postoperative complications
- minimise risk for adverse events
- reduce length of hospital stay
- reduce readmissions following surgery

Steps to achieve the above outcomes include 'preoperative patient evaluation, risk assessment and preparation, intraoperative care, postoperative care, communication and handover to primary care or referrer, coordination of personnel and systems, and shared decision[-]making' (22).

11.1.2 What are the components of perioperative medicines management?

Components of perioperative medicines management include:

- comprehensive and accurate documentation of the patient's medication history
- appropriate consultation of medical providers regarding medication suspension and recommencement postoperatively
- accurate decision-making regarding medication management preoperatively
- perioperative monitoring of patient wellbeing and possible adverse effects
- safe and effective prescribing of discharge medication

The decision regarding whether to suspend medication prior to a surgical procedure is complex and must be made based on good evidence, wide consultation and discussion with the patient.

Sometimes, patients are advised to suspend their essential regular medicines inappropriately, which can destabilise or exacerbate their medical conditions or cause adverse effects from abrupt drug withdrawal. It is not justified to simply omit an oral medication without first clarifying the instruction from a prescriber, an anaesthetist or clinical pharmacist (23). It may be more appropriate to continue the oral medicine, change to an alternative medicine, or administer it via an alternative route (23).

There are several types of medicines that should be discontinued in advance of dental procedures to reduce the risk to the patient and improve postoperative outcomes. Unfortunately, there are currently few peer-reviewed guidelines for the dental profession that give clear instructions on this. Therefore, this chapter aims to address this situation by drawing on available medical guidelines as well as existing dental guidelines.

11.1.3 The importance of an accurate medication history

As mentioned in previous chapters, optimum medication management starts with taking a comprehensive and accurate medication history from the patient and other useful sources such as their pharmacy and GP.

The period leading up to a surgical procedure is perhaps the most important time to ensure a patient's medication history (MHx) is up to date and comprehensively documented. As outlined in Section 13.5, the MHx must include:

- prescription and non-prescription drugs, including over-the-counter (OTC) products, supplements and herbal remedies
- regular and as-required medicines
- recently stopped or withheld medications
- relevant medicines used in the past, such as bisphosphonates or corticosteroids
- history of adverse drug reactions and allergies.

Each drug's name, dose, duration of treatment and reason for use should be documented as illustrated in Table 11.1. Each of the patient's adverse drug reactions (ADRs) and drug allergies should be recorded with the details as in Table 11.2.

Table 11.1 Recommended MHx form.

Drug name	Dose and frequency	Duration of Tx	Reason for use

Table 11.2 Recommended ADR and allergy history form.

Allergy/ADR	Description of reaction	How long ago?

11.2 Patients on anticoagulants and antiplatelet agents

11.2.1 Background

Although most dental procedures are classified by perioperative guidelines as carrying a low bleeding risk, a wide range of medicines can increase bleeding risk and change the level of risk for the patient from low to high. More complex interventions such as flap-raising procedures or dental reconstruction surgery carry a higher bleeding risk, so detailed preoperative medication assessment needs to be undertaken prior to these procedures.

Medicines well known for conferring bleeding risk are anticoagulants and antiplatelet agents, but there are many medicines from other classes that also have antithrombotic (usually antiplatelet) effects such as NSAIDs, SSRIs and herbal remedies. The collective term for drugs that slow down coagulation is 'antithrombotic' drugs. Due to the increasing life expectancy and ageing of our population, there is an increasing use of antithrombotic agents in the community and perioperative management of these medicines is a frequent issue.

Quantification of bleeding risk is a key strategy for minimising intra-operative and postoperative blood loss. In general, the use of blood tests to assess bleeding risk is discouraged in dentistry as no single blood test reflects all aspects of coagulation and dentists are not usually trained to accurately interpret blood test results.

Bleeding risk quantification is approached somewhat arbitrarily by evaluating the three main sources of bleeding: the patient, the medicines, and the procedure. The level of bleeding risk is then expressed as unlikely, low, moderate, or high—each of which guide how the risk is managed.

11.2.2 Quantifying bleeding risk

The three sources of bleeding risk are as follows:

1. **Patient-related bleeding risk factors**

A range of patient-related factors contribute to increased bleeding risk, some of which include:

- advanced age
- decreased preoperative red blood cell volume or anaemia
- medical conditions impacting haemostasis including hereditary bleeding disorders and acquired medical conditions such as chronic kidney or liver disease
- lifestyle factors such as problematic alcohol consumption

2. **Drug-related bleeding risk factors**

A wide range of drugs contribute to delayed haemostasis (see Chapter 9). These include:

- anticoagulants: warfarin, heparin, low molecular-weight heparins
- direct-acting anticoagulants: apixaban, dabigatran, rivaroxaban
- antiplatelet agents: clopidogrel, dipyridamole, ticagrelor, low dose aspirin
- non-selective NSAIDs: diclofenac, ibuprofen, naproxen, piroxicam, etc.
- SSRI antidepressants: citalopram, escitalopram, sertraline, paroxetine, fluoxetine, fluvoxamine, etc.
- complementary medicines: vitamins, herbal remedies, high dose fish oil, turmeric, etc.

3. **Procedure-related bleeding risk factors**

Each dental procedure carries its own level of bleeding risk. The Scottish Dental Clinical Effectiveness Programme published a classification assigning levels of bleeding risk from unlikely, then low to high as outlined in Table 11.3 (2). See Table 11.4 for calculation of overall bleeding risk as derived from patient-, procedure- and drug-related factors. See Table 11.5 for suggested management of each level of overall bleeding risk.

11.3 Managing people on glucocorticoids and 'steroid cover'

11.3.1 Background

People with impaired adrenal gland function are at risk of glucocorticoid deficiency during episodes of physiological stress such as surgery, which can cause the potentially life-threatening complication of 'adrenal crisis'. Dentists may encounter this in patients who have been on long-term corticosteroid treatment and are undergoing prolonged or complex dental procedures. Dentists are required to identify which patients are at risk of adrenal crisis preoperatively, determine their current level of risk, and if necessary prescribe a remedial glucocorticoid dose known as 'steroid cover' prior to or during the procedure.

Table 11.3 Guide to degree of bleeding risk associated with dental procedures* (2).

Dental procedures that are **unlikely to cause bleeding**	Dental procedures that are **likely to cause bleeding**	
	Low risk of postoperative bleeding complications	**Higher risk** of postoperative bleeding complications
Local anaesthesia by infiltration, intraligamentary or mental nerve block[a] Local anaesthesia by inferior dental block or other regional nerve blocks[a, b] Basic periodontal examination (BPE)[c] Supragingival removal of plaque, calculus and stain Direct or indirect restorations with supragingival margins Endodontics—orthograde Impressions and other prosthetics procedures Fitting and adjustments of orthodontic appliances	Simple extractions[d] (1–3 teeth with restricted wound size) Incision and drainage of intra-oral swellings Detailed six-point full periodontal examination Root surface debridement (RSD) Direct or indirect restoration with subgingival margins	Complex extractions[e], adjacent extractions that will cause a large wound or more than 3 extractions at once Flap raising procedures[f] including: • elective surgical extractions • periodontal surgery • preprosthetic surgery • periradicular surgery • crown lengthening • dental implant surgery Gingival recontouring[f] Biopsies[f]

Notes:

* Note that clinical judgement is required to assess the degree of bleeding risk for each case, as there will be variation in invasiveness of procedures and some overlap between the categories (2).

[a] Local anaesthesia should be delivered using an aspirating syringe and should include a vasoconstrictor, unless contraindicated. Note that other methods of local anaesthetic delivery are preferred over regional nerve blocks, whether the patient is taking an anticoagulant or not.

[b] There is no evidence to suggest that an inferior dental block performed on an anticoagulated patient poses a significant risk of bleeding. However, for patients taking warfarin, an international normalized ratio blood test (INR) should always be requested before the procedure as per the protocol from *Therapeutic Guidelines Oral and Dental (Version 3)*.

[c] Although a BPE can result in some bleeding from gingival margins, this is considered extremely unlikely to lead to complications.

[d] Simple extractions refers to those that are expected to be straightforward without surgical complications.

[e] Complex extractions refers to those that may be likely to have surgical complications.

[f] Consideration should be given to the extent and invasiveness of the procedure. Some may be less invasive and could be treated as low risk.

Table 11.4 Calculation of bleeding risk. Adapted from (2, 3).

Overall degree of bleeding risk	Patient-related factors[1]	Procedure-related bleeding risk	Drugs that contribute to bleeding risk
Unlikely	Nil	Unlikely	Generally, drugs do not influence this level of bleeding risk, except triple antithrombotic therapy[2]
Low	Nil	Low	One or two oral antiplatelet or one oral anticoagulant drug(s)
Medium	Nil	High	One oral antiplatelet drug
	One or more factors[3]	Low	One oral anticoagulant or two oral antiplatelet drugs
	Nil	High	One oral anticoagulant or two oral antiplatelet drugs
	Nil	Low or high	One oral anticoagulant and one oral antiplatelet drug
High	Nil	Unlikely, low or high	Three or more antithrombotic drugs
	Patient risk factors (e.g. von Willebrand's disease, inherited clotting disorders[4])	Unlikely, low or high	Generally, the number of antithrombotic drugs does not influence this level of bleeding[4]

Notes:

[1] In addition to patient risk factors, this includes any other drugs that contribute to bleeding risk, including non-selective NSAIDs, drugs that cause thrombocytopenia, serotonergic antidepressants and some complementary medicines. For patients with any patient-related bleeding risk factors, consider specialist referral. Clinical judgement is required to assess the degree of bleeding risk for each case.

[2] If a patient is undergoing a procedure with an unlikely risk of bleeding, they will automatically be classified as having an 'unlikely' level of risk, except if they are on triple antithrombotic therapy. Clinical judgement is required to assess the degree of bleeding risk for each case.

[3] Clinical judgement is required depending on the patient risk factor; for example, an inherited clotting disorder will automatically classify the patient at being at high risk of bleeding. Consult with the patient's prescribing doctor for advice.

[4] When a patient has risk factors, such as an inherited clotting disorder, they are automatically classified as being at high risk of bleeding, regardless of their medications or the procedure risk. Clinical judgement is required to assess the degree of bleeding risk for each case.

Table 11.5 Suggested management of each level of bleeding risk. Based on (2, 3).

Overall degree of bleeding risk	Perioperative management
Unlikely	• Interruption of patient's medication not required • Clinically unnecessary medicines with bleeding risk should be ceased 10–14 days prior to procedure • Treatment can otherwise be carried out according to standard protocols
Low	**As above, for 'unlikely' bleeding risk, but also:** • These patients may display slightly increased or prolonged bleeding, which should be manageable with local haemostatic measures, such as pressure, packing the socket with oxidised cellulose or collagen sponge, or suturing where appropriate • Consider this bleeding risk in treatment planning • Delay elective or non-urgent procedures if possible if the patient is taking antithrombotic therapy for a limited duration • If multiple procedures are required, consider dividing into separate visits to limit procedure-related bleeding risk • Schedule as early morning appointments so arising complications can be managed during the day • If patient is on warfarin, follow recommended protocols (see Section 9.7 or the most recent edition of the *Therapeutic Guidelines Oral and Dental* for the full protocol) • Prescribe only paracetamol for postoperative pain management, unless contraindicated, rather than NSAIDs • Verbal and written instructions about managing haemostasis should be provided to the patient and/or carer • If bleeding recurs after the patient leaves the clinic and they cannot achieve haemostasis by applying pressure, advise patients to contact the practice or seek medical assistance • It is recommended to follow up the patient within 24 hours regarding potential bleeding and manage as appropriate
Medium	• Short-term preoperative suspension of the patient's medication may be required • Consult with the patient's prescribing doctor for advice • Ensure the recommended suspension is commensurate with current perioperative guidelines • Specialist referral may be required depending on the patient's bleeding risk • Clinically unnecessary medicines with bleeding risk should be ceased 10–14 days prior to the procedure • These patients may experience more and prolonged intra-operative or postoperative bleeding. Local haemostatic measures should suffice to achieve haemostasis, such as pressure, packing the socket with oxidised cellulose or collagen sponge, or suturing where appropriate • Delay elective or non-urgent procedures if possible if the patient is taking antithrombotic therapy for a limited duration • If multiple procedures are required, consider dividing into separate visits to limit procedure-related bleeding risk • Schedule as early morning appointments so arising complications can be managed during the day

Table 11.5 (cont.)

Overall degree of bleeding risk	Perioperative management
	• If patient is on warfarin, follow recommended protocols (see Section 9.7 or the most recent edition of the *Therapeutic Guidelines Oral and Dental* for the full protocol) • Prescribe only paracetamol for postoperative pain management, unless contraindicated, rather than NSAIDs • Verbal and written instructions about managing haemostasis should be provided to the patient and/or carer • If bleeding recurs after the patient leaves the clinic and they cannot achieve haemostasis by applying pressure, advise patients to contact the practice or seek medical assistance • It is recommended to follow up the patient within 24 hours regarding potential bleeding and manage as appropriate
High	• With this level of potential bleeding risk, the patient is at significant risk of bleeding and specialist referral is recommended • For patients with medical conditions that predispose to increased bleeding risk, consult with the patient's physician regarding their eligibility for invasive dental treatment and how the bleeding risk can be managed • Consult with the patient's physician for procedures with an unlikely risk of bleeding for advice prior to treatment • Prescribe paracetamol only for pain relief, unless contraindicated, rather than NSAIDs

Note that the physiological 'stress' referred to here is not emotional stress but the metabolic and endocrine stress of the body's response to surgery, major physical injury, or severe medical illness. The body responds to significant injury with a massive surge in adrenocorticotropic hormone (ACTH) and cortisol secretion, up to 20 times the normal daily levels and lasting up to several days, in order to maintain homeostasis and mobilise healing (4). However, this response is impaired in people with adrenal insufficiency.

It is also important to clarify the drug terminology used in this context. The term 'corticosteroid' refers to the two types of steroid hormones produced in the adrenal cortex. First, glucocorticoids (e.g. cortisol, hydrocortisone) which have anti-inflammatory and immunosuppressant actions. Second, mineralocorticoids (e.g. aldosterone) which act on sodium and fluid homeostasis. Drugs such as prednisolone are often referred to as corticosteroids but, having little mineralocorticoid effect, are more accurately referred to as glucocorticoids.

11.3.2 Who is at risk of adrenal suppression?

There are two groups of patients at risk of impaired adrenal function: those with drug-induced adrenal suppression and those with primary adrenal insuffiency. Patients who have received long-term, high-dose glucocorticoid treatment will be subject to drug-induced adrenal gland suppression. Guidelines generally recommend that a daily dose of 10mg or more of oral prednisolone, or an equivalent daily dose of another glucocorticoid (see Table 11.6) for 3 continuous weeks or longer is sufficient to cause adrenal gland suppression. For these patients, normal adrenal function will gradually return to once the exogenous glucocorticoid medication is withdrawn. However, in the meantime, a preoperative glucocorticoid dose is usually required to avoid adrenal crisis.

Table 11.6 Comparison of commonly used glucocorticoids. Based on (4, 5, 23).

Glucocorticoid (oral use only)	Relative glucocorticoid potency	Plasma half-life	Tissue half-life	Approx. equivalent oral daily dose
Cortisone acetate	0.8	0.5 hours	8–12 hours	25mg
Hydrocortisone	1	1.5–2 hours	8–12 hours	20mg
Prednisone/ prednisolone	4	2–4 hours	18–36 hours	5mg
Dexamethasone	25–50	3.5–5 hours	36–54 hours	0.5mg

For patients on doses between 5mg and 10mg per day, adrenal gland response is variable so medical advice should be sought and the patient possibly referred for adrenal function testing (e.g. an ACTH stimulation test). Current literature provides the following recommendation outlined in Table 11.7 regarding a range of doses and risk of adrenal suppression (3–5).

Table 11.7 Risk of adrenal suppression from oral prednisolone. Based on (3–5).

Oral prednisolone dose and duration	Likelihood of adrenal suppression
≥10mg per day for 3 weeks or longer	Expected to cause adrenal suppression
5–10mg per day for 3 weeks or more	Seek medical advice. Patient may require referral for adrenal function testing
5mg or less per day for any duration	Unlikely to cause adrenal suppression

The second patient group who have impaired adrenal function are those with primary adrenal insufficiency, also known as Addison's disease. This medical condition is caused by inadequate production of adrenal hormones and is treated with long-term corticosteroids in replacement doses, not treatment doses. In Addison's disease, adrenal gland function is unlikely to ever return to normal, so daily corticosteroid supplementation is lifelong and preoperative steroid cover is required for significant surgical procedures or severe medical illness.

11.3.3 What causes adrenal crisis and how is it prevented?

The physiological stress of significant medical illness or major surgery requires increased cortisol production from the adrenal glands. People with reduced or absent adrenal function cannot respond adequately and are therefore at risk of an adrenal or Addisonian crisis. Acute adrenal crisis is a medical emergency caused by the lack of the hormone cortisol, and the main symptoms experienced are those due to circulatory failure—e.g. light-headedness, dizziness, weakness, sweating, or loss of consciousness—and gastrointestinal symptoms including abdominal pain, nausea, and vomiting (5).

The risk of adrenal crisis associated with surgery can be ameliorated by administering the at-risk patient a supplementary dose of a glucocorticoid on the day of surgery.

11.3.4 For which surgical procedures is steroid cover required?

Not all surgical procedures cause sufficient physiological trauma and stress to require 'steroid cover'.

In the medical literature, recommendations are made for different types of surgical or medical 'stress', the doses of perioperative steroid required, and for how long it should be administered (4, 5).

Unfortunately, there is limited evidence to inform glucocorticoid dose adjustment for dental procedures for patients with likely adrenal suppression. However, recommendations were published in *Therapeutic Guidelines Oral and Dental* (*Version 3*) in 2019 and are presented in Table 11.8 (3).

Table 11.8 Various dental procedures and steroid cover recommendation. Adapted from (3).

Type of dental procedure	Dosage recommendation for patients at risk of adrenocortical suppression
Non-invasive dental procedures (e.g. dental check, impressions, X-rays)	The dose of corticosteroid does not need to be increased Ensure patients are advised to take their usual dose on the day of treatment
Invasive dental procedures <1 hour in an outpatient setting (e.g. professional teeth cleaning, restorative treatment, tooth extraction, periodontal treatment, implant placement)	Patients at risk of adrenocortical suppression require an increased dose of corticosteroid Some patients will already have a dosing strategy (action plan) from their own physician for managing periods of medical or surgical stress. For surgery, the 'stress' dose is usually started on the morning of the procedure and administered for 2–3 days afterwards If the patient does not have a dosing strategy in place, consult their medical practitioner
Invasive dental procedures >1 hour or dental procedures requiring sedation, general anaesthesia or fasting	For patients at risk of adrenocortical suppression, seek specialist advice regarding perioperative management

Note: These recommendations are based on the consensus view of the Oral and Dental Expert Group from the *Therapeutic Guidelines Oral and Dental (Version 3)*. There is limited evidence to inform the approach to corticosteroid dose adjustment for dental procedures in patients at risk of adrenocortical suppression.

11.3.5 What is a 'stress dose' of glucocorticoid and what drug is prescribed?

The dose of glucocorticoid required for 'steroid cover' should parallel the amount of physiologic steroid the normal adrenal gland would produce in response to surgical stress or severe medical illness. The regimen prescribed depends on the health of the patient, the drug and dose the patient has been taking prior to surgery and the type of operative procedure planned.

11.3.6 Is a supplementary glucocorticoid always needed?

Since the decision to recommend 'steroid cover' can be a difficult one, dentists are encouraged to consult with the patient's medical practitioner or an anaesthetist about the need to administer supplementary glucocorticoid to their patient prior to an invasive procedure. This is important because the supplementary dose may not be needed at all. As glucocorticoids have many significant adverse effects, even very short-term use may only serve to adversely impact the patient and procedure. Short-term adverse effects, which can occur within a few days of treatment, include immunosuppression, impaired wound healing, increased risk of infection, insomnia, hyperglycaemia and mood instability. Therefore, the benefit of prescribing steroid cover should always be weighed against the potential for adverse effects.

11.4 Managing patients on medicines for diabetes

11.4.1 Preoperative considerations

Perioperative care of people living with diabetes is complex for many reasons. The primary concern is preoperative glycaemic control, as hyperglycaemia is an independent predictor of poor surgical outcomes due to its contribution to delayed wound healing, infection risk and anaesthetic complications, all of which may prevent the procedure from going ahead (6–8, 10).

An important preoperative consideration is ensuring the diabetic patient can manage their food intake and control of blood sugar throughout the day of the procedure, as per their usual routine. The patient should be advised to bring their own glucometer machine and interventions for emergency management (e.g. insulin, glucose) in case they experience hyper- or hypoglycaemia during treatment.

Strategies should also be in place to manage the patient's hydration, nausea and vomiting, should they occur. Overall, the goals of perioperative diabetes management includes avoidance of hyper- or hypoglycaemia, prevention of ketoacidosis, and maintenance of appropriate fluid and electrolyte balance (3, 8).

Finally, the patient's medications must be appropriately documented and reviewed, as some medicines may require temporary cessation (3).

11.4.2 Preoperative assessment

Preoperative assessment of the diabetic patient requires a thorough medical and medication history. Particular attention should be paid to identifying the patient's most recent measurement of glycosylated haemoglobin (HbA1c) (9). HbA1c measures the amount of glucose attached to haemoglobin and reflects blood glucose control over the preceding three months. Current guidelines recommend a result of 53mmol/mol (7%) or less. HbA1c higher than 7% indicates exposure to elevated blood sugar over the preceding three months (3, 8).

Although there are no specific HbA1c cut-off values for permitting surgical procedures, some literature suggests it is plausible to postpone elective surgery if HbA1c is higher than 10% (11). However, urgent procedures should not be delayed by this target. The focus should instead be on optimising perioperative glucose control (8, 11).

Once the type and extent of the dental procedure has been decided the patient should schedule the procedure around their food intake and medication regimen. Extensive procedures and prolonged appointments should be avoided. The patient should be given a morning appointment for their procedure, so if adverse events occur there is time during the day for resolution.

If the procedure is likely to be prolonged or extensive, the patient's diabetes specialist should be contacted to obtain advice regarding withholding diabetic medicines before the procedure, when the medications should be restarted, and any dietary requirements to consider on recommencement of food intake.

Arrangements should also be made for how the dental clinic will check the patient's blood sugar and manage emergent symptoms of hypo- or hyperglycaemia during the procedure.

For diabetic patients on SGLT2 inhibitors (see Section 11.4.4) who have a significant risk of hypoglycaemia, the patient should skip the dose of their SGLT2 inhibitor on the day or the night before the procedure, and recommence the medication when they resume normal eating.

11.4.3 Medications for diabetes

A vast array of medicines is used for management of type 1 (T1D) and type 2 diabetes (T2D) (see Table 11.9). T1D is largely managed with different types of insulin, based on frequently measured blood glucose levels throughout the day. T2D is managed with oral hypoglycaemic agents, newer injectable agents and less frequent blood glucose testing. Most T2D gradually progresses in severity as pancreatic function declines and, over this time, the patient is transitioned from oral to injectable agents (see Table 11.9), including insulin and insulin-analogues.

For both types of diabetes, HbA1C results are also sought to reflect long-term blood glucose control.

11.4.4 Precautions regarding SGLT2 inhibitors ('flozins')

SGLT2 inhibitors carry a small but significant risk of causing intra-operative and postoperative euglycaemic diabetic ketoacidosis (eDKA) in patients with T1D or T2D (13, 14). Diabetic ketoacidosis (DKA) is a well-known, potentially life-threatening complication of diabetes characterised by metabolic acidosis, high serum ketones and hyperglycaemia. When the patient has DKA, eDKA occurs when their blood glucose levels are not elevated due to the presence of the SGLT2 inhibitor keeping serum glucose levels down (14, 15). The absence of hyperglycaemia makes the condition difficult to diagnose as the blood sugar levels will not suggest DKA.

Table 11.9 Drugs used to manage diabetes. Based on (12, 13).

Drug class	Examples of drugs	Route of administration	Mechanism of action
Sulfonylureas	Glibenclamide Gliclazide Glimepiride Glipizide	Oral	Increases the release of insulin from the beta cells of the pancreas; also reduce gluconeogenesis in the liver
Biguanide	Metformin	Oral	Prevents absorption of glucose, protein and fat through the gut; increases utilisation of glucose in the periphery and suppresses gluconeogenesis in the liver
Dipeptidyl peptidase-4 (DPP-4) inhibitors	Alogliptin Linagliptin Saxagliptin Sitalgiptan Vildagliptin	Oral	Inhibits DPP-4 in the gut, resulting in increased incretin hormones that reduce glucagon production and increase glucose-dependent insulin secretion from the pancreas
Glucagon-like peptide 1 (GLP-1) analogues	Dulaglutide Exenatide Liraglutide Semaglutide Tirzepatide	Subcutaneous injection	Increases insulin response to food intake, suppresses glucagon secretion, improves beta-cell function
Sodium-glucose co-transporter 2 (SGLT2) inhibitors ('flozins')	Dapagliflozin Empagliflozin Ertugliflozin	Oral	Inhibits SGLT2 co-transporters in renal proximal tubules that normally reabsorb glucose back into the blood stream. Blockade of SGLT2 transporters increases glucose and fluid excretion, which reduces blood sugar levels and decreases systemic fluid load
Alpha glucosidase inhibitors	Acarbose	Oral	Reduces absorption of simple sugars in the gut
Thiazolidinediones	Pioglitazone	Oral	Interacts with genes that regulate fat and glucose metabolism
Insulin and insulin analogues	Ultra-short, short- and long-acting insulins Long-acting insulin analogues Combinations of short- and long-acting mixed insulins and analogues	Subcutaneous injections	Promotes cellular uptake of glucose Used when endogenous insulin production is insufficient

Risk factors for eDKA are being fasted, dehydrated and/or hypoglycaemia. As this often affects people preparing for surgical procedures, dentists should anticipate that this syndrome could occur in the dental setting.

Symptoms suggestive of eDKA are thirst, abdominal pain, nausea, vomiting, fatigue, rapid breathing, fruity smelling breath (due to ketosis), tachycardia, hypotension and confusion (15). Management of eDKA is IV fluids and administration of insulin/glucose by infusion.

SGLT2 inhibitors are not only used in the management of diabetes, but for management of heart failure and chronic kidney disease in non-diabetic patients. Fortunately, the risk of eDKA is considerably less if the patient does not have diabetes.

As mentioned in Section 11.4.2, if the dental procedure is likely to involve prolonged or extensive treatment with a risk of hypoglycaemia, the patient's specialist should be contacted to obtain advice regarding withholding diabetic medicines before the procedure, when the medications should be restarted, and dietary requirements to consider on recommencement of food intake.

For patients on SGLT2 inhibitors undergoing stressful or complex dental procedures, guidelines recommend the patient skips the dose of their SGLT2 inhibitor on the day of the procedure, or the night before if they take their medication at night. Dosing can recommence once they resume their normal food intake (24).

11.4.5 On the day of the procedure

Ensure the patient has complied with the pretreatment plan regarding food intake, blood sugar management and suspension of medicines. Double check whether the patient has eaten prior to the procedure, as some patients may fast despite being warned otherwise.

If a patient has not eaten prior to the procedure, arrange for them to eat something and delay treatment by 30 minutes if possible, or reschedule their appointment for another time (3). This is especially important if they have taken their diabetic medication without eating, as this will increase the risk of hypoglycaemia during the procedure. If the patient has eaten but not taken their medication, then this could increase the risk of hyperglycaemia during the procedure.

11.4.6 After the procedure

Provide advice on when patients can resume their usual food intake and activity levels, and exactly when to resume medications, even if their mouth is sore. Provide advice on soft foods if the patient are likely to have trouble eating or chewing.

Give written postoperative instructions and advice regarding symptoms suggestive of diabetic ketoacidosis, such as nausea and vomiting. If symptoms develop, patients should seek urgent medical advice.

11.5 Managing patients undergoing cancer treatment

11.5.1 Background to cancer treatment

Dentists are increasingly required to provide care to patients undergoing cancer treatment. This is partly due to our ageing population living longer with a cancer diagnosis and the fact that more cancers are being treated in the community setting with oral and non-cytotoxic medicines (16).

There are over 120 different types of cancer. The four main types are: carcinomas, sarcomas, leukemias and lymphomas (16). Cancers can be managed with a variety of interventions, but the most common are surgery, radiation, and drug treatment or 'chemotherapy'. Chemotherapy is no longer limited to conventional cytotoxic drugs, which indiscriminately kill rapidly dividing cells including cancer cells. Newer, more tailored treatments include targeted, hormonal, and immunotherapies that are not only better tolerated but are often more effective than cytotoxics.

11.5.2 Types and goals of chemotherapy

There are over 100 different drugs used as chemotherapy. The main chemotherapy groups are: alkylating agents, antimetabolites, cytotoxic antibiotics, hormone antagonists, topoisomerase inhibitors, mitotic inhibitors and plant alkaloids. Targeted therapies include inhibitors of programmed cell death, vascular endothelial growth factor and tyrosine kinase inhibitors (see Table 11.10). These drugs are often combined into specific regimens to attack cancers in complementary ways to increase treatment efficacy.

Table 11.10 An overview of anticancer drugs. Adapted from (21).

Type	Group	Examples	Main mechanism
Alkylating and related cytotoxic agents	Nitrogen mustards	Cyclophosphamide, ifosfamide	Disruption of intra-strand DNA cross-linkage
	Platinum compounds	Carboplatin, cisplatin, oxaliplatin	
	Other	Busulfan, thiotepa, dacarbazine, temozolomide	
Antimetabolites	Folate antagonists	Methotrexate, pemetrexed	Blocking synthesis of DNA and RNA
	Pyrimidine pathway	Fluorouracil, capecitabine, cytarabine, gemcitabine	
	Purine pathway	Fludarabine, cladribine, mercaptopurine	
Cytotoxic antibiotics	Anthracyclines	Doxorubicin, epirubicin, idarubicin	Multiple effects on DNA/RNA synthesis and topoisomerase activity
	Other	Bleomycin, dactinomycin, mitomycin	
Plant derivatives	Taxanes	Paclitaxel, docetaxel	Disruption of microtubule assembly. Inhibition of spindle formation and topoisomerases
	Vinca alkaloids	Vinblastine, vincristine	
	Campothecins	Irinotecan, topotecan	
	Other	Etoposide	

Table 11.10 (cont.)

Type	Group	Examples	Main mechanism
Hormones/ antagonists	Hormones/analogues	Medroxyprogesterone, megestrol, goserelin, leuprorelin, octreotide	Disruption of hormone-dependent tumour growth
	Hormone antagonists	Tamoxifen, fulvestrant, cyproterone, flutamide, bicalutamide	
	Aromatase inhibitors	Anastrazole, letrozole, exemestane	
Protein kinase inhibitors	Tyrosine kinase inhibitors	Dasatinib, erlotinib, imatinib, nilotinib, osimertinib, sunitnib	Inhibition of kinases involved in growth factor receptor transduction
	Pan kinase inhibitors	Sorafenib	
Monoclonal antibodies	Anti-EGF, EGF2	Trastuzumab, pertuzumab	Blocks tumour cell and lymphocyte proliferation Prevent angiogenesis
	Anti-CD20/CD52	Rituximab, obinutuzumab	
	Anti-VEGF	Bevacizumab	
Small molecule inhibitors	CDK inhibitors	Palbociclib, ribociclib	Block cyclin-dependent kinase inside cancer cells

Depending on the stage of the cancer at diagnosis, chemotherapy is administered in three phases: induction, which is short and intensive, usually lasting about a month; consolidation, which involves intensification and occurs over a few months; followed by maintenance (post-consolidation), which is less intensive and lasts for about two years.

The goals of chemotherapy depend on the cancer type, whether it has spread, and if it is combined with other treatments. 'Curative chemotherapy' is a regimen that aims to eliminate all the cancer and prevent its return. 'Neoadjuvant chemotherapy' aims to shrink the tumour prior to surgery or radiation, and 'adjuvant chemotherapy' is given after surgery or radiation and aims to destroy any lingering cancer cells. 'Palliative chemotherapy' cannot eliminate the cancer but aims to slow its progression and improve patient symptoms (17).

11.5.3 Preoperative considerations for cancer patients

Cancer patients will usually require a dental review prior to starting cancer treatment to ensure their oral health is stable. While undergoing active cancer treatment, patients should ideally only attend for dental treatment when their white blood cell and platelet count is adequate. Invasive elective procedures should be avoided if a patient is undergoing cancer treatment. Non-invasive and emergency treatments may be undertaken, as long as the the dentist contacts the patient's oncology or haematology team to find out whether it is safe to do so.

The main purpose of contacting the patient's cancer team is to determine the form of cancer the patient is undergoing treatment for, whether the patient is immunocompetent, and whether the patient has an adequate platelet count to avoid excessive bleeding. The discussion can also include optimal timing of dental procedures and whether antibiotic prophylaxis is required.

As with all patients, a comprehensive medication history is needed for cancer patients so the dentist knows exactly what chemotherapy drugs are being used, which supportive medicines are being taken, as well as the patient's regular and complementary medicines.

11.5.4 Preoperative assessment

Cancer patients often receive treatments that have adverse effects on oral health and dental care. Therefore, consideration should be given to each cancer patient's dental care prior to and during cancer treatment. Decisions regarding dental treatment should be handled individually, considering the patient's medical and cancer history, the treatments they have had or are still having, and what the patient can currently tolerate.

The main risk of cytotoxic chemotherapy is bone marrow suppression, which can impair the formation of white blood cells, red blood cells and platelets, resulting in increased risk of infection, risk of anaemia, and bleeding, respectively (18). For this reason, a cancer patient should not undergo invasive dental treatment unless their current full blood count—mainly neutrophil and platelet count—has been assessed by their treating doctor and they have been deemed fit for dental treatment.

As cytotoxic chemotherapy drugs target rapidly dividing cells, many of their adverse reactions occur in the oral cavity. The main oral adverse effects relevant to dental procedures include oral ulceration, mucositis (see Chapter 15), glossitis and taste disturbance. Other reported oral mucosal effects include stomatitis with mTOR inhibitors and pigmentary changes and lichenoid reactions with imatinib (19).

Cancer patients are also often treated with high dose bisphosphonates or denosumab to reduce skeletal adverse events from bony metastases. However, these drugs are well known to significantly increase the risk of medication-related osteonecrosis of the jaw (MRONJ) (see Chapter 10).

An important characteristic of a tumour cell is its ability to metastasise. Tumours release angiogenic factors to grow their own blood vessels to connect to the body's circulatory system. This allows the tumour to obtain nutrients for growth but also to metastasise and spread. Several targeted anticancer drugs specifically block angiogenic factors to inhibit tumour angiogenesis, and limit the growth and spread of the tumour. Chemotherapy drugs that have anti-angiogenic properties are also associated with increased MRONJ risk (see Chapter 10).

11.5.5 Postoperative management

As cancer patients may have an abrupt change in their medical status at any time, it is vital to manage any oral health concerns proactively yet conservatively. Should an invasive procedure be deemed appropriate after careful preoperative assessment, postoperative care should consider the bleeding, infection and wound healing risks created by the drugs taken by these patients.

11.6 Managing patients on immunosuppressants

11.6.1 Background

The umbrella term for drugs that alter immune function is 'immunomodulators'. There are two types of immunomodulators: immunostimulants and immunosuppressants. Immunostimulants are drugs that enhance the immune response against infectious diseases such as vaccines, primary or secondary immunodeficiency, and certain types of cancers. Immunosuppressive drugs are used to reduce the immune response against transplanted organs, autoimmune diseases and inflammation. Table 11.11 outlines commonly encountered immunosuppressant drugs, their mechanisms of action, and common indications.

Biologically manufactured drugs used to inhibit pathways in the immune system are often referred to as 'biologics'. Some biologics include:

- monoclonal and polyclonal antibodies (with names ending in -mab), such as infliximab and tocilizumab
- cytokine inhibitors, such as interleukin and tumour necrosis factor (TNF) blockers

It is important to remember that just because monoclonal antibodies have similar names, their molecular targets are different and thus have very different actions and side effects. For example, the immunosuppressant drug adalimumab is a TNF-α inhibitor and is used to treat rheumatoid arthritis, whereas the drug denosumab is a RANK-ligand inhibitor and is used to treat osteoporosis.

Cytokine inhibitors and modulators are drugs that block one or more of the many chemical messengers in the immune system that cause chronic inflammation in disorders such as rheumatoid arthritis (RA), Crohn's disease, ankylosing spondylitis and psoriasis. These drugs reduce inflammation and promote tissue repair, but they can also increase the recurrence of serious infections such as tuberculosis, hepatitis B, pneumococcal and fungal infections. Examples of TNF-α inhibitors include certolizumab (Cimzia), adalimumab (Humira), infliximab (Remicade), and etanercept (Enbrel). Secukinumab (Cosentyx) is a cytokine modulator that works by inhibiting interleukin-17A, used to treat psoriatic arthritis and ankylosing spondylitis (see Table 11.11).

The most well-known immunosuppressants in Western medicine are the corticosteroids. These medicines have glucocorticoid effects that include immunosuppression. There are wide range of drugs in this family, with a range of anti-inflammatory and immunosuppressant potency. As discussed earlier in this chapter, another perioperative consideration is their ability to suppress adrenal function when taken in supraphysiological doses for an extended period.

Table 11.11 Commonly used immunosuppressant drugs. Based on (13).

Drug class	Mechanism of action	Common uses	Examples
Corticosteroids	Inhibit glucocorticoid receptor and gene replication of immune reactants	Acute and chronic inflammation of any kind	Betamethasone Dexamethasone Hydrocortisone Prednisolone
Calcineurin inhibitors	Prevention production of IL-2 and other cytokines	Auto-immune conditions. Prevention of transplant rejection	Ciclosporin Tacrolimus
Anti-metabolite	Immuno-modulatory effects	Rheumatoid arthritis, psoriasis and other auto-immune conditions	Azathioprine Mercaptopurine Methotrexate Leflunomide
Immunosuppressant antibodies	Inhibits T lymphocyte activation and proliferation	Prevention or treatment of transplant rejection	Basiliximab
mTOR inhibitors	Blocks the action of mTOR kinase, inhibits B and T cell development	Prevention of transplant rejection Cancer treatment	Everolimus Sirolimus
Cytokine modulators	Inhibits the activity of interleukins 17A,12 and 23	Reduce inflammation and immune reactions in dermatological disease	Secukinumb Ustekinumab
TNF-α antagonists	Inhibits TNF-α; TNF-α is involved in inflammatory and immune responses	Rheumatological disease (e.g. SLE, rheumatoid arthritis, ankylosing spondylitis)	Adalimumab Certolizumab Etanercept Infliximab Tocilizumab
Anti-IgE antibody	Prevents IgE from activating allergic-type asthma	Asthma, allergic rhinitis	Omalizumab

Note: SLE: system lupus erythematosus.

11.6.2 Adverse effects and dental considerations

Older immunosuppressants such as methotrexate, hydroxychloroquine, leflunomide and corticosteroids are well known for their wide range of adverse effects. The most important perioperative consideration for these medicines is their risk of myelosuppression that can result in reduced red cells, white cells and platelets. Regular monitoring and preoperative assessment is required. Corticosteroids also impair collagen synthesis and wound repair, thereby increasing the risk of infection and delayed healing.

Biologic medicines are unlikely to cause myelosuppression, but due to their potent suppression of inflammation they can mask signs of infection and are associated with rebound of latent serious infections such as tuberculosis and hepatitis B (16).

Some anti-TNF-α medicines such as methotrexate, adalimumab, and rituximab have been associated with case reports of MRONJ. It is thought that the MRONJ risk arises from these drugs' anti-angiogenic properties, which impairs wound repair and healing after dental procedures such as extractions (see Chapter 10).

11.6.3 Preoperative considerations

There are three main issues to consider when assessing patients on immunosuppressant medication and their eligibility to undergo dental procedures:

1. Whether the patient is medically stable and able to withstand the rigours of an invasive procedure
2. Whether the patient is subject to side effects of their medications that require management, such as adrenal suppression requiring steroid cover, or immunosuppression that may require antibiotic cover
3. The effects the patient's drug therapy may have on the procedure, as many of these drugs increase risk of infection, bleeding, poor wound healing and MRONJ

A frequently asked question is whether immunosuppressants and biologics should be suspended prior to invasive dental procedures. Although this might be considered for major surgery, such as joint replacement, it is generally thought to be unnecessary for dental procedures as the risk of destabilising the patient's autoimmune condition from withholding their medication outweighs the risk of adverse effects of dental treatment (20). The Australian Rheumatology Association has published guidelines on perioperative management of antirheumatic medicines (21).

Nevertheless, each patient and their dental needs should be discussed with the patient's specialist prescriber, including the potential need for antibiotic prophylaxis (22).

11.6.4 Postoperative considerations

Postoperative pain management can be a challenge in patients on immunosuppressants, as they are often living with chronic disease and are already taking regular and 'when required' pain medication. They may also be self-medicating with over-the-counter medicines in addition to their prescription medications. It is recommended that dentists consult with the patient's medical practitioner or pain management specialist for advice on managing postoperative pain in these complex patients.

Patients on immunosuppressants for chronic musculoskeletal disorders often have prosthetic joint replacements, so it is important to remember that a joint prostheses is not a specific indication for surgical antibiotic prophylaxis before dental procedures (3).

FURTHER READING

Australian Diabetes Society and New Zealand Society for the Study of Diabetes. *ALERT UPDATE. Periprocedural Diabetic ketoacidosis (DKA) with SGLT2 inhibitor Use in People with Diabetes.* 2022. https://www.diabetessociety.com.au/downloads/20220726%20ADS%20ADEA%20 ANZCA%20NZSSD_DKA_SGLT2i_Alert_Ver%20July%202022.pdf

NSW Clinical Excellence Commission. *Guidelines on perioperative management of anticoagulant and antiplatelet agents.* 2018. https://www.cec.health.nsw.gov.au/__data/assets/ pdf_file/0006/458988/Guidelines-on-perioperative-management-of-anticoagulant-and-antiplatelet-agents.pdf

Statman BJ. Perioperative Management of Oral Antithrombotics in Dentistry and Oral Surgery: Part 1. *Anesthesia Progress.* 2022;69(3):40–74.

UK Clinical Pharmacy Association. *The Handbook of Perioperative Medicines.* Accessed March 26, 2023. https://www.ukcpa-periophandbook.co.uk/

REFERENCES

1. Australian and New Zealand College of Anaesthetists. *What is perioperative medicine?* Accessed February 25, 2023. https://www.anzca.edu.au/patient-information/about-perioperative-medicine#:~:text=Perioperative%20medicine%20emphasises%20the%20 importance,any%20surgical%20procedure%20involving%20anaesthesia.

2. Scottish Dental Clinical Effectiveness Programme. *Management of Dental Patients Taking Anticoagulants or Antiplatelet Drugs.* 2nd edition. 2022. https://www.sdcep.org.uk/media/ ypnl2cpz/sdcep-management-of-dental-patients-taking-anticoagulants-or-antiplatelet-drugs-2nd-edition.pdf

3. Oral and Dental Expert Group. *Therapeutic Guideline Oral and Dental (Version 3).* Therapeutic Guidelines Pty Ltd; 2019.

4. Jung C, Inder WJ. Management of adrenal insufficiency during the stress of medical illness and surgery. *Med J Aust.* 2008;188(7):409–413.

5. Hamrahian AH, Roman S, Milan S. The management of the surgical patient taking glucocorticoids. *UpToDate Inc*; 2019.

6. Kotagal M, Symons RG, Hirsch IB et al. SCOAP-CERTAIN Collaborative. Perioperative hyperglycemia and risk of adverse events among patients with and without diabetes. *Ann Surg.* 2015 Jan;261(1):97–103.

7. Kwon S, Thompson R, Dellinger P, Yanez D, Farrohki E, Flum D. Importance of perioperative glycemic control in general surgery: a report from the Surgical Care and Outcomes Assessment Program. *Ann Surg.* 2013 Jan;257(1):8–14.

8. Dogra P, Jialal I. *Diabetic Perioperative Management.* StatPearls Publishing; 2022. https://www.ncbi.nlm.nih.gov/books/NBK540965/

9. Phillips P. HbA1c and monitoring glycaemia. *Aust Fam Phys.* 2012;41(1). https://www.racgp .org.au/afp/2012/january-february/hba1c-and-monitoring-glycaemia

10. Cornelius BW. Patients With Type 2 Diabetes: Anesthetic Management in the Ambulatory Setting: Part 2: Pharmacology and Guidelines for Perioperative Management. *Anesth Prog.* 2017 Spring;64(1):39–44.

11. Kuwajerwala NK, Schwer WA. *Perioperative Medication Management.* Medscape; 2018. https://emedicine.medscape.com/article/284801-overview

12. Li J, Lian H. Recent development of single preparations and fixed-dose combination tablets for the treatment of non-insulin-dependent diabetes mellitus: A comprehensive summary for antidiabetic drugs. *Arch Pharm Res.* 2016 Jun;39(6):731–746.

13. Rossie S (ed). *Australian Medicines Handbook*. Australian Medicines Handbook Pty Ltd; 2022.

14. Douros A, Lix LM, Fralick M et al. Canadian Network for Observational Drug Effect Studies (CNODES) Investigators. Sodium-Glucose Cotransporter-2 Inhibitors and the Risk for Diabetic Ketoacidosis: A Multicenter cohort Study. *Ann Intern Med*. 2020;173(6):417–425.

15. Bryant PMC, King-Thiele R. *Euglycemia Diabetic Ketoacidosis*. StatPearls Publishing; 2022. https://www.ncbi.nlm.nih.gov/books/NBK554570/

16. Cancer.Net. *Living with Chronic Cancer*. https://www.cancer.net/survivorship/living-with-chronic-cancer

17. Cancer.Net. What is Chemotherapy? Accessed July 31, 2022. https://www.cancer.net/navigating-cancer-care/how-cancer-treated/chemotherapy/what-chemotherapy

18. McEntee J. *How should adults with cancer be managed by general dental practitioners if they need dental treatment?* UK Specialist Pharmacy Service. Accessed March 23, 2020. https://www.sps.nhs.uk/ articles/how-should-adults-with-cancer-be-managed-by-general-dental-practitioners-if-they-need-dental-treatment/

19. Vigarios E, Epstein JB, Sibaud V. Oral mucosal changes induced by anticancer targeted therapies and immune checkpoint inhibitors. *Support Care Cancer*. 2017;25(5):1713–1739.

20. Goodman SM, George MD. Should we stop or continue conventional synthetic (including glucocorticoids) and targeted DMARDs before surgery in patients with inflammatory rheumatic diseases? *RMD Open*. 2020;6(2):e001214.

21. Australian Rheumatology Association. *Recommendations on biologic and targeted synthetic disease modifying anti-rheumatic drugs (b/ts dmards) for the treatment of rheumatic diseases*. 2022. Accessed May 20, 2023. https://rheumatology.org.au/Portals/2/Documents/Public/Professionals/Position%20Statements/2022_03_16%20Recommendations%20for%20the%20use%20of%20b%20and%20tsDMARDs_March22_FINAL%20updated.pdf?ver=2022-05-07-120804-747

22. Bui T, Fitzptrick B, Forrester T et al. Standard of practice in surgery and perioperative medicine for pharmacy services. *J Pharm Pract Res*. 2022;52:139–158. doi:10.1002/jppr.1805

23. AusDI. *Corticosteroids—Independent Monograph*. Health Communication Network Pty Limited; 2023.

24. Australian Diabetes Society. *Alert update: Periprocedural Diabetic Ketoacidosis (DKA) with SGLT2 Inhibitor Use In People with Diabetes*. ADS; May 2023. https://www.diabetessociety.com.au/wp-content/uploads/2023/05/ADS-ADEA-ANZCA-NZSSD_DKA_SGLT2i_Alert_Ver-May-2023.pdf

PRESCRIBING FOR CHILDREN

12

KEY POINTS

- Prescribing for infants and children is more complex than prescribing for adults.
- Changes in anatomy and physiology that occur during child development influence the pharmacokinetics and pharmacodynamics of medicines.
- Specific skills are required for safe prescribing for paediatric patients regarding drug and product selection, dosage, route of administration, consent, adverse reaction monitoring, adherence, and error prevention.
- Adverse drug reactions in children often manifest differently from those in adults.
- Paediatric prescriptions require additional annotations such as the child's date of birth, age and weight.
- Drug doses for paediatric patients should be sourced from the most recent editions of references such as *Therapeutic Guidelines Oral and Dental* or *Australian Medicines Handbook Children's Dosing Companion* (AMH-CDC), rather than commercial product information.

12.1 Introduction

Despite recent advances in the development and regulation of medicines for children, unavoidable factors specific to the care of this age group will always make prescribing for infants and children challenging. These factors (see Figure 12.1) include:

- the changes in anatomy and physiology that occur during child development that impact on drug pharmacokinetics and pharmacodynamics
- the general lack of research on drug safety and efficacy in children due to practical and ethical reasons
- the need to individualise drug dosage based on parameters such as the child's age, weight or surface area
- the limited availability of medicinal products specifically formulated for children
- the vagaries of administering medicines to infants and children
- the general difficulties of communicating with children
- the challenge of diagnosing and recognising adverse reactions in children
- the higher risk for medication error in paediatrics
- the frequency of off-label prescribing in paediatrics and associated medicolegal issues
- recognition that treatment of infants and children involves managing their parents and/or carers as well

Figure 12.1 Factors that complicate paediatric prescribing (1).

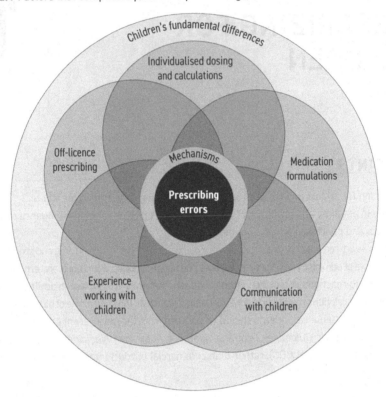

12.2 Limited drug and formulation development

Children are often referred to as 'therapeutic orphans' because medicines are infrequently developed for treatment of paediatric disease or paediatric patients (2). The outcomes of this are twofold. First, adult medicines are used for treating children, which raises the issue of off-label prescribing (see Section 12.3). Second, dosage forms that children find easier to swallow, such as liquids, are made by modifying adult dosage forms (e.g. by crushing tablets or giving injection fluid by mouth) which carries risks of inaccurate dose calculation and instability of altered dose formulations.

12.3 Off-label prescribing in paediatrics

The term 'off-label' is applied when a medicine is prescribed or administered in ways other than specified in the approved product information, including when the medicine is used:

- for another indication
- in a different dose
- via a different route of administration
- in a different patient group, age group or gender group

Until recently, regulatory authorities did little to mandate that manufacturers submit data regarding use of their products in children. This has changed slightly in the last decade, as new drugs must now overtly state whether their product has been trialled in a paediatric population. Despite this, most drugs marketed today have not been tested in a paediatric population and therefore do not carry a legally approved indication for children aged up to 12 years. As a result, 40–90% of paediatric prescribing in Australia is off-label (3).

Off-label prescribing is even more common in dentistry since few drugs, other than dental local anaesthetics, carry a legally approved dental indication. Luckily, drugs most frequently prescribed for children in dentistry are well-established antibiotics and analgesics that have been on the market for so long that paediatric formulations abound. However, it is wise to be aware that this is not always the case. For example, in Australia, clindamycin is not available in a paediatric formulation despite it being on the market for decades and being the main antibiotic used for penicillin-allergic patients.

Medicines are rarely developed for infants and children due to the wide range of ethical, clinical, and logistical difficulties of involving this age group in clinical trials. Therefore, understanding the safety and efficacy of drugs in children is delayed by years until clinicians working with children use the drug off-label, often in a research setting, to eventually establish the efficacy, safety, and appropriate dosing of the drug in this age group (4).

Off-label prescribing is not illegal and not synonymous with 'off-evidence' and may be clinically appropriate providing there is sufficient preliminary evidence to support its use. Practitioners should also understand the clinical, safety and ethical issues involved in off-label prescribing, ensuring it is supported by high-quality evidence and an informed consent process (2–5).

See Chapter 2 for more detail on off-label prescribing.

12.4 Childhood growth and pharmacology

12.4.1 Definitions of paediatric stages

Children are not simply small adults. Differences in the physiology and anatomy at different ages and stages of development can significantly affect the pharmacokinetics and pharmacodynamics of certain drugs. These differences mean that drug data from adult studies cannot be automatically applied to children.

In the past, poor understanding of how different paediatric pharmacodynamics and pharmacokinetics could be from adults led to several well-documented drug disasters (6, 7), including:

- grey baby syndrome, caused by excessively high serum levels of chloramphenicol given to premature and newborn infants, whose diminished ability to conjugate chloramphenicol and renally excrete the active form led to toxic accumulation (8)
- severe respiratory depression in children aged up to 6 years caused by sedating antihistamines, such as promethazine or chlorpheniramine, as children in

this age group are less able to protect their own airway than older children and adults (9)

- increased risk of depression and suicidal ideation among children taking selective serotonin reuptake inhibitor antidepressants (10)

In order to appreciate the differences in pharmacology at different ages, practitioners should first be familiar with the definitions of paediatric developmental stages corresponding to different ages. Neonates are those aged 0–28 days, followed by infants (from 28 days to 12 months), and toddlers (from 12 months to 23 months). Preschool children are 2–5 years old, and school aged children are 6–11 years old. The final paediatric classification is adolescent from 12–18 years old. This classification is based on definitions developed by the US National institute of Child Health and Human Development (12), modified for the Australian environment by Clarke et al. (13).

Rapid changes in body size, composition and organ function take place during the first few years of life that influence drug prescribing and administration to infants and children. These changes continue until about 12 years of age, as the child reaches adolescence, when drug handling and dosing is generally considered to be the same as adults (11, 12).

Although paediatric drug doses are calculated based on the patient's age, weight or body surface area, dosing can be complicated by factors such as obesity. Not only are obese children at greater risk of certain medical conditions, such as type-2 diabetes and hypertension, they are also at greater risk of medication overdose if actual body weight is used for dose calculations. In general, drug doses for obese children should be calculated based on ideal body weight or average weight for age (see Section 12.9 for further detail on dosage calculation).

12.4.2 Pharmacokinetics in paediatric patients

12.4.2.1 Oral drug absorption

Immaturity of the gastrointestinal (GI) tract in infancy and until about 2 years of age, significantly impairs oral absorption of drugs. Newborns and infants have reduced gastric acidity and slower gastric emptying. This is one reason why liquid preparations are preferred in this group: as the drug is in a pre-dissolved form making passage through the gut easier and facilitating drug exposure to the surface area of the gut (14). Solid dosage forms do not dissolve as easily in the stomachs of infants and toddlers and are less readily propelled out of the stomach and along the GI tract due to weaker peristalsis and slower GI transit times.

Swallowing difficulties are another reason why infants' and children's medicines are formulated as liquids because tablets and capsules are difficult to swallow whole. However, GI function reaches adult activity by about 5 years of age, so children at this age can be taught to swallow solid dosage forms (14).

Administration of medicines with food should be appropriately tailored to children of different ages and circumstances. Although most medications can be given with food to improve adherence, food can reduce absorption and delay the onset of some medicines, such as ibuprofen and paracetamol (15).

12.4.2.2 Non-oral drug absorption

Non-oral routes of drug administration include transdermal, transmucosal, sublingual, intranasal and rectal. These routes are often utilised in young children when oral administration is difficult due to sickness, unpleasant taste, poor tolerability or lack of cooperation. However, physiological differences with children may require consideration before these non-oral routes of drug administration are prescribed.

Absorption of some drugs through the skin can be greatly increased in infants and children due their thinner stratum corneum, increased skin hydration and higher surface area to volume ratio (17, 18). Enhanced absorption through the skin is one reason why infants are at increased risk of methaemoglobinaemia with some topically applied local anaesthetics, such as benzocaine, lidocaine and prilocaine (19, 20).

Infants and toddlers also have higher subcutaneous fat concentrations than adults and, as such, fat-soluble drugs administered via the skin can accumulate in the dermis and take longer to reach the systemic circulation. For this reason, few transdermal patches have been researched or are marketed for paediatric indications (18).

Rectal administration of medicines such as paracetamol or anticonvulsants can be useful for young children in emergencies or if they are too sick to swallow medication orally. However, suppositories may be unsuitable for newborns and infants, as they are often expelled from the rectal canal due to immaturity of the anal sphincter (14, 15). Site of placement in the rectal cavity can also significantly alter drug absorption due to differences in venous drainage.

Suppositories can be administered to children from 6 months of age, but rectal drug therapy is generally only appropriate if the intravenous or oral route is not available.

12.4.3 Drug distribution

Age-related changes to body composition (i.e. fat, muscle, water) strongly influence the rate and extent of drug distribution. As children grow, their body's percentage of total body water (TBW) decreases compared with fat and muscle. For example, TBW in newborns is about 70%, but decreases to 60% by 5 months, then levels off to about 65% by age 15 and 60% by adulthood. This decreases further to 45–50% for the elderly (17, 18). The percentage of total body fat doubles from birth to the age of 4 to 5 months, then plateaus at around 20–30% by adulthood (18). See Table 12.1 for percentages of body water, protein, fat and mineral composition from infancy to advanced age.

Clinically, this translates to increased volume of distribution and increased dosing requirements for water-soluble medicines, such as penicillin and cephalosporin antibiotics. Larger initial doses, on a mg/kg body weight basis, need to be given to children up to 2 years of age to achieve plasma concentrations similar to those obtained in adults. In contrast, highly fat-soluble compounds such as sedative/hypnotic agents exhibit relatively smaller volumes of distribution and require reduced dosing. This highlights the importance of dosing according to expert guidelines and paediatric pharmacopoeias as these compensatory adjustments are embedded in the doses recommended.

12.4.4 Drug metabolism and clearance

During the neonatal period, hepatic enzyme and plasma/tissue esterase activity are reduced, making drug half-lives up to 2–3 times longer. However, metabolic enzyme

Table 12.1 Changes in body composition from infancy to advanced age. Adapted from (33).

Age	Weight (kg)	Water (%)	Protein (%)	Fat (%)	Minerals (%)
Premature	2	80	12	6	2
Full term	3.5	70	13.4	13.4	3.2
1 year	10	61.2	13.4	22.4	3
10 years	31	64.8	17.3	13.7	4.2
15 years	60	64.6	18.1	13	4.3
Adult	70	60	16.5	18	5.5
Elder	65	54	12	30	4

activity rapidly increases by the time the child reaches 6 months of age and then exceeds adult levels until the age of about 3 years (14, 18). At this age, the child's capacity for drug metabolism is the greatest it will ever be, sometimes requiring paediatric doses to be higher than adult doses. Liver function slows down in older children and reaches adult levels by age 12.

Genetic polymorphisms of metabolic enzyme systems may be expressed erratically during infancy and childhood (17, 18). As this aspect of drug metabolism is unpredictable and prone to change in early childhood, it is important to be aware of this issue, especially in the event of unexpected drug effects. For example, conversion of codeine to morphine via CYP2D6 is more difficult to predict in infants and children, and combined with reduced clearance leads to less reliable analgesia, greater risk of morphine accumulation and risk of lethal CNS and respiratory depression. For this reason, codeine is contraindicated in children younger than 12 years and in older children aged 12–18 years whose respiratory function is potentially compromised, including post-tonsillectomy and/or adenoidectomy for obstructive sleep apnoea (14).

Small molecules and drug metabolites are generally cleared via the bile or the kidneys. Biliary excretion in the liver and glomerular filtration in the kidneys increases dramatically in the first week of life, from relatively low rates to normal rates by 4–5 weeks of age, reaching maximum capacity by 6–12 months. Glomerular filtration at this age exceeds that in adults and but declines to adult rates by about 1 year of age (17, 18). Clinically this means that infants aged 6–12 months may require shorter drug dosage intervals to account for more rapid drug elimination, but once renal function approximates adult levels at 1 year of age, dosing intervals are the same as for adults (14, 18).

12.5 Pharmacodynamics in infants and children

The pharmacodynamic effects of some medicines are different for infants and children, compared to adults, due to differences in drug targets such as receptors, transporters, channels, and metabolic enzymes.

For example, there is evidence that beta-agonist medication such as salbutamol ('Ventolin') is less effective to treat bronchospasm in infants and children than it is in adults due to fewer beta receptors in the lungs (16). It is well documented that infants and children are more susceptible than adults to respiratory depression and paradoxical excitation from benzodiazepines and sedating antihistamines such as promethazine (9, 14).

12.6 Adverse drug reactions in paediatric patients

It is perhaps easier to appreciate how differently children react to medicines from the perspective of their idiosyncratic adverse reactions. Children are not necessarily at more risk of adverse drug reactions (ADRs) but many ADRs manifest differently in children than in adults, and children are more at risk of harm from ADRs. Some well-documented examples of increased risk of ADRs in children include:

- methaemoglobinaemia associated with medical and dental use of local anaesthetics such as benzocaine, lidocaine, and prilocaine (19, 20)
- acute dystonic reactions, particularly oculogyric crisis, in young children after exposure to the anti-emetics including metoclopramide and prochlorperazine (14, 20)

Another difficulty with ADRs in infants and children is that this cohort is less able to communicate when they are experiencing adverse effects (17). It is more difficult to anticipate what sort of adverse reactions to monitor, as most medicines have not undergone clinical trials in paediatric patients, so extensive information about side effects and tolerability in younger patients is often unavailable.

A number of generic risk factors for ADRs occur across all populations. These include a history of prior ADRs, being at extremes of age, having impaired liver or kidney function, and being on polypharmacy—especially medicines for off-label drug use (2). When considering all of these risk factors, the children at greatest risk for ADRs are the very young (infants and toddlers) and children with chronic disease on polypharmacy.

In summary, clinicians prescribing to paediatric patients (especially in an off-label setting) should keep an open mind about the potential for side effects and have a high index of suspicion that any unusual or unexpected symptoms could be drug-induced. Parents and carers should be encouraged to report any unusual symptoms in order to receive prompt medical advice and intervention if necessary. Wherever possible, clinicians should report adverse drugs reactions occurring in children to the Therapeutic Goods Administration (TGA) to contribute to postmarking surveillance of drugs in this population.

12.7 Medication errors in paediatrics

Medication errors are one of the most common and preventable adverse events in healthcare settings (21). Unlike ADRs that occur due the pharmacology of a drug, medication errors primarily occur due to human error. The increased complexity of caring and prescribing for younger patients also creates a higher risk of medication errors. The Australian Commission on Safety and Quality in Health Care states that 'a worldwide systematic review has estimated 100 to 400 prescribing errors occur per 1,000 paediatric patients' (22, 31).

In addition to the greater vulnerability of paediatric patients who are unable to care and advocate for themselves, they are at more risk of harm from errors (23). A study of hospitalised children showed that although medication errors occurred at similar rates to adults (4.3–5.7% of drug orders), they had three times greater potential to cause harm (24, 25). Of the medication errors encountered in children, dose calculation errors were the most frequent type (31).

Factors that contribute to medication errors in paediatric patients include:

- unavailability of age-appropriate prescribing guidelines
- absence of paediatric formulations/dosage forms
- the wrong route of administration
- calculation errors based on mg/kg
- reformulation of adult medicines to a form more suitable for children
- difficulty with dose measurement
- lack of cooperation from children
- poor communication with parents and carers (25)

Prevention of medication errors require more than just being 'careful'. Clinicians are encouraged to consider the processes involved in prescribing as described in Section 12.8, recognise all opportunities for error, and proactively address them in order to prevent errors from occurring.

12.8 Steps to safer prescribing for children

As mentioned in Chapter 2, to best understand the process of prescribing for children it is first necessary to differentiate the terms 'prescribing' and 'prescription'. 'Prescribing' is the intellectual process of treatment consideration, determining all therapeutic options for a given diagnosis (including no treatment at all), evaluating the advantages and disadvantages of each option, making a selection, then tailoring that treatment to the individual and their circumstances (21, 22, 32).

'Prescription' is the act of writing/communicating a treatment order to a dispenser that satisfies legal, professional, ethical, and practical requirements so the treatment can be properly dispensed (22, 32). Therefore, when considering the risk of prescribing errors, it is important to recognise that they could arise from the intellectual process of prescribing or the act of generating the prescription or both.

Step 1: Medical and medication history. Caring for patients of any age should always begin with taking an up-to-date, accurate and comprehensive medical and medication history (MHx). This should be conducted at each visit, as children change so much as they grow. A comprehensive MHx of a paediatric patient includes the child's current age and weight, medical diagnoses, full medication list, and up to date allergy and adverse reaction history as these can change from month to month.

Step 2: Drug selection. Drug selection is based on the treatment plan and expected therapeutic goal in the context of individual patient characteristics. Drug selection is limited in paediatrics, however, as only a small proportion of available drugs are suitable for use in children. This is either because they are not registered for use in children, have not been trialed for use in paediatric conditions, or are not marketed in a paediatric dosage form. Therefore, the clinician must carefully consider the drug selection for treating children and whether the drug will be used off-label, in which case a portfolio of evidence should substantiate such use and parent/carer consent be obtained.

Step 3: Dose selection and documentation. Once a drug is selected, it is important to decide how the dose will be calculated and to document the basis for the calculation, such as it being based on weight, age or surface area. The reference from which the paediatric dose has been sourced should also be documented in the patient notes. Such references should include authoritative Australian guides such as the most recent editions of the *Therapeutic Guidelines Oral and Dental* or the AMH-CDC, depending on which reference covers the indication being treated.

Step 4: Dose calculation. Children are usually dosed on a mg/kg per dose basis. Calculate the dose to be administered in milligrams by multiplying the child's weight by the mg/kg dose. Make sure their weight is current. Consider using the ideal body weight (IBW) for obese children. If the calculated dose exceeds the adult dose, prescribe the adult dose instead.

For example, the dose of ibuprofen is 10mg/kg per dose, so for an 8-year-old child weighing 25kg the dose is 250mg, which can be given as 1x 200mg tablet or measured out as 12.5mL of the 100mg/5mL liquid = the 250mg dose. If the child weighs 45kg, then the dose calculates to 450mg; but the adult dose is 400mg so give the child 400mg.

Children whose weight differs significantly from the average weight for age, such as in obesity, should generally be dosed by IBW not actual weight, as the latter has led to overdose and fatal outcomes with drugs such as paracetamol. However, dosage alteration for overweight and obesity is medication-specific, so references such as the AMH-CDC should be consulted for guidance. This reference provides a table with average weights-for-age and weight as shown in Table 12.2.

The most widely accepted definition of obesity in adults relates to body mass index (BMI), which is calculated as weight (kg)/height^2 (metres) (26, 27). In children, however, height and body composition continually change as they grow, so a separate classification has been developed for overweight and obesity in children and adolescents up to the age of 18 years based on age and sex. According to work by Cole et al., children above the 85th percentile for BMI are classified as overweight and those above the 95th percentile are classified as obese (26). The United States Centre for Disease Control and Prevention has developed a graphical tool for depicting paediatric BMI by age and gender:

- Boys BMI-for-age: https://www.cdc.gov/growthcharts/data/set1clinical/cj41l023.pdf
- Girls BMI-for-age: https://www.cdc.gov/growthcharts/data/set1clinical/cj41l024.pdf.

Table 12.2 Average weight and height according to age (29).

Age	Weight (kg)	Height (cm)
Birth (at term)	3.3	50
1 month	4.4	55
2 months	5.4	58
3 months	6.1	61
4 months	6.7	63
6 months	7.6	67
1 year	9	75
2 years	12	87
3 years	14	96
4 years	16	103
5 years	18	110
6 years	21	115
8 years	25	127
10 years	33	139
12 years	41	150
14 year-old boy	51	164
14 year-old girl	50	160

Step 5: Formulation selection. Liquid medicines are favoured over solid dosage forms as the formulation of choice for children as they are easier to swallow and are absorbed better in the gut. Measuring a fraction of a dose is much easier with liquids and many liquids are flavoured sweetly, which can encourage patient compliance. Be aware that liquids are inappropriate for children or babies with swallowing difficulties, as they can be aspirated in the lungs. Older children should be transitioned from liquids to solid dosage forms by about the age of 6, once they can manage swallowing tablets and capsules, as the volume of liquid required becomes impractical and persistence with liquids can lead to long-term reluctance to swallow tablets whole.

When prescribing a liquid dosage form, express the dose in milligrams (mg) and the volume (mL) of liquid to be administered. If the dose's volume exceeds 15–20mL, prescribe a higher strength formulation where possible.

Always round the dose up or down to more easily measured volumes, depending on the measuring device being used, such as an oral syringe or spoon, considering how much medicine is retained in the device after the dose is administered.

Step 6: Writing the prescription. On the prescription, specify the dose, the frequency, the number of days the child should be treated and the strength and volume of medicine to be dispensed (e.g. amoxicillin 125mg/5mL liquid, 6mL every 8 hours for 5 days). Supply 100mL (discard unused portion).

The prescriber must specify the formulation to be dispensed (e.g. amoxicillin 125mg/5mL liquid, 100ml). A generic drug cannot be prescribed leaving product/formulation selection to the dispensing pharmacist.

> **Example 1: Amoxicillin prescription for a 20kg child for treatment of an odontogenic infection.**
> Amoxicillin dose for a child: 15mg/kg, up to 500mg per dose, every 8 hours (28).
> Child is 20kg: 15mg × 20kg = 300mg per dose.
> The strength of amoxicillin liquid is 250mg/5mL
> 300mg = 6mL of liquid
> Directions: Amoxicillin 250mg/5mL liquid. Give 6mL 3 times daily for 5 days. Supply 100mL. Discard unused portion.
>
> **Example 2: Clindamycin prescription for a child of 14kg for treatment of an odontogenic infection.**
> Clindamycin dose for a child: 7.5mg/kg, up to 300mg per dose, every 8 hours (27).
> Clindamycin does not come in a paediatric liquid formulation, so needs to be made up by the patient/carer. Each capsule is 150mg. Instruct the patient/carer to empty the contents of one 150mg capsule into 3mL of water to make a 50mg/mL solution.
> Child is 14kg: 14kg × 7.5mg = 105mg per dose
> The solution is 50mg/mL; dose of 2mLs (round down to 100mg/dose).
> Directions: Clindamycin 150mg capsules. Dissolve the contents of 1 capsule in 3mL of water to make a 50mg/mL solution. Give 2mL 3 times a day (every 8 hours) for 5 days. Discard remaining solution after each dose. Supply 15 capsules.

12.9 Prescribing common medications for children in dental practice

Antibiotics are the most commonly prescribed drug class in dental practice. The folllowing tables suggest doses and prescriptions for paediatric prescriptions according to body weight and dosage recommendations in the most recent edition of the *Therapeutic Guidelines Oral and Dental* (28). Note that some suggested volumes have been rounded up or down for ease of administration.

For more information on individual antibiotics, see Chapter 4.

Table 12.3 Recommended doses and paediatric prescriptions for amoxicillin to treat infection, based on body weight. Based on (28–30).

Child's weight (kg)	Volume (mL) of amoxicillin liquid required of 250mg/5mL liquid per dose (for 3 times daily dosing)*	Total volume (mL) of amoxicillin required for prescription^
12	4–6	100
13–14	4–7	100
15	5–7	100
16–17	5–8	100–200
18	5–9	100–200
19	6–9	100–200
20–21	6–10	100–200
22–24	7–10	100–200
25–28	8–10	200
29–31	9–10	200
32+	10	200

Notes:

* The paediatric dosage range is provided based on recommendations from the most recent edition of the *Therapeutic Guidelines Oral and Dental* and *Australian Medicines Handbook* (see Section 4.7.6) (28, 29). Clinical judgement is required for which dose to choose; for milder infections, the lower end of the dosage range can be used, and the higher end for more serious infections.

^ The total volume required will depend on the dose. Volumes will be either 100mL or 200mL and cannot be in between. A volume of 200mL should be written as a non-PBS 'private' prescription, as this volume exceeds the limit that can be prescribed on the PBS by dentists.

Suggested prescription format: Supply amoxicillin 250mg/5mL liquid, total volume mL. Give (dose) mL, 3 times daily (every 8 hours) for 5 days. Discard unused liquid.

    Example for a child of 23kg for a severe infection: Supply amoxicillin 250mg/5mL liquid, 2 × 100mL. Give 10mL, 3 times daily (every 8 hours) for 5 days. Discard unused liquid.

Table 12.4 Recommended doses and paediatric prescriptions for phenoxymethylpenicillin (PMP) to treat infection, based on body weight. Based on (28–30).

Child's weight (kg)	Volume (mL) of 250mg/5mL PMP liquid per dose (for 4 times daily dosing)*	Total volume required for prescription (mL)
12–13	3	100
14–17	4	100
18–21	5	100
22–25	6	200
26–29	7	200
30–33	8	200
34–37	9	200
38+	10	200

Note:

* Dose is based on that recommended in the most recent edition of the *Therapeutic Guidelines Oral and Dental*, calculated based on body weight (28). Volumes have been rounded up or down to an easily measured volume.

Suggested prescription format: Supply phenoxymethylpenicillin 200mg/5mL liquid, total volume mL. Give (dose) mL, 4 times daily (every 6 hours), half an hour before food, for 5 days. Discard unused liquid.

    Example for a child of 20kg: Supply phenoxymethylpenicillin 250mg/5mL liquid, 100mL. Give 5mL, 4 times daily (every 6 hours), half an hour before food, for 5 days. Discard unused liquid.

Table 12.5 Recommended paediatric doses for co-amoxiclav to treat infection, based on body weight. Based on (28–30).

Child's weight (kg)	Volume (mL) of co-amoxiclav liquid required of 400/57/5mL liquid per dose (for twice daily dosing)*	Total volume (mL) of co-amoxiclav required for prescription^
11–13	3	60
14–16	4	60
17–20	5	60
21–23	6	60
24–27	7	120
28–30	8	120
31–34	9	120
35–38	10	120
39+	11	120

Notes:

* Dose is based on that recommended in the most recent edition of the *Therapeutic Guidelines Oral and Dental*, calculated based on body weight (28). Volumes should be rounded up or down to an easily measured volume, depending on the severity of the infection, clinical judgement and measuring device used.

^ The total volume required will depend on the dose. Volumes will be either 60mL or 120mL and cannot be in between. A volume of 120mL should be written as a non-PBS 'private' prescription, as this volume exceeds the limit that can be prescribed on the PBS by dentists.

Suggested prescription format: Supply co-amoxiclav 400mg/57/5mL liquid, total volume mL. Give (dose) mL, twice daily (every 12 hours), for 5 days. Discard unused liquid.

Example for a child of 26kg: Supply co-amoxiclav 400mg/57mg/5mL liquid, 120mL. Give 7mL, twice daily (every 12 hours), for 5 days. Discard unused liquid.

Table 12.6 Recommended paediatric doses for metronidazole to treat infection, based on body weight. Based on (28–30).

Child's weight (kg)	Volume (mL) of metronidazole liquid required of 200mg/5mL liquid per dose (for twice daily dosing)*	Total volume (mL) of metronidazole required for the prescription
12–13	3	100
14–17	4	100
18–21	5	100
22–25	6	100
26–29	7	100
30–33	8	100
34–37	9	100
38+	10	100

Note:

* Dose is based on that recommended in the most recent edition of the *Therapeutic Guidelines Oral and Dental*, calculated based on body weight (28). Volumes should be rounded up or down to an easily measured volume, depending on the severity of the infection, clinical judgement and measuring device used.

Suggested prescription: Supply metronidazole 200mg/5mL liquid, total volume mL. Give (dose) mL, twice daily (every 12 hours), for 5 days, supply (volume) mL. Discard unused liquid.

   Example for a child of 28kg: Supply metronidazole 200mg/5mL liquid, 100mL. Give 7mL, twice daily (every 12 hours), for 5 days. Discard unused liquid.

Table 12.7 Recommended paediatric doses for clindamycin to treat infection, based on body weight. Based on (28–30).

Child's weight (kg)	Number of clindamycin 150mg capsules required to make each dose	Volume (mL) of water required to dissolve the capsule(s) to make a 50mg/mL solution	Volume (mL) clindamycin 50mg/mL liquid per dose (for 3 times daily dosing)*	Total number of clindamycin capsules required for prescription^
10–11	1	3	1.5	15
12–15	1	3	2	15
16–18	1	3	2.5	15
19–22	1	3	3	15
23–24	2	6	3.5	30
25–28	2	6	4	30
29–31	2	6	4.5	30
32–34	2	6	5	30
35–38	2	6	5.5	30
39+	2	6	6	30

Notes:

* Dose is formulated by dissolving the contents of one 150mg capsule in 3mL of water. Dose is based on that recommended in the most recent edition of the *Therapeutic Guidelines Oral and Dental*, calculated based on body weight (28). Volumes should be rounded up or down to an easily measured volume, depending on the severity of the infection, clinical judgement and measuring device used.
^ The total number of tablets required will depend on the dose. A quantity of 30 tablets should be written as a non-PBS 'private' prescription, as this quantity exceeds the limit that can be prescribed on the PBS by dentists.

Suggested prescription format: Supply clindamycin 150mg capsules × total required. Open (number) capsules and dissolve the contents in (volume) of water to make a 50mg/1mL solution. Give (volume) mL of this solution 3 times daily (every 8 hours) for 5 days. Discard unused portion after each dose.

Example for a child of 34kg: Supply clindamycin 150mg capsules × 30. Open 2 capsules and dissolve the contents in 6mL of water to make a 50mg/1mL solution. Give 5mL of this solution 3 times daily (every 8 hours) for 5 days. Discard unused portion after each dose.

FURTHER READING

Australian Commission on Safety and Quality in Health Care. *Position statement on paediatric prescribing*. 2018. https://www.safetyandquality.gov.au/sites/default/files/migrated/Paediatric-prescribing-position-statement-Apr-2018.pdf

Editorial Advisory Committee. *AMH Children's Dosing Companion*. Australian Medicines Handbook Pty Ltd; 2020.

Royal Children's Hospital Melbourne. *Clinical Practice Guidelines*. https://www.rch.org.au/clinicalguide/about_rch_cpgs/Welcome_to_the_Clinical_Practice_Guidelines/

REFERENCES

1. McAlinden J, Masson C. Keep within sight and reach: teaching paediatric prescribing. *Prescriber*. 2021 Oct;32(10):28–33. doi/10.1002/psb.1948

2. Gazarian M. Why are children still therapeutic orphans? *Aust Prescr*. 2003;26:122–123. doi:10.18773/austprescr.20

3. Schaffer AL, Bruno C, Buckley NA et al. Prescribed medicine use, and extent of off-label use according to age in a nationwide sample of Australian children. *Paediatr Perinat Epidemiol*. 2022;36(5):726–737. doi:10.1111/ppe.12870

4. Yackey K, Stanley R. Off-label prescribing in children remains high: A call for prioritized research. *Pediatrics* 2019;144(4):e20191571.

5. Council of Australian Therapeutic Advisory Groups (CATAG). *Rethinking medicines decision-making in Australian Hospitals. Guiding Principles for the Quality Use of Off-label Medicines*. NSW Therapeutic Advisory Group; 2013. http://www.catag.org.au/rethinking-medicines-decision-making/

6. Wiffen P, Mitchell M, Snelling M, Stoner N (eds). *Oxford Handbook of Clinical Pharmacy*. 3rd edition. Oxford University Press; 2017.

7. Yashwant S, Cranswick NE. How to use medicines in children: principles of paediatric pharmacology. *J Paed Child Health*. 2007;43:107–111.

8. Lischner H, Seligman S, Krammer A, Parmelee A. An outbreak of neonatal deaths among term infants associated with administration of chloramphenicol. *J. Pediatr*. 1961;59:21–34.

9. MedSafe. Children and sedating antihistamines. *Prescriber Update*. 2013;34(1):11–12.

10. Jureidini JN, Doecke CJ, Mansfield PR, Haby MM, Menkes DB, Tonkin AL. Efficacy and safety of antidepressants for children and adolescents. *BMJ*. 2004;328:879–883.

11. O'Hara K. Paediatric pharmacokinetics and drug doses. *Aust Prescr*. 2016;39:208–210. doi:10.18773/austprescr.2016.071

12. Williams K, Thomson D, Seto I et al. Standard 6: Age Groups for Pediatric Trials. *Pediatrics* 2012;129(Supp 3):S153–S160. doi:10.1542/peds.2012-0055I

13. Clark R, Locke M, Bialocerkowski A. Paediatric terminology in the Australian health and health-education context: a systematic review. *Devel Med Child Neurol*. 2015 Nov;57911:1011–1118. doi:10.1111/dmcn.12803

14. Helms Q. *Textbook of Therapeutics: Drugs and Disease Management*. 8th edition. Lippincott Williams & Wilkins; 2006.

15. Moore RA, Derry S, Wiffen PJ, Straube S. Effects of food on pharmacokinetics of immediate release oral formulations of aspirin, dipyrone, paracetamol and NSAIDs—a systematic review. *Br J Clin Pharmacol*. 2015;80(3):381–388. doi:10.1111/bcp.12628

16. Ku L, Smith P. Dosing in neonates: special considerations in physiology and trial design. *Pediatr Res*. 2015;77:2–9. doi:10.1038/pr.2014.143

17. Fernandez E, Perez R, Hernandez A et al. Factors and Mechanisms for Pharmacokinetic Differences between Pediatric Population and Adults. *Pharmaceutics*. 2011;3(1):53–72. doi:10.3390/pharmaceutics3010053

18. Gulu M, Haykir N, Boran P, Gulnyr T. How safe is prilocaine as a local anesthetic in children younger than 2 years of age: a case series. *South Clin Ist Euras*. 2018;29(1):63–67. doi:10.14744/scie.2018.79106

19. Rieder M. Adverse Drug Reactions in Children: Pediatric Pharmacy and Drug Safety. *J Pediatr Pharmacol Ther*. 2019;24(1):4–9. doi:10.5863/1551-6776-24.1.4

20. Joint Commission. Preventing pediatric medication errors. *Sentinel Event Alert*. 2008;(39). Revised April 14, 2021.

21. Aronson JK. Medication errors: definitions and classification. *Br J Clin Pharmacol.* 2009;67(6):599–604.

22. Miller MR, Robinson KA, Lubomski LH et al. Medication errors in paediatric care: a systematic review of epidemiology and an evaluation of evidence supporting reduction strategy recommendations. *Qual Saf Health Care.* 2007;16(2):116–216.

23. Kaushal R, Bates DW, Landrigan C et al. Medication errors and adverse drug events in pediatric inpatients. *JAMA.* 2001;285(16):2114–2120.

24. Levine SR, Cohen MR, Blanchard NR, Frederico F. Guidelines for preventing medication errors in pediatrics. *J Pediatr Pharmacol Ther.* 2001;6:246–262.

25. Australian Commission on Safety and Quality in Health Care. *Position statement on paediatric prescribing.* 2018. https://www.safetyandquality.gov.au/sites/default/files/ migrated/Paediatric-prescribing-position-statement-Apr-2018.pdf

26. Cole TJ, Bellizzi MC, Flegal KM, Dietz WH. Establishing a standard definition for child overweight and obesity worldwide: international survey. *BMJ.* 2000;320:1240. doi:10.1136/ bmj.320.7244.1240

27. US Centre for Disease Control and Prevention. *Using the BMI-for-Age Growth Charts.* https://www.cdc.gov/nccdphp/dnpa/growthcharts/training/modules/module1/text/ module1print.pdf

28. Oral and Dental Expert Group. *Therapeutic Guidelines Oral and Dental* (Version 3). Therapeutic Guidelines Pty Ltd; 2019.

29. Rossi S (ed). *Australian Medicines Handbook.* Australian Medicines Handbook Pty Ltd; 2022.

30. AusDI by Medical Director. Accessed June 20, 2022. https://ausdi.hcn.com.au/quickSearch .hcn [Subscription only]

31. Australian Commission on Safety and Quality in Health Care. *Position statement on paediatric prescribing.* 2018. https://www.safetyandquality.gov.au/sites/default/files/ migrated/Paediatric-prescribing-position-statement-Apr-2018.pdf

32. Teoh L, McCullogh MJ, Moses G. Preventing medication errors in dental practice: An Australian perspective. *Journal of Dentistry.* 2022;119:1–6.

33. MSD Manual: Professional version. *Changes in body composition with growth and aging.* https://www.msdmanuals.com/professional/multimedia/figure/changes-in-body-composition-with-growth-and-aging

DRUGS IN THE ELDERLY

13

KEY POINTS

- Physiological changes associated with ageing alter the pharmacokinetics and pharmacodynamics of medicines in older people.
- Due to our ageing population, an increasing proportion of dental patients are in their later years (>75 years) and medication use is more complex.
- Care of patients in aged care facilities is frequently complicated by the additional factor of frailty.
- Safe prescribing for older people requires that their medical and medication history is comprehensive, accurate and up to date.
- Prescribing guidelines for older patients not only provide more appropriate doses and frequencies but also identify drugs that are best avoided.
- Prescribing for older patients is best approached conservatively by following the adage 'start low and go slow'.

13.1 Introduction

A hallmark of the 21st century is that people are living longer, making it increasingly likely that many dental patients are in their later years. In 2020, the proportion of Australians aged 65 years and older reached 16.3%, increasing from 12.4% in 2000, and this proportion is predicted to reach approximately 25% by 2050 (1). Meanwhile, people aged 85 years and over are in the fastest growing sector, increasing by 2.5% in 2020 alone and by 110% over the preceding 20 years, compared with growth of only 35% for the total population over the same 20-year period (1).

Caring for older patients is an increasing challenge for dental practitioners. In addition to living longer, older Australians are retaining their own teeth for longer (2). Changes in the oral cavity due to ageing reflect changes throughout the rest of the body, such as loss of elasticity, decreased muscle tone and degradation of hard and soft tissues due to wear and tear. Healthcare of older patients is more complex due to the increased likelihood of medical diagnoses and prescription of medications.

Medicines are relevant to care of dental patients of any age for the following reasons:

- **Current and past medicines** may cause or influence the presentation of an oral health condition, cause oral side effects, alter the preparedness of a patient for a procedure, or influence the approach and outcome of the procedure.

- **Reactions to drugs taken in the past**, such as adverse and allergic reactions, inform current clinical decisions and treatment choices.
- **Medications used during treatment** may need to be tailored to the patient's co-morbidities and current pharmacotherapy.
- **Medicines prescribed after treatment is completed** may also need to be tailored to the patient's current functional status, co-morbidities and current medication in order to avoid drug interactions.

In addition, many age-related changes in physiology alter the pharmacokinetics and pharmacodynamics of medicines in older patients. For these reasons, the safe use of medicines in older dental patients is a special skill required by all dental professionals.

13.2 Who are 'the elderly'?

The age at which people are defined as 'elderly' or 'geriatric' is quite controversial as there is no widely accepted definition (3). Textbooks on geriatric medicine often describe people aged 65 years or more (over 50 years for Aboriginal and Torres Strait Islander peoples) as older, aged, geriatric or elderly but this convention was established in the 1950s when 65 years was the age at which many people retired.

Presently, many people aged 65 or older are still working and in good health, demonstrating how chronological age alone is not a reliable indicator of health or function (4).

If a specific age is required to define when age-related changes can alter patient care, then 75 years is often used in clinical practice. Always remember that the focus should be on age plus aspects of functional and physiological decline that together indicate clinically relevant aspects of ageing.

13.3 What is frailty and how is it relevant?

Healthy diet, regular exercise and conscientious hygiene have not only increased life expectancy in developed countries but also improved the likelihood that older people will remain active well into their later years. While this applies to many older people, others experience complex problems associated with disease, dependence and disability, requiring more frequent and attentive healthcare. 'Frailty' is a term used to describe this group, capturing their difference in health status.

Frailty is defined as 'a recognizable state of increased vulnerability amongst older patients resulting from age-associated decline in functional reserve, reducing their ability to maintain homeostasis and cope with acute stressors' (5). There are many methods for assessing frailty; the most popular is the Fried's Frailty Phenotype that consists of five components: weak grip strength, slow walking speed, unintentional weight loss (5% or more), exhaustion, and low physical activity (6, 9). Individuals are classified as robust, pre-frail, frail or most-frail depending on the number of components by which they are affected: zero, one or two, three, four or more respectively (9) (see Table 13.1).

Approximately 10% of people aged over 65 years are frail and this increases to as much as 50% for people aged over 85 (7). Between 73% and 85% of residents of aged care facilities have been assessed as being either frail or most-frail (8, 9).

Table 13.1 Fried's Frailty Phenotype and defining features. Based on (6).

Fried's Frailty Phenotype	Fried's defining features
Frail = when patient demonstrates three or more of these five features	Weak grip strength
	Slow walking speed
	Unintentional weight loss (5% or more)
	Exhaustion, low endurance
	Low physical activity

High prevalence of frailty is one of the main features that differentiates care of the elderly from care of the 'old-old'. The term is intended to identify people at greatest risk of adverse events, institutionalisation, hospitalisation and decreased life expectancy, and to recognise their higher care needs (9).

Dental professionals caring for the elderly, especially in aged care facilities, will frequently encounter frailty. Extra attention should be paid when assessing and treating these vulnerable patients, and even more so when considering prescription of medicines. For example, administration of standard doses of sedatives, such as benzodiazepines, to frail elderly patients can result in a state of acute confusion and delirium rather than sedation.

13.4 Medications for the elderly and risks of polypharmacy

Older people are increasingly living with complex healthcare needs, involving multiple chronic diseases managed with multiple medicines. The Australian Bureau of Statistics (ABS) National Health Survey in 2017–18 estimated that 47% of Australians had chronic health conditions. Of those people over 65 years, 29% had one chronic condition, just over 23% had two conditions, and 28% (1 million people) had three or more (10).

Older people have also been shown to take more medicines. The NPS MedicineWise Census of Medicines in 2012 found that 65% of Australians aged 75 years or more were taking at least one medicine regularly and 50% of those aged over 85 years were taking six or more medicines regularly (11). A study of the prevalence of continuous polypharmacy (i.e. five or more unique medicines for six months or more) showed that 6.1% of older Australians were affected (12). Rates 'were higher among women than men (36.6% versus 35.4%) and highest among those aged 80–84 years (43.9%) or 85–89 years (46.0%)' (12).

In addition, older people are enthusiastic users of complementary medicines. A study of over 10,000 healthy community-living Australians over 70 years of age found that 74.3% of respondents reported using complementary medicines daily or occasionally (13). These included fish oil (44.5%), glucosamine (26.7%) and calcium supplements (22.7%). The problem here is that complementary medicine contribute to polypharmacy (13).

Polypharmacy places older people at risk of harm from medication errors, adverse drug reactions (ADRs) and drug interactions and is associated with poor clinical outcomes, including geriatric syndromes such as falls, frailty, impaired cognition, constipation, urinary incontinence and more frequent hospitalisations (12, 14). As the number of medicines increases, so does the risk of non-adherence due to problems such as memory or vision impairment, poor manual dexterity, lack of interest and inability to obtain or afford medications (14).

13.5 The vital importance of an accurate medication history

A medication history is defined as an accurate recording of a patient's medicines. It comprises a list of all current medicines, including prescription and non-prescription medicines, complementary healthcare products and medicines used intermittently; recent changes to medicines; past history of ADRs including allergies; and recreational drug use (15).

A core competency of a prescriber is accurate documentation of the patient's medication history. This is even more important for older patients who are likely to have long medical histories involving multiple conditions and polypharmacy. Ensuring that past and current medicines are accurately documented is critical for safe prescribing for every patient, not just those in their later years. An accurate medication history provides deep insight into a person's medical history, medication-related issues, history of drug intolerances and provides an important foundation for future care planning.

A sample form is given in Figure 13.1.

Figure 13.1 Form for recording patient medications.

Please list any medications you may be taking (including herbal remedies, vitamins, supplements, cold/flu treatments, sleeping pills, pain relievers, injections, implants, etc.) so we can take appropriate precautions and avoid drug interactions.

Drug name	Dose	Duration of treatment	Purpose

Date_____   Signature_____

To collect all the necessary details for a medication history, the following steps should be taken:

1. Use a table with at least four columns that prompt the patient to provide the necessary details.
2. Document the patient's name, sex, date of birth, weight and frailty score.

3. Ask about regular medicines, including:
    - prescription medicines
    - medicines from a pharmacy or pharmacist
    - over-the-counter (OTC) medicines
    - medicines purchased online or by mail-order
    - vitamins, supplements, herbal remedies
    - inhalers and puffers
    - eyedrops, ear drops, nasal sprays
    - injections or implants
    - patches, dermatological preparations.

4. Ask about medicines taken as required, PRN or only occasionally, including:
    - prescription medicines
    - medicines from a pharmacy or pharmacist
    - OTC medicines
    - medicines purchased online or by mail-order
    - vitamins, supplements, herbal remedies
    - inhalers and puffers
    - eyedrops, ear drops, nasal sprays
    - injections or implants
    - patches, dermatological preparations.

5. Specifically ask about self-selected medicines, including:
    - sleeping tablets
    - indigestion/gastric reflux medicines
    - erectile or sexual dysfunction treatment
    - menopause treatment
    - hair loss or excess hair treatments
    - weight loss remedies.

6. Ask about social drugs that are easily neglected, including:
    - caffeine
    - alcohol
    - tobacco
    - marijuana
    - other recreational drugs (e.g. cocaine, amphetamines)

It is inadequate to only document the names of the patient's medicines. Each drug must have its generic and brand name, strength, formulation, dose taken and duration of treatment documented. A column can be added for the purpose of each drug if necessary. An example of a well-written, comprehensive medication history is in Table 13.2.

Several difficulties can arise when taking medication histories from older adults that make this task challenging. These include:

- communication problems due to impaired hearing and vision
- denial of medicine use due to health beliefs or cognitive impairment
- inaccuracy of medication recall due to memory impairment or confusion
- unfamiliarity with medicine names when responsibility is deferred to caregivers
- absence of medical records to confirm findings

Table 13.2 Sample medication history.

Patient name: Mrs Sample	DOB: 11/09/52		Date of this list
Drug name, strength and formulation	Dose	Duration	Purpose
Methotrexate 15mg tabs	1× weekly (on Mondays)	3 years	Rheumatoid arthritis
Prednisone 10mg tabs	1× morning	6 months	Rheumatoid arthritis
Folic acid 5mg tabs	1× weekly (on Tuesdays)	3 years	Rheumatoid arthritis
Mirtazapine 30mg tabs (Avanza)	1× bedtime	3 months	Depression
Irbesartan/hydrochlorothiazide 150mg/12.5mg tabs (Avapro)	1× morning	2 years	Hypertension
Paracetamol 665mg tabs (Panadol osteo)	1–2× tabs (up to 2–3× daily)	6 years	Pain management
Pregabalin 75mg caps (Lyrica)	1× bedtime	2 years	Pain management
Oxycodone SR 10mg tabs (Oxycontin)	1× twice daily	3 months	Pain management
Oxycodone 5mg tabs (Endone)	1× up to q6h PRN	12 months	Pain management
Rivaroxaban 20mg (Xarelto)	1× twice daily	1 month	Stroke prevention
Fish Oil triple strength caps 1500mg (Carusos)	1× daily	12 months	Non-specific benefit
Turmeric tabs (Fusion) 368mg	2× daily	6 months	Anti-inflammatory
Ibuprofen 200mg tabs ('Nurofen Zavance')	2× as required most days	10 years	Back pain to help sleep
Alcohol	1–2 wines with dinner every night	10 years	–
Smoking	Non-smoker	–	–
Caffeine	6–8 cups instant coffee per day	35 years	–

Despite these potential problems, health professionals should make every effort to collect medication history information from the patient or their carer. Reconciliation with other sources such as the patient's GP, their pharmacy or electronic health record (*My Health Record* in Australia) may be valuable. The importance of documenting the patient's use of non-prescription medicines and supplements cannot be overstressed, as these drugs may not only cause side effects but also interact with other drugs prescribed.

Patients and caregivers should be asked specifically about well-known risk factors for medication misadventure, such as treatment from multiple physicians with multiple medications or adherence problems due to impaired hearing, vision, and/or cognition, inability to open medication containers and/or swallowing difficulties.

The medication history should conclude with information about past allergic and adverse drug reactions (ADRs). It is preferable to document past reactions with plenty of detail (see Figure 13.2). Figure 13.2 presents information in three columns. It is inadequate to simply write 'Allergy: penicillin' or 'Ibuprofen: GI upset' as this does not provide enough detail to support clinical decision-making.

Figure 13.2 Form for documenting allergic and ADRs.

Please list any known allergies or adverse reactions to drugs (especially antibiotics e.g. penicillin), medicines, antiseptics, local anaesthetics, preservatives, etc. that we should know about.

Drug name	Nature of reaction	How long ago

Once a comprehensive medication history has been compiled, consider whether the patient's medicines have contributed to their presentation and what new treatments can be safely added and/or prescribed.

13.6 Medication compliance and adherence

It is often assumed that older patients comply poorly with their drug therapy; however, current evidence does not support this (20). Studies in Northern Ireland and Europe demonstrate that elderly patients are as adherent to their drug therapy as younger people, provided they want to take the medication and do not have confounding disease to adversely impact their adherence, such as dementia (14, 20). Nevertheless, medication non-adherence is associated with poor therapeutic outcomes, progression of disease, increased healthcare utilisation, and billions of dollars per year in avoidable direct healthcare costs.

Medication non-adherence can be divided into two broad categories: primary and secondary. Primary non-adherence occurs when a new medication is prescribed for a patient, but the medication is not dispensed or commenced within an acceptable period (16, 42). Secondary non-adherence is defined as a patient acquiring medication but not taking it as intended or prescribed (17).

Non-adherence can also be categorised according to the patient's intent to take the medication, known as intentional and unintentional non-adherence. These types of non-adherence are managed according to the underlying factors involved. Intentional non-adherence refers to the patient's deliberate action to avoid the medication, typically associated with their motivation, attitudes and beliefs. Unintentional non-adherence is driven by a lack of patient ability to access, remember or take their medication (17).

Dental professionals need to appreciate the different types of non-adherence as the key to resolving adherence issues is understanding the underlying causes—not all medication non-adherence is simply due to the patient forgetting to take it. Only by understanding why a patient is non-adherent can we find strategies to change behaviour, improve patient health and promote independent daily living. This understanding also increases the likelihood that medication prescribed by the dentist will be taken as recommended (18).

13.7 Effects of ageing on pharmacokinetics

Medication use in older adults is made even more challenging by the physiological changes that occur due to ageing. These changes alter how a drug works (pharmacodynamics) and the way it is handled by the body (pharmacokinetics). Prescribers need to be competent to prescribe medicines in a way that is considerate of these idiosyncrasies of older age.

Ageing affects almost every aspect of drug processing in the body. First, we consider pharmacokinetics, which is divided into four stages: absorption, distribution, metabolism and excretion (see Table 13.3 for a summary of these changes). Then, we examine the effects of ageing on pharmacodynamics, which are the pharmacological actions and effects of drugs.

13.7.1 Absorption

Many age-related changes to the gastrointestinal (GI) tract can influence the absorption of medicines. These include decreased gastric acid secretion, reduced GI motility, declining intestinal surface area, and reduced splanchnic blood flow (43). Despite these changes, oral absorption of most medicines is not significantly altered (43). Certain disease states and medications can alter drug absorption by changing the GI environment and older people are more likely to experience both (19).

For example, proton pump inhibitors (PPIs) such as esomeprazole (Nexium), are popular amongst older people for the treatment of gastroesophageal reflux. PPIs work by reducing gastric acid secretion, which, when reduced completely, is known as 'achlorhydria' and results in persistently elevated gastric pH. This can significantly alter bioavailability of drugs whose solubility and absorption relies on low gastric pH; for example, digoxin. PPIs can also reduce the absorption of nutrients from food and supplements: these include iron, calcium, magnesium and vitamin B12. An increasing proportion of iron deficiency anaemia is thought to be PPI-induced (41).

Antacid medications and mineral supplements containing magnesium, calcium and aluminium salts are commonly used by older patients. These can reduce oral absorption of other medications, such as bisphosphonates and tetracyclines, by chelating with them. Antacids work by neutralising the gastric acid they encounter, and only work for a very short period, so they do not alter gastric pH significantly.

Drugs that slow GI activity and prolong transit time can increase oral absorption of some drugs. An example of this is long-term use of opioids for persistent pain, which not only causes chronic constipation but can also cause increased absorption of certain drugs over time.

Swallowing difficulties are often experienced by older people, from dysphagia to oesophageal dysmotility, and can complicate administration and absorption of oral medications. Although switching from tablets and capsules to liquid formulations may seem like the obvious solution, it can sometimes make things worse by putting the patient at risk of aspiration of liquids, especially if they are often lying down. Therefore, consideration may need to be given to administering medicines by non-oral routes.

13.7.2 Firstpass metabolism

After absorption into the blood stream, drugs are transported by the portal circulation to the liver where many are extensively metabolised (sometimes up to 95%). This is called 'first pass metabolism' and can dramatically reduce oral bioavailability. Impaired first pass metabolism has been demonstrated in the elderly, where even minor reductions in first pass metabolism can lead to increased serum levels and clinical effects of these drugs (20).

13.7.3 Non-oral drug absorption

Absorption of drugs from non-oral routes, such as via the skin, can be affected by ageing. Decreased subcutaneous fat and increased keratinisation can prevent the passage of drugs through the skin. However, transdermal drug administration has several advantages over the oral route: it avoids gastrointestinal absorption and hepatic first-pass metabolism, minimises adverse effects arising from peak plasma drug concentrations, is non-invasive so carries no risk of infection and improves patient compliance (21). For elderly people, who are often on multiple oral medicines, transdermal drug delivery can be a useful route of administration to help reduce their medication burden. Transdermal patches are commonly used in clinical practice to treat Parkinson's disease, bladder dysfunction, persistent pain, and as hormone replacement therapy (21).

Administration of medicines via the respiratory tract using puffers and inhalers can be impaired due to weak grip strength, poor inhaler technique and difficulty coordinating actuation of the puffer with inhalation. Older people may also have insufficient respiratory strength to breathe in the drug when in powder form.

Problems with managing medicines and administering them correctly is a major reason why medicines for the elderly are increasingly formulated as long-lasting injections and implants to eliminate the need for daily consumption and improve adherence. Intramuscular injections are, however, often avoided in the elderly due to the loss of muscle mass from sarcopenia.

13.7.4 Distribution

Distribution is the pharmacokinetic step where drugs are delivered around the body and into various compartments. In general, ageing causes a relative decrease in total body water (TBW), reduced lean body mass, and a relative increase in percentage body fat. The relative increase in fat and decreased TBW in older people increases the volume of distribution of lipophilic drugs and decreases it for hydrophilic drugs.

The result is that water-soluble medications have higher serum concentrations in older people and lipid-soluble drugs have lower serum concentrations but prolonged tissue half-lives (20).

These effects are illustrated by what happens when an older patient takes a long-acting, fat-soluble drug such as diazepam. Diazepam has a long half-life, but its metabolites last even longer. This temporarily decreases diazepam serum levels but prolongs the half-life from an average of 20 hours in a younger person to >50 hours in an older person. With repeated dosing, diazepam accumulates throughout the body, leading to persistent drug effects, especially in the central nervous system. This can result in prolonged sedation, respiratory depression, and high risk of falls and fractures (22).

13.7.5 Metabolism

Metabolism of drugs occurs twice as they circulate around the body. First, when drugs travel through the gut and liver on their 'first pass' into the body; second, when the drugs return to the liver for elimination. As first pass metabolism is responsible for impeding some drugs' absorption, reduction of first pass metabolism can increase drug exposure and potential toxicity.

Age-related changes in the liver function significantly contribute to variable drug response in older people (46). Liver changes include reductions in liver mass, hepatic blood flow and decreased liver cell regeneration—all of which can reduce drug metabolism via Phase I or oxidative metabolism (i.e. via CYP enzymes); however, Phase II (conjugative) reactions (e.g. glucuronidation enzymes) are said to be preserved (45). Long-term fatty liver disease, hepatitis and cirrhosis all directly damage hepatocytes and will further complicate the liver's ability to metabolise and eliminate medications with age.

Overall, Phase I liver metabolism declines with age but Phase II stays relatively intact. So medications that rely on Phase 1 metabolism for their breakdown and clearance (check prescribing information for this detail) should be either avoided or used in lower doses in older patients (20–23).

13.7.6 Elimination

Drugs are eliminated from the body primarily by the liver or the kidneys. Age- and disease-related factors affecting drug elimination via the liver have been described in Section 13.7.5. In general, liver elimination of drugs is preserved in the elderly except in those with chronic liver disease (45). However, due to the decline in renal function that frequently accompanies ageing, alteration of drug dosing in renal impairment is an everyday consideration for elderly patients.

Nearly one in four older people who are prescribed medicines that are cleared by the kidneys are prescribed an excessive dose (24). Thus, one of the most important pharmacokinetic changes associated with ageing is decreased renal elimination of drugs (44).

As early as age 40, renal function, as measured by creatinine clearance, declines on average by 8 mL/min/1.73m^2 per decade. However, this varies substantially from person to person. Epidemiologic studies suggest that this decline is not so much from ageing itself but from long-term exposure to systemic hypertension, smoking, dyslipidaemia, diabetes, atherosclerotic disease, chronic inflammation and obesity (20, 25). Regardless, diminished kidney function is common in older patients potentially causing accumulation of renally excreted drugs.

The clinical implications of this depend on the extent to which renal elimination contributes to total elimination of the drug and the drug's therapeutic index (ratio of maximum tolerated dose to minimum effective dose) (44). For drugs that rely heavily on renal elimination, the dose should be lower and/or the frequency reduced (44). Examples of dental drugs that are renally eliminated include amoxicillin, cefalexin, codeine, morphine (from codeine) and oxycodone. Refer to Table 13.4 for guidance (25).

An accurate and readily available measure of renal function is the estimated glomerular filtration rate or 'eGFR', which is automatically calculated by the pathology companies using age, gender and serum creatinine level, and is reported in the frequently performed blood test called 'urea and electrolytes' (U&E). A normal eGFR reading is >90mL/min and significantly reduced renal function is defined as <60mL/min. Less than 60mL/min has been chosen by experts as the point where referral to a renal clinic or specialist should be considered.

As renal function is dynamic, only very recent results should be used to guide drug dosing. Renal function results more than one month old may be unreliable. Drug prescribing resources such as the *AMH Aged Care Companion* (26) or the *Australian Medicines Handbook* (28) can be consulted for instructions on reducing drug doses in line with the patient's current renal function.

Table 13.3 Effects of ageing on pharmacokinetics. Based on (6–8).

Pharmacokinetic step	Effect with ageing	Significance
Absorption	Unchanged GI absorption Increased transdermal absorption Reduced first pass metabolism	Same amount of oral medication absorbed Increased bioavailability of drugs subject to first pass metabolism
Distribution	Increased body fat Decreased body water Lower serum albumin in frail or unwell elderly	Prolonged half-life of fat-soluble drugs Increased serum concentrations of water-soluble drugs
Metabolism	Reduced oxidative metabolism Unchanged conjugative metabolism	Prolonged half-life and increased steady-state concentrations of drugs metabolised by oxidative metabolism
Elimination	Preserved liver elimination except in severe chronic liver disease Reduced renal blood flow, glomerular filtration rate and tubular secretion	Prolonged half-life and increased steady-state concentrations of renally eliminated drugs

Table 13.4 Age-related pharmacokinetic changes to drugs commonly used in dentistry. Based on (19–22, 39, 40).

Dental drug	Pharmacokinetic changes	Dosage change required
Antibiotics		
Amoxicillin	Prolonged half-life due to decreased renal elimination	Reduce dose or frequency if CrCl <30mL/min. Seek medical advice
Co-amoxiclav	Prolonged half-life due to declining renal elimination	Dosage reduction required if CrCl <30mL/min. Seek medical advice Patients with a history of penicillin-induced cholestatic hepatitis should not be prescribed co-amoxiclav Patients aged >55 years, or patients taking prolonged courses of >2 weeks are at increased risk of hepatitis
Cephalexin	Prolonged half-life due to decreased renal elimination	Reduce dose or frequency if CrCl <30mL/min. Seek medical advice
Clindamycin	Reduced Phase I metabolism, increased risk of nephrotoxicity	Due to the risk of acute kidney injury, clindamycin should be avoided by patients with kidney disease Seek medical advice regarding an alternative antibiotic Dosage interval should be prolonged in patients with moderate to severe hepatic impairment. Seek medical advice for patients with liver disease
Metronidazole	Liver metabolised, renal and liver excretion	Dose reduction or avoidance required for patients with severe liver disease or impairment. Seek medical advice
Phenoxymethylpenicillin	Prolonged half-life due to decreased renal elimination	Dose as per normal renal function
Analgesics		
Paracetamol	Liver metabolism preserved	Increased risk of liver damage in patients with chronic liver disease Seek medical advice
NSAIDs (e.g. ibuprofen and COX-2 inhibitors)	Reduced renal excretion and greater vulnerability to renal adverse effects	Avoid where possible in renal impairment. Seek medical advice Contraindicated in severe liver impairment. Seek medical advice for patients with liver disease Avoid completely in patients with heart failure or eGFR <60mL/min

Table 13.4 (cont.)

Dental drug	Pharmacokinetic changes	Dosage change required
Codeine/morphine	Reduced renal excretion of morphine and its active metabolites	Avoid use in renal impairment. Seek medical advice Dose reduction required in moderate to severe liver impairment. Seek medical advice For eGFR 30–60mL/min reduce dose by 25% and if <30mL/min reduce dose by 50%
Oxycodone	Reduced renal excretion	Dose reduction required in renal impairment. Seek medical advice Dose reduction required in moderate to severe liver impairment. Seek medical advice
Local anaesthetics		
All amide local anaesthetics	Metabolism and elimination preserved	No dosage change required in elderly as dental doses are small
Sedatives		
Diazepam	Reduced Phase I liver metabolism and renal excretion Prolonged half-life of active metabolites	Do not use diazepam in the elderly due to extremely long half-life
Lorazepam	Liver metabolism preserved, reduced renal excretion of glucuronide metabolites	Reduce usual adult dose by at least 50%
Oxazepam	Reduced renal excretion of glucuronide metabolites	Reduce usual adult dose by at least 50%
Temazepam	Reduced Phase I liver metabolism and renal excretion Prolonged half-life of active metabolites	Reduce usual adult dose by at least 50%

Note: CrCl: creatinine clearance.

13.8 Age-related changes in pharmacodynamics

Pharmacodynamics is defined as the response of the body to a drug. Older people often react to drugs differently than younger people due to their reduced ability to maintain physiological homeostasis in the presence of a drug and alterations in drug receptor numbers and sensitivity. The additional context of polypharmacy and multi-morbidity makes pharmacological treatment of older people different to treating younger patients, despite the use of a similar drug in similar doses and concentrations. Under-appreciation of the differences in older patients can contribute to inappropriate dosing, inadequate monitoring and increased risk of adverse drug reactions (ADRs) (22).

13.8.1 Altered drug receptor status

Many of the changes to pharmacodynamics in the elderly are due to altered drug receptor status, which include decreased receptor numbers, downregulation of receptor sensitivity, or decreased cellular response to receptor activation. A common example is decreased responsiveness to β-2 adrenoceptor agonists, such as salbutamol ('Ventolin') in the treatment of asthma and chronic obstructive pulmonary disease. β-2 receptors are fewer in number and have reduced sensitivity in older people, so standard doses of β-2 agonist medicines are less effective (19).

13.8.2 Increased risk of orthostatic hypotension

Reflex mechanisms that maintain homeostasis in the body are often impaired in the elderly. In particular, the baroreceptor reflex that induces vasoconstriction and reflex tachycardia in response to dropped blood pressure, such as that which occurs on standing up too quickly, is impaired. This results in a condition known as orthostatic hypotension (OH), which is a significant risk factor for falls and fractures. OH is often made worse by medicines that further impair homeostatic mechanisms or contribute to hypotension. Drugs that carry greater risk for OH include sedatives, tricyclic antidepressants, antihypertensives, sedating antihistamines and muscle relaxants (20). Dentists should consider that OH can occur when elderly patients arise from a supine position, such as from examination in the dental chair.

13.8.3 Increased risk of central nervous system effects

Older people are more sensitive to the sedative effects of medicines on the central nervous system (CNS) such as anxiolytics, opioid analgesics, antidepressants and muscle relaxants. This increased sensitivity is a result of structural and neurochemical changes in the CNS, including neuronal loss, increased permeability of the blood–brain barrier and depletion of central neurotransmitters (e.g. dopamine, acetylcholine and serotonin). As a result, older people are more susceptible to the sedation, cognitive impairment, mood- and respiratory-depressant effects of CNS-active drugs. Therefore, these drugs should be avoided as much as possible in this population and, if they are necessary, much lower doses should be used (20, 22).

13.8.4 Increased risk of anticholinergic burden

Older people are particularly sensitive to the anticholinergic effects of medicines. Many drugs such as tricyclic antidepressants, sedating antihistamines, antimuscarinic agents for bladder problems, some antipsychotic drugs, and many non-prescription sleep aids and cough/cold preparations contain anticholinergic drugs. Older adults, particularly those with cognitive impairment, are more prone to the adverse effects of such drugs and will become more confused, drowsy or delirious on these medicines (44). Anticholinergic drugs also commonly cause dry mouth, blurred vision, constipation, urinary retention (especially in older men with benign prostatic hyperplasia) and orthostatic hypotension (44). Therefore, older adults should avoid drugs with anticholinergic effects whenever possible (19, 29).

13.9 ADRs in the elderly and geriatric syndromes

It is recognised that ADRs occur more frequently in the elderly. Up to 30% of urgent hospital admissions for older adults are attributed to ADRs (24, 30). In high-income countries, approximately three times more ADRs are reported per million inhabitants per year in adults aged 65–74 years compared with adults aged 5–19 years (31).

Many factors contribute to older people's predisposition to ADRs: from the interaction of multimorbidity and polypharmacy, combined with renal and liver impairment causing prolonged drug half-lives and higher serum levels, to increased drug sensitivity. This is all in the context of decreased homeostasis, frailty, and general vulnerability (30, 31).

Geriatric syndromes and their management are also a frequent consideration in caring for the elderly. These syndromes involve a range of symptoms that are often regarded as an unavoidable consequence of ageing, but in reality they are often, avoidably, drug-induced. The five most common geriatric syndromes are pressure sores, incontinence, falls, functional decline, and delirium. Whenever these occur in the aged-care setting, the first consideration should be that they are drug-induced and the offending drug's dose reduced or removed altogether (32, 33).

A well-known adage in geriatric medicine is that 'any new symptom in an older patient should be considered a possible drug side effect until proven otherwise' (45). This is because, once recognised, a drug side effect can be reversible by stopping the offending prescription or lowering the dose (34).

13.10 Avoiding potentially inappropriate medicines

Medications are potentially inappropriate in the elderly when the risk of ADRs exceed the expected clinical benefit, even when better-tolerated alternatives are available (34). There are two well-known lists of potentially inappropriate medicines (PIMs) used in care of the elderly: the Beers Criteria (35, 36) and the STOPP START criteria (37).

STOPP (Screening Tool of Older Persons' Prescriptions) and START (Screening Tool to Alert to Right Treatment) are lists of criteria used to review potentially inappropriate medications in older adults. These criteria have been endorsed as a best practice by many organisations. Applying STOPP/START criteria improves clinical outcomes for older people on polypharmacy. Benzodiazepines, Z-drugs, antihistamines, anticholinergics, and cardiac glycosides are the common inappropriate medicines for geriatric patients. Table 13.5 lists drugs often prescribed by dentists that would be considered inappropriate for the elderly.

Table 13.5 Drugs used in dentistry that can be inappropriate for the elderly. Based on (35–37).

Potentially inappropriate medicines	Risk in the elderly
Anti-nauseants • cinnarizine • cyclizine • dimenhydrinate • diphenhydramine • prochlorperazine • metoclopramide • ondansetron	**CNS depression:** confusion, sedation, delirium, falls and fractures **Extra-pyramidal effects:** drug-induced parkinsonism, involuntary movements, dyskinesias **QT prolongation:** cardiac dysrhythmia
Benzodiazepines and Z-drugs • diazepam, oxazepam • lorazepam, midazolam, alprazolam, temazepam • zolpidem, zopiclone	**CNS depression:** confusion, delirium, depressed mood, respiratory depression **Muscle weakness:** increased risk of falls and fractures **Rebound anxiety and rebound insomnia** when each dose wears off
Sedating antihistamines • cinnarizine • cetirizine chlorpheniramine • cyproheptadine • dexchlorpheniramine • diphenhydramine • promethazine	**CNS depression:** sedation, confusion, delirium, depressed mood, respiratory depression **Muscle weakness:** increased risk of falls and fractures **QT prolongation** **Anticholinergic effects:** dry mouth, dry eyes, confusion, constipation, weight gain, delirium
NSAIDS: non-selective • diclofenac • ibuprofen • indomethacin • naproxen	Increased blood pressure Decreased renal function Fluid retention Aggravation of heart failure Risk of GI bleeding
NSAIDS, COX-2 selective • celecoxib • etoricoxib • meloxicam	Increased blood pressure Decreased renal function Fluid retention Aggravation of heart failure
Opioid analgesics • codeine • hydromorphone • morphine • oxycodone • tapentadol • tramadol	**CNS depression:** sedation, confusion, delirium, depressed mood, respiratory depression **Muscle weakness:** increased risk of falls and fractures **QT prolongation** **Anticholinergic effects:** dry mouth, dry eyes, confusion, constipation, weight gain, delirium

13.11 Safe prescribing for older patients

Prescribing for older patients presents unique challenges. Premarketing clinical trials often exclude geriatric patients, so recommended doses in the approved product information may not be appropriate for older adults (19). It is important for dental practitioners to pay close attention to the complexity of medication use in older patients.

Selection of drug treatment must be considerate of age-related issues and certain drugs should be avoided completely as they may be inappropriate in aged patients (see Tables 13.4 and 13.5). Be considerate of the added vulnerability of older patients to altered efficacy and increased risk of ADRs.

A golden rule for prescribing to older patients is 'Start low and go slow'. Start with low doses wherever possible (without compromising efficacy), escalate doses slowly and carefully titrate to the desired effect. Find out the patient's renal function and, if necessary, alter the medicine's dosage or frequency according to guidelines to take reduced renal function into account.

Always take time to assess the risk of drug–drug and drug–disease interactions as this population is more likely to have multiple medical conditions and be on other medications. If a considerable proportion of your patients are in their later years, it is worthwhile to invest in a drug reference such as the *AMH Aged Care Companion* (27) and consult a drug information service if you need help.

General principles that promote safe medication use by older people include:

- Non-medication treatments should be used wherever possible.
- Treat adequately to achieve goals of therapy.
- With new medications: start low and go slow. Increase slowly, checking for tolerability and response.
- Use the lowest effective maintenance dose.
- Prescribe the least number of medications, with the simplest dose regimens.
- Consider the patient's functional and cognitive ability when prescribing.
- Whenever there is a decline in physical or cognitive functions or self-care abilities, consider medication adverse effects as a possible cause.
- Prescribe formulations that are considerate of the patient's swallowing ability.
- Be familiar with common geriatric syndromes and the possibility that prescribing medicines may cause or exacerbate them.
- Avoid inappropriate drugs such as benzodiazepines, NSAIDs and opioids wherever possible. If they are necessary, start with the lowest dose possible and titrate slowly to affect.
- Provide patient education such as the Consumer Medicine Information or simple verbal and written instructions for each medication to reinforce adherence.
- Regularly review treatment and the patient's ability to manage the medications.
- Be considerate of all the medicines the patient uses, including prescription, non-prescription and complementary medicines (38).

FURTHER READING

Deutsch A, Jay E. Optimising oral health in frail older people. *Aust Prescr.* 2021;44:153–160. doi:10.18773/austprescr.2021.037

Hilmer SN, Gnjidic D. Prescribing for frail older people. *Aust Prescr.* 2017;40:174–178. doi:10.18773/austprescr.2017.055

Page A, Potter K, Naganathan V et al. Polypharmacy and medicine regimens in older adults in residential aged care. *Arch Geront Geriatrics.* 2023;105. doi:10.1016/j.archger.2022.104849

REFERENCES

1. Australian Bureau of Statistics. *Twenty years of population change*. 2020. Accessed April 20, 2022. https://www.abs.gov.au/articles/twenty-years-population-change#ageing-population

2. Australian Institute of Health and Welfare, Dental Statistics and Research Unit. *Oral Health and Access to Dental Care—Older Adults in Australia*. Research Report. November 2000. https://www.aihw.gov.au/getmedia/9fa75681-9f85-4b0e-b0b7-a612802e241e/den-72-report-11.pdf.aspx?inline=true

3. Singh S, Bajorek B. Defining 'elderly' in clinical practice guidelines for pharmacotherapy. *Pharmacy Practice*. 2014;12(4):489.

4. Hekmat-panah J. "Elderly"—an outdated and potentially harmful term. *BMJ*. 2019;Opinion March 1.

5. Xue, Qian-Li. The frailty syndrome: definition and natural history. *Clinics in Geriatric Medicine*. 2011;27(1):1–15. PMC3028599

6. Bieniek J, Wilczyński K, Szewieczek J. Fried frailty phenotype assessment components as applied to geriatric inpatients. *Clin Interv Aging*. 2016;11:453–459. doi:10.2147/CIA.S101369

7. Turner G. Fit for Frailty—Introduction to Frailty. Part 1. *British Geriatrics Society*. 2014. https://www.bgs.org.uk/resources/introduction-to-frailty

8. Jadczak AD, Robson L, Cooper T et al. The Frailty In Residential Sector over Time (FIRST) study: methods and baseline cohort description. *BMC Geriatr*. 2021;21:99. doi:10.1186/s12877-020-01974-1

9. Alves S, Teixeira L, Ribeiro O, Paúl C. Examining Frailty Phenotype Dimensions in the Oldest Old. *Frontiers in Psycholog*. 2020;11(9).

10. Australian Bureau of Statistics. *National Health Survey: first results, 2017–18, Australia*. 2018. Accessed April 22, 2022. https://www.abs.gov.au/statistics/health/health-conditions-and-risks/national-health-survey-first-results/latest-release

11. Morgan TK, Williamson M, Pirotta M et al. A national census of medicines use: a 24-hour snapshot of Australians aged 50 years and older. *Med J Aust*. 2012;196(1):50–53. doi:10.5694/mja11.10698

12. Page AT, Falster MO, Litchfield M et al. Polypharmacy among older Australians, 2006–2017: a population-based study. *Med J Aust*. 2019;211(2):71–75. doi:10.5694/mja2.5024

13. Lefevre A, Hopper I, McNeil J et al. Complementary medicine use by community-dwelling older Australians. *Med J Aust*. 2021;214(3):140–141. doi:10.5694/mja2.50884

14. Khairullah A, Platt B, Chater RW. Medication nonadherence in older adults: patient engagement solutions and pharmacist impact. *Pharmacy Times*. November 7, 2018. Accessed April 29, 2022. https://www.pharmacytimes.com/view/medication-nonadherence-in-older-adults-patient-engagement-solutions-and-pharmacist-impact

15. Australian Commission on Safety and Quality in Healthcare. *Documentation of patient Information*. Accessed April 29, 2022. https://www.safetyandquality.gov.au/standards/nsqhs-standards/medication-safety-standard/documentation-patient-information

16. Tamblyn R, Eguale T, Huang A et al. The incidence and determinants of primary nonadherence with prescribed medication in primary care: a cohort study. *Ann Intern Med*. 2014;160(7):441–450. doi:10.7326/M13-1705

17. Raebel MA, Schmittdiel J, Karter AJ et al. Standardizing terminology and definitions of medication adherence and persistence in research employing electronic databases. *Med Care*. 2013;51(8 Suppl 3):S11–S21. doi:10.1097/MLR.0b013e31829b1d2a

18. Molloy GJ, Messerli-Bürgy N, Hutton G, Wikman A, Perkins-Porras L, Steptoe A. Intentional and unintentional non-adherence to medications following an acute coronary

syndrome: A longitudinal study. *Journal of Psychosomatic Research.* 2014;76(5):430–432. doi:10.1016/j.jpsychores.2014.02.007

19. Sansom L. (ed.) *Australian Pharmaceutical Formulary and Handbook. Medicines in Older People.* Pharmaceutical Society of Australia; 2018.

20. Shetty HGM, Woodhouse K. Geriatrics. In Walker R, Whittlesea C (eds). *Clinical Pharmacy and Therapeutics.* 4th edition. Elsevier; 2007.

21. Kaestli LZ, Wasilewski-Rasca AF, Bonnabry P, Vogt-Ferrier N. Use of transdermal drug formulations in the elderly. *Drugs Aging.* 2008;25(4):269–280.

22. Holbeach E. Prescribing in the Elderly. *Australian Family Physician.* 2010;39(10):728–733.

23. Pea F. Pharmacokinetics and drug metabolism of antibiotics in the elderly. *Exp Opin Drug Metab.* 2018;14(10):1087–1100.

24. Pharmaceutical Society of Australia. *Medicine Safety: Take care.* Canberra PSA; 2019. https://www.psa.org.au/wp-content/uploads/2019/01/PSA-Medicine-Safety-Report.pdf

25. Weinstein JR, Anderson S. The aging kidney: physiological changes. *Adv Chronic Kidney Dis.* 2010;17(4):302–307.

26. Editorial Advisory Committee. *AMH Aged Care Companion.* Australian Medicines Handbook Pty Ltd; April 2023.

27. Ouanounou A, Haas DA. Pharmacotherapy for the elderly dental patient. *J Can Dent Assoc.* 2015;80:f18.

28. Rossi S. (ed.) *Australian Medicines Handbook.* AMH Pty Ltd; 2023.

29. NPS MedicineWise. *Anticholinergic burden: the unintended consequences for older people.* 2022. https://www.nps.org.au/professionals/anticholinergic-burden#hp

30. Pedros C, Formiga F, Corbella X, Arnau J. Adverse drug reactions leading to urgent hospital admission in an elderly population: prevalence and main features. *Eur J Clin Pharmacol.* 2016;72(2):219–226.

31. Aagaard L, Strandell J, Melskens L, Petersen PS, Holme HE. Global patterns of adverse drug reactions over a decade: analyses of spontaneous reports to VigiBase™. *Drug Saf.* 2012;35(12):1171–1182.

32. Brown-O'Hara T. Geriatric syndromes and their implications for nursing. *Nursing.* Jan 2013;4391:1–3.

33. Sanford AM, Morley JE, Berg-Weger M et al. High prevalence of geriatric syndromes in older adults. *PLoS ONE.* 2020;15(6):e0233857. doi:10.1371/journal.pone.0233857

34. Avorn J, Shrank WH. Adverse Drug Reactions in Elderly People: A substantial cause of preventable illness. *BMJ.* 2008;336(7650):956–957. doi:10.1136/bmj.39520.671053.94

35. Fixen DR. *AGS Beers Criteria for Older Adults.* Pharmacy Today; November 2019.

36. American Geriatrics Society. 2019 Updated AGS Beers Criteria® for potentially Inappropriate Medication Use in Older Adults. *J Am Geriatric Soc.* 2019;Apr (6794):674–694.

37. O'Mahony D, O'Sullivan D, Byrne S, O'Connor MN, Ryan C, Gallagher P. STOPP/START criteria for potentially inappropriate prescribing in older people: Version 2. *Age Ageing.* 2015;44(2):213–218. doi:10.1093/ageing/afu145

38. Royal Australian College of General Practitioners. *RACGP Aged Care Clinical Guide (Silver Book).* 5th edition. 2019. https://www.racgp.org.au/clinical-resources/clinical-guidelines/key-racgp-guidelines/view-all-racgp-guidelines/silver-book/part-a/medication-management

39. Ashley C, Dunleavy A. *The Renal Drug Handbook.* CRC Press; 2018.

40. Editorial Advisory Committee. *Australian Medicines Handbook.* AMH Pty Ltd; 2022.

41. Tran-Duy A, Connell NJ, Vanmolkot FH et al. Use of proton-pump inhibitors and risk of iron deficiency: a population-based case-control study. *J Int Medicine.* 2019;285(2):205–214.

42. Laius O, Pisarev H, Volmer D, Kõks S, Märtson A, Maasalu K. Use of a national database as a tool to identify primary medication non-adherence: The Estonian ePrescription system. *Research in Social and Administrative Pharmacy.* 2018;14(8):776–783.

43. Lee HC, Huang KTL, Shen WK. Use of antiarrhythmic drugs in elderly patients. *J Geriatr Cardiol.* 2011;8(3):184–194. doi:10.3724/SP.J.1263.2011.00184

44. Ruscin JM, Linnebur SA. *Pharmacokinetics in Older Adults.* MSD Manual. 2021. https://www.msdmanuals.com/professional/geriatrics/drug-therapy-in-older-adults/pharmacokinetics-in-older-adults?query=pharmacokinetics4

45. Avom J, Shrank WH, Spinewine A. Adverse Drug Reactions in Elderly People. *BMJ.* 2008;336(7650):956–957.

46. Jansen PL. Liver disease in the elderly. *Best Pract Res Clin Gastroenterol.* 2002;16(1):149–158. doi:10.1053/bega.2002.0271

DRUGS IN PREGNANCY AND LACTATION

14

KEY POINTS

- The safety of drugs in pregnancy varies depending on the stage of pregnancy the exposure occurs.
- The two main considerations regarding drugs in pregnancy are the effect of the drugs on the mother and fetus, and the effect of the pregnancy on the pharmacokinetics of the drug.
- The traditional alphabetical categories of drug safety in pregnancy are oversimplified and are being abandoned for systems that fully explain the safety issues.
- The safety of drugs in lactation is determined by the degree to which the drug distributes into breastmilk, its possible adverse effects, its oral bioavailability and to what extent exposure can be reduced by juggling feeds around the dose.
- The final decision of whether to use a medicine during pregnancy or lactation should be evidence-based and made by the pregnant woman in consultation with health professionals.

14.1 Introduction

Dental practitioners are often faced with questions about the safety of dental interventions during pregnancy and breastfeeding. Questions often focus on the safety of the drugs involved, such as local anaesthetics, sedatives, analgesics, fluoride and antibiotics. Despite the general wisdom that it is best to avoid all drugs during pregnancy and lactation, situations do arise where drug treatment is unavoidable. Therefore, it is necessary that dental professionals competently address these queries with up to date, accurate and evidence-based advice or appropriate referral to expert resources. This chapter addresses the common areas of concern for pregnant and breastfeeding women relating to drugs used in dental practice.

14.2 Drugs in pregnancy

The use of drugs for dental treatment of pregnant women is common. These drugs may interact with other drugs the patient is taking, as most women take at least one form of medication during pregnancy—the average number ranging from 1.2 to 3.2 (1, 2). Medical indications for drug use in pregnancy range from chronic illness, such as epilepsy or depression, to problems associated with pregnancy, such as urinary tract infections, musculoskeletal pain, and gastrointestinal complaints. Therefore, careful attention to the safety of dental drugs in pregnancy is critical.

14.2.1 Pregnancy stages

The gestation period of human pregnancy is approximately 40 weeks from the last menstrual period (38 weeks post-conception) and conventionally divided into the first, second and third trimesters, each lasting thee calendar months. Even though this model of pregnancy is convenient and easy to follow, it is not the most appropriate for assessing drug safety in pregnancy. The approach used in the medical literature expresses drug exposure in terms of stages of fetal development (3).

Conception is the first step in the biological process that leads to pregnancy and is defined as the point at which sperm and ovum are united and fertilisation takes place. The three stages of fetal development thereafter are:

- **The pre-embryonic stage** is the first 17 days post-conception and involves implantation of the fertilised ovum.
- **The embryonic stage** takes place from days 18–56, when the major organs systems are formed.
- **The fetal stage** (weeks 8–38) involves maturation, development, and growth of the fetus.

14.2.2 Placental drug transfer

Most drugs diffuse easily across the placenta and enter the fetal circulation to some extent. However, specific drug characteristics limit placental transfer, including molecular size, lipid solubility and degree of ionisation. Small drugs with a molecular weight of <500 Da, such as amoxicillin or ibuprofen, cross the placenta easily but larger molecules with a molecular weight >1000 Da, such as insulin, have negligible transfer (4). Lipophilic, unionised drugs such as benzodiazepines readily cross the placenta but hydrophilic ionised drugs such as local anaesthetics do not. Weakly basic lipophilic drugs, such as opioids, not only diffuse across the placenta but also can become 'trapped' in the fetal circulation due to their slightly lower pH than maternal plasma (3). Drug transporters and enzymes present in the placenta also influence drug transfer. Despite this knowledge, the extent of placental drug transfer is seldom employed to evaluate drug safety during pregnancy. Knowledge of the drug's pharmacological and toxic effects on the mother and fetus, as well as experience of the drug's use during all stages of pregnancy, is more important (3–7).

14.2.3 Considerations of drugs in pregnancy

Ideally, all unnecessary drug therapy should cease prior to conception. However, as approximately half of all pregnancies are unplanned, inadvertent drug exposure frequently occurs (4). Therefore, it is important to make careful and informed choices when prescribing for women of childbearing age who are potentially pregnant.

It should be remembered that drugs are never tested in pregnant humans due to the safety and ethical problems of such experimentation. Therefore, data on drug safety in pregnancy is gathered from the experience of women who have taken medicines either by accident or deliberately during pregnancy, and the data collected by clinicians working in obstetrics and published or collated into registries that compare the outcomes with matched controls (6, 7).

The two major issues to consider regarding drug use in pregnancy are: first, the effect of the drug on the pregnancy, the mother, the fetus, or the neonate: and second, the influence of the pregnancy on the pharmacokinetics of the drug.

When evaluating the effects of a drug on pregnancy, there are two further considerations. First is whether the drug is teratogenic, especially in early pregnancy. All pregnancies have a 3–5% chance of a birth defect (5). This is called the 'background risk'. Teratogenic risk associated with drug exposure should therefore be expressed in relation to this background risk. In other words, for a birth defect to be considered drug-related, the frequency with which it occurs needs to be greater than the background risk (27). Second, one should consider the potential adverse pharmacological effects of the drug on the mother or fetus, as opposed to its teratogenicity.

There are only a few known teratogens, examples of which are listed below (4). For a drug to be classified as a teratogen, the criteria are:

1. being present in fetal circulation at the critical time of the affected body part or system's development
2. a repeated pattern of reported abnormalities
3. likely pharmacological mechanisms for the malformation (7)

The establishment of pregnancy registries and databases operated by the worldwide Organization of Teratology Information Specialists and others document reports of drug exposures during pregnancy and compare the outcomes with case-matched controls. This has significantly strengthened the evidence on which these associations are made (6).

Some well-established teratogens are:

- alcohol/ethanol
- carbamazepine
- fluconazole
- lithium
- methotrexate
- sodium valproate
- testosterone and other anabolic steroids
- vitamin A and its derivatives (e.g. isotretinoin)
- warfarin (8, 9)

Drug use during the first trimester, especially during the embryonic stage, carries the greatest risk of malformations as this is when fetal organs are being formed. Congenital defects such as spina bifida and hydrocephalus are increasingly being detected prior to birth through high-resolution imaging and may even be remedied *in utero*. However, most fetal anomalies are detected at birth and others may take many years to be identified, such as the behavioural and intellectual disorders associated with fetal exposure to alcohol (4, 5, 7).

14.2.4 Adverse pharmacological effects

Drugs ingested by the mother may adversely affect the developing fetus due to the pharmacological effects, without causing malformation. For example, high doses of corticosteroids (>10mg prednisolone daily) can cause fetal adrenal suppression. Benzodiazepines taken by the mother can linger in the baby's circulation causing 'floppy infant syndrome' and benzodiazepine withdrawal effects in the baby after it is delivered (6–8).

14.2.5 Timing of drug exposure

The stage of pregnancy at which a drug is administered contributes significantly to the likelihood, severity, and nature of adverse effects on the fetus. Of note, drug exposure during the pre-embryonic stage is understood to undergo an 'all or nothing' effect, in that any damage to the embryo incurred by drug exposure at this critical time leads either to death of the embryo or complete recovery without residual harm (4, 6). Malformations from drugs taken at this stage are considered unlikely unless the drug has a long enough half-life to extend into the embryonic stage.

Organogenesis mostly takes place during the embryonic stage and, except for certain aspects of the brain, eyes, teeth, external genitalia and ears, formation is largely complete by the end of the tenth week (3). Exposure to drugs during the embryonic stage represents the greatest risk for major malformation and forms the basis for the general principle of avoiding or minimising all drug use during the first trimester. If a careful risk–benefit assessment has been undertaken, however, even known teratogens may be used in the second and third trimesters once organogenesis is complete.

In the fetal stage, drugs continue to have their potential adverse effects on the fetus. NSAIDs, such as ibuprofen, impair prostaglandin production which can increase risk of miscarriage if taken early in pregnancy, and are associated with premature closure of the fetal ductus arteriosus, fetal renal impairment, and delay of labour and birth if taken in the third trimester (8).

14.2.6 Pharmacokinetic changes

During pregnancy, women experience weight gain, blood volume expansion and increased total body water and fat. Liver metabolism of many drugs is increased during pregnancy and, combined with increased renal excretion, drugs may be cleared more quickly (4). These factors alter the distribution of drugs around a pregnant woman's body and may require increased loading and maintenance doses and altered frequency.

Despite this, the dose of any drug should remain as low as possible to minimise the risk of adverse effects to the mother or fetus. Therefore, it is recommended that clinicians start with the usual effective dose of the medicine, providing the drug is safe is pregnancy, and seek expert assistance if there are concerns about the efficacy of the dose.

14.2.7 Drug selection

There are few drugs, if any, for which safety in pregnancy can be assured. Conversely, only a handful of drugs used in pregnancy have been shown conclusively to be teratogenic. The most cautious approach is for prescribers to select drugs that have been used extensively by large numbers of pregnant women without reported or apparent problems. These drugs should be prescribed in preference to newer drugs for which there is less experience. For example, the drug of choice for treating hypertension in pregnancy is methyldopa due to its long history of safe use in pregnancy, even though it is rarely used to treat hypertension in non-pregnant people.

Table 14.1 Definitions of the Australian categories for prescribing medicines in pregnancy (9).

Pregnancy category	Definition
Category A	Drugs which have been taken by a large number of pregnant women and women of childbearing age without any proven increase in the frequency of malformations or other direct or indirect harmful effects on the fetus having been observed
Category B1	Drugs which have been taken by only a limited number of pregnant women and women of childbearing age without an increase in the frequency of malformation or other direct or indirect harmful effects on the human fetus having been observed Studies in animals have not shown evidence of an increased occurrence of fetal damage
Category B2	Drugs which have been taken by only a limited number of pregnant women and women of childbearing age, without an increase in the frequency of malformation or other direct or indirect harmful effects on the human fetus having been observed Studies in animals are inadequate or may be lacking, but available data show no evidence of an increased occurrence of fetal damage
Category B3	Drugs which have been taken by only a limited number of pregnant women and women of childbearing age without an increase in the frequency of malformation or other direct or indirect harmful effects on the human fetus having been observed Studies in animals have shown evidence of an increased occurrence of fetal damage, the significance of which is considered uncertain in humans
Category C	Drugs which, owing to their pharmacological effects, have caused or may be suspected of causing, harmful effects on the human fetus or neonate without causing malformations. These effects may be reversible. Accompanying texts should be consulted for further details
Category D	Drugs which have caused, are suspected to have caused, or may be expected to cause an increased incidence of human fetal malformations or irreversible damage. These drugs may also have adverse pharmacological effects. Accompanying texts should be consulted for further details
Category X	Drugs which have such a high risk of causing permanent damage to the fetus that they should not be used in pregnancy or when there is a possibility of pregnancy

14.2.8 Strengths and weaknesses of alphabetical classification

After the thalidomide tragedy in the 1960s, a system for classifying the safety of drugs in pregnancy using letters of the alphabet was developed by the Federal Drug Administration (FDA) in the US. This was modified by the Australian Drug Evaluation Committee in the late 1980s who published an Australian version of the Risk of Drugs in Pregnancy Categorisation (A, B1, B2, B3, C, D, X) in 1989 (see Table 14.1.)

This alphabetical system has been simple to understand and easy to find in prescribing guides, so has been widely used by professionals and consumers. However, concerns have been raised in recent years that it dangerously oversimplifies the safety issues in pregnancy, which can lead to misinterpretation of risk (5).

The first problem is the alphabetical nature of the A–X categorisation incorrectly implies that there is a hierarchy of risk, with Category A being the safest, Category C being 'worse' than Category B, etc., which is not the case. Category D drugs carry a higher risk of adverse effects but can be taken in pregnancy as long the risks are managed and the benefits outweigh the risks.

These categories have also led to the incorrect assumption that medicines within the same category carry the same level of risk in pregnancy. For example, the anticonvulsants lamotrigine ('lamictal') and sodium valproate ('epilim') are both Category D drugs, but valproate carries much greater teratogenic potential than lamotrigine (2).

The most relevant issue for dental practitioners is that the categorisation makes little allowance for different doses, route of administration or contexts of use. For example, the tiny doses of local anaesthetic used in dentistry are not differentiated from very large doses used in orthopaedic surgery. Minimal exposure from topical administration of a drug is not differentiated from the same drug given systemically. Notably, fluconazole is a drug that has different classifications for different doses. The single oral dose of fluconazole used for vaginal candidiasis is not considered teratogenic so is classified Category A; however, multi-dosed oral or intravenous fluconazole is associated with craniofacial and skeletal malformations so is classified Category D.

Most importantly, the alphabetical categories rarely differentiate the safety of drug by the stage of pregnancy in which it is taken; for example, tetracyclines are given a Category D listing, but they only cause tooth discoloration if taken after 18 weeks of pregnancy and often cause unnecessary concern for first-trimester exposure (5, 8).

Categories B1–B3 relate to safety data from animal testing. However, these statements can be alarming and are not very instructive as animal data may not translate to humans. After all, thalidomide did not cause adverse pregnancy outcomes in several animal species (10). It should be noted that product information from sponsors and manufacturers often give a recommendation such as 'Do not use in pregnancy unless the benefits outweigh the risks' which is reasonable from a medico-legal perspective but offers little in terms of risk assessment. It is recommended that safety information of drugs in pregnancy is sought from other resources, such as drugs in pregnancy databases, textbooks, the *Australian Medicines Handbook* or expert advisers.

14.2.9 How is advice on drugs in pregnancy changing?

Problems with the alphabetical pregnancy categories are so well recognised that many countries have been phasing them out and replacing them with advice in narrative format. In the US, the FDA started phasing out the alphabetical system from July 2016 (11). The new system of classification provides detail on the risks of each drug as it relates to fertility, each separate trimester of pregnancy, postnatal issues, and lactation (12). To see how the new rating system works in the US, see www.drugs.com. A similar system is to be gradually introduced in Australia over the coming years by the Therapeutic Goods Administration (TGA).

14.2.10 Questions to ask regarding drugs in pregnancy

When investigating the safety of a drug in pregnancy, dentists should ask the following questions:

- **How long has the patient been pregnant?** Safety of a drug depends on the stage of pregnancy, including the antenatal and postnatal periods. If the patient is pregnant, check whether her gestation is calculated from the date of first missed period or from conception.
- **What is the drug and dosing schedule?** Commonly used antibiotics, local anaesthetics and analgesics in dentistry pose little risk to a pregnant patient.
- **What do a range of resources say about safety in pregnancy?** Don't just read the product information, consult widely.
- **Could a safer or non-pharmacological treatment be found?** Consider whether treatment could be delayed until the pregnany, or at least the first trimester, is complete.

See Table 14.2 for recommendations of drugs commonly used in pregnancy and when breastfeeding.

Medication use in pregnancy should be guided by the principle that the potential benefits outweigh the potential risks. When investigating the safety of drugs in pregnancy, do not rely solely on the A, B, C, D and X categories. Consult widely, see what the studies say, and determine whether the drug doses and routes of administration match those in your patient's situation. The bottom line is that most drugs used in dentistry are low risk in pregnancy.

14.3 Drugs in lactation

Safe medication use during breastfeeding is important, as approximately 50% of Australian women breastfeed their babies for at least 6 months and women often seek medical or dental care during the postpartum period (12–14). One Dutch study found that 66% of breastfeeding women used some form of medicine on a limited or long-term basis while breastfeeding (15).

Unfortunately, many mothers are inappropriately advised to avoid taking medications during breastfeeding or to interrupt/discontinue breastfeeding because of fears of adverse effects on the breastfed infant (16, 17). This cautious approach is often unnecessary because only a small range of medications are truly contraindicated during lactation or associated with adverse effects on the infant. For these reasons, accurate information about the extent of excretion for a particular drug into human milk and the effects on the infant and the mother is greatly needed (17).

When researching the safety of medicines in breastfeeding, it is important to recognise that a safety classification like that used for drugs in pregnancy (Categories A, B, C, D and X) has not been created. Obviously, the pregnancy categories do not apply to drug use in lactation (14, 16).

When considering drug treatment for a breastfeeding woman, it is worth emphasising that this is a challenging time for most new mothers who are seeking accurate and authoritative advice on their healthcare. The patient may be unwell, sleep-deprived and emotionally drained as she is feeding and caring for a dependent newborn child and perhaps other children as well. It is important to avoid medicines such as sedatives, which have adverse effects that may compromise the mother's ability to care for her baby. Tiny amounts of sedative might be tolerable for the newborn infant via breastmilk but are best avoided by a breastfeeding mother as she often cannot sleep off the sedative effect overnight due to the baby's feeding demands, and will likely cause her to experience lingering sedation and impairment the next day.

14.3.1 Guiding principles of safe drug use in breastfeeding

To weigh up the risks and benefits of taking medication during breastfeeding, clinicians need to consider multiple factors:

- the need for the drug by the mother
- the risk of adverse effects on the mother and her ability to care for her baby
- the potential effects of the drug on breastmilk production
- the amount of drug excreted into breastmilk
- the extent of oral absorption of the drug by the breastfed infant
- the potential for adverse drug effects on the breastfed infant

Not all drugs distribute into breastmilk. Even those that do pass into breastmilk rarely build up to clinically significant amounts. As a rule, the amount of drug received by the breastfed infant is usually less than 10% of the maternal dose (17, 18). Determining whether this amount of drug would be tolerable for the baby must be assessed on a case-by-case basis.

Transfer of a drug into the breastmilk is governed by its chemical characteristics. Drugs more likely to pass into breastmilk have low ionisation, low molecular weight (<200 Da), low volume of distribution, low maternal serum protein binding and high lipid solubility (18). For example, a drug that does not pass easily into breastmilk is heparin, whose molecular weight of 3000–30,000 Da prevents it from passing through the small pores in the mammary epithelium (3, 17).

Even if drugs do distribute into breastmilk, and they are not eliminated in a feed, they will distribute back into the mother's circulation, the timing of which is determined by the drug's half-life. Drugs with short half-lives, such as inhaled anaesthetics and ultra-short-acting sedatives, will distribute in and out of milk very quickly, so breastfeeding may be resumed shortly after use (17). However, drugs with long half-lives (e.g. >12 hours) and active metabolites will persist in milk and accumulate with repeated dosing (20).

14.3.2 What testing is conducted for drugs in breastfeeding?

Unlike in pregnancy, clinical testing of drugs in lactation is often conducted to determine how much of each drug passes into breastmilk, when peak breastmilk concentrations occur, and the ratio of milk/plasma concentrations, which determines whether the drug is favouring milk or plasma (17). Knowing when peak drug concentrations occur in breast milk allows the mother to schedule her breastfeeding to minimise the infant's drug exposure. This is best done by avoiding peak milk levels, which is usually within 1–2 hours of the dose, and coinciding with the time drug levels are lowest in breastmilk, which is just before the next dose (17) (see Section 14.3.4).

Human data is not available for all drugs in lactation and may be limited to animal data only. As in pregnancy, these data should be viewed sceptically as they may not correlate with human experience (3, 17). Note that manufacturers' product information will invariably discourage use in lactation if human data is unavailable, but this advice may not be accurate and may not concur with medical advice.

14.3.3 Is the drug safe for the baby?

A handy rule of thumb is that if a drug is already used safely directly in infants, then it will also be safe in breastfeeding, since the amount delivered via breast milk is unlikely to exceed the normal neonatal/paediatric dose (6). For example, amoxicillin is frequently used to treat infections in neonates, so is therefore considered safe in breastfeeding. Of course, monitoring for potential side effects of a drug such as gastrointestinal upset or candida infection in both mother and infant must still be maintained.

Even if some of the drug is consumed by the nursing infant, only orally active drugs need to be considered, as drugs with little or no oral bioavailability, such as local anaesthetics and nitrous oxide, will have no systemic effects on the baby (17).

14.3.4 Reducing infant exposure—juggling feeds

Another strategy often recommended for reducing infant exposure to substances ingested by the breastfeeding mother is to feed the baby first, then give the maternal dose immediately afterward. This technique works well if the baby doesn't feed for the next 3–4 hours, during which time the mother's medication will be absorbed, distribute into her milk, reach peak milk concentrations, and then decline to less significant concentrations by the time the next feed is due. (Peak breast milk concentrations generally occur at the same time as peak plasma concentrations.) This tactic is only practical for babies who feed every 3–4 hours, and if the drug has a short half-life (e.g. 0.5–2 hours), so must be applied judiciously.

Other methods for reducing infant drug exposure include using drugs with a once daily dosing regimen and administering that dose at night time to coincide with the time it is more likely the baby will sleep through peak milk concentrations. In addition, consideration should be given to using topical instead of systemic routes of drug administration, such as topical steroid creams or nasal decongestants instead of tablets, to minimise systemic concentrations.

14.4 Recommendations for drugs commonly used in dentistry during pregnancy and breastfeeding

Recommendations have been gathered from a wide range of expert resources on drug safety in both pregnancy and lactation and summarised in Table 14.2 for drugs commonly used in dentistry. Where specific published research has been used, separate references are cited within the table.

Table 14.2 Recommendations for drugs commonly used in dentistry during pregnancy and breastfeeding. Based on 7, 8, 19, 21, 23, 24–26.

Drugs used commonly in dentistry	Safety in pregnancy	Safety in breastfeeding
NSAIDS (non-selective) diclofenac ibuprofen indomethacin naproxen	Best avoided throughout pregnancy. Use in first trimester may increase risk of miscarriage and, in the third trimester, premature closure of patent ductus	Non-selective NSAIDs are safe to use
COX-2 inhibitors celecoxib etoricoxib meloxicam	Best avoided throughout pregnancy, especially in first and third trimesters as per non-selective NSAIDs	Selective NSAIDs (COX–2 inhibitors) have limited data but appear safe
Paracetamol	Safe throughout pregnancy	Safe in breastfeeding
Opioids codeine hydromorphone morphine oxycodone tapentadol tramadol	Opioids may be used during pregnancy; however, lowest dose for shortest period is advised. May cause respiratory depression and neonatal abstinence syndrome in newborn infant Due to its predictable kinetics, and more extensive experience in pregnancy, oxycodone is the preferred opioid for use in pregnancy	Codeine is contraindicated in breastfeeding due to the possibility of morphine metabolites accumulating in the breastmilk of CYP2D6 fast metabolisers, risking overdose in the breastfed infant Occasional doses of other opioids are permitted, but avoid repeated dosing, especially if infant is <4 weeks old. Monitor infant and mother for sedation
Carbamazepine (CBZ) **Oxcarbazepine (OXC)**	CBZ use in pregnancy is associated with increased risk of neural tube defects, cleft palate, cardiovascular and urinary tract abnormalities. If use is unavoidable, close monitoring is required throughout pregnancy. Seek expert medical advice OXC has limited data available on use in human pregnancy. May cause vitamin K deficiency in the fetus. If use is unavoidable, close monitoring is required throughout pregnancy	Both drugs safe to use in breastfeeding. Monitor infant for drowsiness and poor suckling Ensure breastfeeding mother is sufficiently alert to care for her baby

Table 14.2 (cont.)

Drugs used commonly in dentistry	Safety in pregnancy	Safety in breastfeeding
Amitriptyline	Considered safe in pregnancy. However, use in late pregnancy can cause neonatal withdrawal syndrome for up to 2 weeks after delivery	Small amounts of amitriptyline and its active metabolite, nortriptyline, are distributed into breastmilk, but no serious harmful effects have been noted in breastfed infants Monitor infant for excessive drowsiness or impaired feeding
Pregabalin Gabapentin	Limited information available. Several small studies have found an increased risk of congenital malformations after first trimester exposure to pregabalin but findings may have been due to confounders Cases of neonatal withdrawal have also been reported following prolonged *in utero* exposure to gabapentinoids. Consider alternative drug treatment and seek specialist advice	Small amounts of gabapentin are excreted into breastmilk, but these amounts are unlikely to pose harm to the breastfed infant Monitor infant for excessive drowsiness, poor feeding and restlessness. Ensure breastfeeding mother is sufficiently alert to care for her baby
Nitrous oxide	Sporadic exposure is considered safe in pregnancy or during labour However, there is increased risk of central nervous system abnormalities in children born to women exposed to nitrous oxide chronically during pregnancy, either through their occupation or deliberate abuse It is therefore recommended that pregnant patients may use nitrous oxide for a single dental appointment; however, pregnant dental staff should avoid exposure as much as possible	Given the lack of oral bioavailability and very short half-life, nitrous oxide is considered safe for use by breastfeeding women
Methoxyflurane	Rare cases of maternal hepatitis have been reported following use of methoxyflurane in obstetric analgesia and during labour However, due to its short half-life, sporadic use of methoxyflurane is considered safe during pregnancy	Given the lack of oral bioavailability and short half-life, methoxyflurane is considered safe for use by women who are breastfeeding. However, the mother should wait until she has fully recovered from the effects of methoxyflurane before resuming breastfeeding

Table 14.2 (cont.)

Drugs used commonly in dentistry	Safety in pregnancy	Safety in breastfeeding
Antibacterials amoxicillin amoxicillin/clavulanate* azithromycin cefalexin clindamycin dicloxacillin doxycycline** erythromycin*** flucloxacillin metronidazole**** phenoxymethylpenicillin roxithromycin	All are considered safe in throughout pregnancy except: *Avoid co-amoxiclav in pregnant women with premature rupture of membranes, due to increased risk of neonatal necrotising enterocolitis ** Doxycycline safe for the first 18 weeks of pregnancy (16 weeks post-conception) after which may affect the formation of baby's teeth and cause discolouration *** Erythromycin use in pregnancy has been associated with cardiovascular and pyloric stenosis. Studies conflict, but use only when necessary	All are compatible with breastfeeding but may cause diarrhoea and/or oral thrush in breastfed infant ***Likely to cause gastrointestinal distress in lactating mother and breastfed infant ****Metronidazole may give bitter taste to milk; baby may feed less well. Juggle feeds around doses
Antifungals amphotericin clotrimazole fluconazole miconazole nystatin	Nystatin and amphotericin are both considered safe in pregnancy due to minimal systemic absorption Topically administered azole antifungals are safe in pregnancy due to low systemic absorption Multiple doses of systemically administered fluconazole and itraconazole have been associated with malformations so should be avoided throughout pregnancy	All are considered safe to use in breastfeeding, as systemic absorption by breastfed infant is negligible Consider risk of drug interactions with systemically absorbed antifungals
Antivirals aciclovir famciclovir valaciclovir	Topical and systemic aciclovir is considered safe to use, and preferred over famciclovir and valaciclovir due to greater clinical experience Valaciclovir may be used from 36 weeks of pregnancy	Aciclovir and valaciclovir are safe to use in breastfeeding Avoid famciclovir due to insufficient safety data in pregnancy
Local anaesthetics +/− adrenaline articaine felypressin* lidocaine mepivacaine prilocaine	Due to the low doses used for dental indications and the remote route of administration, dental local anaesthetics and their vasoconstrictors are considered safe in pregnancy *Historical safety concerns regarding felypressin in pregnancy are no longer considered evidence-based	All local anaesthetics are minimally distributed into the blood stream or breast milk. Negligible oral bioavailability ensures little effect on the breastfed infant

Table 14.2 (cont.)

Drugs used commonly in dentistry	Safety in pregnancy	Safety in breastfeeding
Benzodiazepines (BZDs) diazepam lorazepam midazolam oxazepam temazepam	Case control studies suggest BZD use in first trimester is associated with fetal cleft lip and cleft palate. However, a single dose is likely to be safe. Avoid in the third trimester, especially near term or during labour, due to risk of neonatal complications including neonatal hypotonia and withdrawal symptoms. Risk benefit needs to be considered. Seek medical advice	BZDs distribute into breastmilk and will accumulate with continuous use. However, single doses can be juggled around feeds. Regular and high dose is not recommended, due to risk of infant sedation, lethargy and poor feeding. Risk of over-sedation of breastfeeding mother should also be considered

FURTHER READING

Anderson PO. Local Anesthesia and Breastfeeding. *Breastfeeding Medicine.* 2021;16(3):173–174. doi.org.ezproxy.library.uq.edu.au/10.1089/bfm.2020.0384

Black E, Khor KE, Kennedy D et al. Medication Use and Pain Management in Pregnancy: A Critical Review. *Pain Pract.* 2019;19(8):875–899. doi:10.1111/papr.12814

Mothersafe, Royal Hospital for Women. *Dental Treatment in Pregnancy and Breastfeeding.* 2020. https://www.seslhd.health.nsw.gov.au/sites/default/files/groups/Royal_Hospital_for_Women/Mothersafe/documents/DentaltreatmentpregbreastNov2020.pdf

REFERENCES

1. Henry A, Crowther C. Patterns of medication use during and prior to pregnancy: the MAP study. *Aust N Z J Obstet Gynaecol.* 2000;40:165–172.
2. Sawicki E, Stewart K, Wong S et al. Medication use for chronic health conditions by pregnant women attending an Australian maternity hospital. *Aust N Z J Obstet Gynaecol.* 2011;51:333–338.
3. Gardiner SJ, Woods DJ. Drugs in Pregnancy and Lactation. In Walker R, Whittlesea C (eds). *Clinical Pharmacy and Therapeutics.* 4th edition. Elsevier Ltd; 2007.
4. International Anesthesia Research Society. Pharmacology of the Placenta. *Open Anesthesia.* Accessed July 22, 2022. https://www.openanesthesia.org/pharmacology_of_the_placenta/#:~:text=Size,molecular%20weights)%20cross%20the%20placenta
5. Kennedy D. Classifying drugs in pregnancy. *Aust Prescr.* 2014;37:38–40.
6. Organization of Teratology Information Specialists (OTIS). *MotherToBaby.* https://mothertobaby.org/about-otis/
7. Briggs G, Freeman RK, Towers CV, Forinash AB. *Brigg Drugs in Pregnancy and Lactation.* 12th edition. Wolters Kluwer; 2022.
8. Rossi S (ed). *Australian Medicines Handbook.* Australian Medicines Handbook Pty Ltd; 2023.
9. TGA. *Prescribing medicines in pregnancy database.* 2022. https://www.tga.gov.au/prescribing-medicines-pregnancy-database

10. England R. *Could the thalidomide tragedy have been averted by more extensive animal testing?* 2015. http://www.safermedicines.org/page/faqs_faq17

11. FDA. *Pregnancy Risk Information: An Update.* 2017. https://www.drugs.com/pregnancy-categories.html

12. Stern A, Elmore J. Medication for Gravid and Nursing Dental Patients. *Dent Clin N Am.* 2016;523–531.

13. Amir LH, Donath SM. Socioeconomic status and rates of breastfeeding in Australia: evidence from three recent national health surveys. *Med J Aust.* 2008;189:254–256.

14. Gunn J, Lumley J, Young D. The role of the general practitioner in postnatal care: a survey from Australia general practice. *Br J Gen Pract.* 1998;48:1570–1574.

15. Schirm E, Schwagermann MP, Tobi H et al. Drug use during breastfeeding. A survey from the Netherlands. *Eur J Clin Nutr.* 2004;58:386–390.

16. Amir LH, Pirotta MV. *Medicines for breastfeeding women: a postal survey of knowledge, attitudes and practices of general practitioners in Victoria.* Report. Melbourne Mother and Child Research, La Trobe University. 2010.

17. McGuire T. Safe Use of Drugs While Breastfeeding. *Breastfeeding Management in Australia.* Australian Breastfeeding Association Melbourne; 2019.

18. Sachs HC. The transfer of drugs and therapeutics into human breast milk: an update on selected topics. *Pediatrics.* 2013;132(3):e796–e809.

19. LactMed® Drugs and Lactation Database. Accessed August 30, 2023. https://www.ncbi.nlm.nih.gov/books/NBK501922/

20. Marks JM, Spatz DL. Medications and Lactation: What PNPs Need to Know. *J Pediatr Health Care.* 2003;17(6):311–317.

21. Loke YC, Vo-Tran H, Wong S (eds). *Pregnancy and Breastfeeding Medicines Guide.* The Royal Women's Hospital, Melbourne; 2023.

22. Favero V, Bacci C, Volpato A et al. Pregnancy and Dentistry: A Literature Review on Risk Management during Dental Surgical Procedures. *Dent J (Basel).* 2021;9(4):46. doi:10.3390/dj9040046

23. Lee JM, Shin TJ. Use of local anesthetics for dental treatment during pregnancy; safety for parturient. *J Dent Anesth Pain Med.* 2017;17(2):81–90.

24. Fan H, Gilbert R, O'Callaghan F, Li L. Associations between macrolide antibiotics prescribing during pregnancy and adverse child outcomes in the UK: population-based cohort study. *BMJ.* 2020;368:m331

25. Andersson NW, Olsen RH, Andersen JT. Association between use of macrolides in pregnancy and risk of major birth defects: nationwide, register based cohort study. *BMJ.* 2021;372:n107.

26. Oral and Dental Expert Group. *Therapeutic Guidelines Oral and Dental (Version 3).* Therapeutic Guidelines Pty Ltd; 2019.

27. MotherToBaby. *Critical Periods of Development.* National Library of Medicine. 1 March 2021. https://www.ncbi.nlm.nih.gov/books/NBK582659/

ORAL ADVERSE DRUG REACTIONS

15

KEY POINTS

- Adverse drug reactions (ADRs) in the oral cavity are frequently encountered in everyday practice and are best diagnosed and managed by dental professionals.
- ADRs are important as they often go unrecognised and are misdiagnosed as iatrogenic disease.
- Common and well-known drug-induced oral adverse effects include bruxism, gingival overgrowth, taste disturbance, tooth discolouration and xerostomia.
- Rare oral adverse reactions include lichenoid reactions, drug-induced lupus and bullous pemphigoid.
- Dental professionals should participate in pharmacovigilance, including voluntary reporting of oral ADRs.

15.1 Introduction

An ADR is defined as 'a response to a medicine that is noxious and unintended, and occurs at doses normally used or tested in humans' (1). Adverse drug events (ADEs) and ADRs are very different terms. ADE is the broader term that refers to any negative outcome associated with medicine use. ADEs encompasses **two subtypes**:

1. ADRs = an adverse drug reaction where no human error was involved. In most literature, the term 'adverse effects' and 'adverse reactions' are synonymous and used interchangeably.
2. Medication error = this may or may not involve patient harm but human error (e.g. a prescribing error) is the issue.

ADRs that manifest in the orofacial region are common, being associated with at least 43 of the top 100 drugs dispensed on the Pharmaceutical Benefits Scheme (PBS) in Australia (2). There is an increasing awareness of oral ADRs amongst dental professionals, with more patients taking medicines, polypharmacy becoming more prevalent and improved understanding of which symptoms can be considered drug-induced. In Australia, 87.1% of the population aged 50 years or more takes at least one medicine regularly, thus making ADRs a risk for a significant proportion of the population (3). Indeed, ADRs are a major public health problem because they occur frequently, incur economic expense and contribute significantly to human suffering.

The *Medication Safety Report* from the Pharmaceutical Society of Australia in 2019 stated that 250,000 Australian hospitalisations per year are caused by ADEs, most of which are due to ADRs, at a cost of approximately AU$1.4 billion per year (4). ADRs occurring in hospital increase the patient's length of stay by 2–4 days (5). In general practice, ADRs result in 400,000 GP visits a year (4). The tragedy of these ADRs is that 50% are preventable and yet little is being done to prevent them (4).

ADRs often go unrecognised or misdiagnosed as iatrogenic disease; for example, long-term benzodiazepine use can cause drug-induced memory dysfunction and be misdiagnosed as dementia. Including adverse drug effects in a differential diagnosis is critical to accurately identifying drug-induced symptoms that could be addressed by ceasing the implicated drug or lowering its dose. Dentists must be continuously upskilled in all aspects of ADRs in order to play their pivotal role in identifying, managing, reporting and preventing oral ADRs.

This chapter summarises ADRs in the orofacial region associated with commonly used drugs to assist with patient management in dental practice. For information on pharmacovigilance and how to report ADRs, see Section 15.18.

15.2 Drug-associated bruxism

15.2.1 Definition

Bruxism is defined as 'a repetitive jaw-muscle activity characterised by clenching or grinding of the teeth and/or by bracing or thrusting of the mandible. Bruxism has two distinct circadian manifestations: it can occur during sleep (indicated as sleep bruxism) or during wakefulness (indicated as awake bruxism)' (6).

15.2.2 Clinical effects

Persistent bruxism can result in pain in the teeth, muscles, or jaw joint; tooth wear, fracture, cracks in teeth, restorations or implants; and hypertrophy of the temporomandibular joint musculature (7).

15.2.3 Incidence

The prevalence of bruxism is reported to be 14–20% in children, approximately 8% in adults and 3% in the elderly (8, 9).

15.2.4 Drugs associated and mechanism

Several neurotransmitters are involved in the pathophysiology of bruxism, including dopamine, noradrenaline, serotonin and, to a lesser extent, histamine. Drugs that act to enhance or suppress levels of these central nervous system (CNS) neurotransmitters are more likely to cause bruxism (10). See Table 15.1 for drugs associated with bruxism.

The role of dopamine in oromandibular movements is well established, so drugs such as the typical and atypical antipsychotics that inhibit dopamine receptor neurotransmission are frequently associated with bruxism, orofacial dystonia and dyskinesia (11). However, the pathogenesis of bruxism is complex, with some drugs acting on multiple pathways resulting in bruxism (10).

Two classes of antidepressants have consistently been associated with bruxism. These are:

1. selective serotonin reuptake inhibitors (SSRIs) including citalopram, escitalopram, fluoxetine, fluvoxamine, paroxetine and sertraline
2. selective serotonin and noradrenaline reuptake inhibitors (SNRIs), which include atomoxetine, venlafaxine and duloxetine

The antidepressants most frequently implicated are fluoxetine, sertraline and venlafaxine (12).

Bruxism appears to be dose-dependent and tends to develop quickly—within 3–4 weeks of commencing the antidepressant or after dose escalation (12). Alleviation of symptoms tends to occur with dose reduction or within 2–3 weeks of drug cessation. However, one case report of fluoxetine detailed spontaneous resolution of bruxism with no intervention after 4 weeks (12).

Table 15.1 Drugs associated with bruxism (13). Adapted from (12).

Drug class	Drug
Antidepressants	Citalopram Escitalopram Duloxetine Fluoxetine Fluvoxamine Paroxetine Sertraline Venlafaxine
Antipsychotics	Chlorpromazine Fluphenazine Haloperidol
Drugs for ADHD	Atomoxetine

15.3 Drug-associated tardive dyskinesia

15.3.1 Definition

Tardive dyskinesia (TD) is a delayed-onset adverse drug effect that manifests as persistent, sometimes reversible, abnormal, involuntary, repetitive movements that can affect the orofacial region, neck, trunk or limbs (11, 14). The frequency of TD occurs at a rate of 2–5% per year, with an incidence between 15–30% in patients being treated with long-term antipsychotics (15).

15.3.2 Clinical effects

Orofacial dyskinesia is the most common and often earliest symptom of TD. It can present as facial grimacing, rapid eye blinking, repetitive tongue protrusion, puckering, smacking and licking of the lips, with lateral movements of the jaw (11). TD can be very distressing for the patient, negatively affect a patient's quality of life and threaten medication adherence (16). Patients with TD may be unaware of their involuntary movements.

TD is not associated with pain, but orofacial pain can arise from trauma caused by abnormal movement such as between dentures and the denture-bearing mucosa (17).

15.3.3 Risk factors

Known risk factors for TD include advanced age, female gender, diabetes, smoking, antidopaminergic therapy, the presence of movement disorders prior to initiation of antidopaminergic therapy, and alcohol abuse/dependence (18).

TD is particularly associated with antipsychotic and anti-emetic medication used long term, as this syndrome rarely manifests before three months of continuous use. However, the duration of drug exposure may be as little as one month in adults aged over 60 years (19).

15.3.4 Drugs associated and mechanism

The proposed mechanism for TD is that these drugs block dopaminergic neurotransmission along mesocortical and nigrostriatal pathways in the brain, which impairs coordination of voluntary and involuntary muscle movement (16).

After long-term use of antidopaminergic medication, signs of TD may persist even after the medication is ceased. Dopamine antagonists—metoclopramide and prochlorperazine—are both associated with a variety of extrapyramidal disorders with TD being the most common; the risk increases with cumulative dose and length of treatment (13, 14, 20, 21).

All antipsychotics are implicated with causing TD, but the first-generation (i.e. older and less specific) antipsychotics (fluphenazine, haloperidol and trifluoperazine) carry the greatest risk of TD and clozapine, being a more modern and targeted drug, has a lower risk (14). Up to 1 in 3 people using 'older' antipsychotics will develop TD after 10 years of use (14). The risk of TD is reduced for the newer antispychotics such as olanzapine, quetiapine and risperidone because their mode of action involves the blockade of serotonin as well as dopamine (22). The better tolerated and more selective antipsychotics, such as lurasidone, carry a small risk of TD.

The first antipsychotic drugs used in clinical practice, such as chlorpromazine ('Largactil') were developed in the 1950s. These were revolutionary medicines in their ability to treat psychosis, but they also caused a lot of unwanted side effects such as drowsiness, weight gain and involuntary movements. Equally effective but much better tolerated drugs were developed in the 1970s and 1980s that dramatically reduced the risk of movement disorders. The older drugs from the 1950s are often termed 'first generation' antipsychotics and the more modern, better tolerated drugs (e.g. risperidone) are referred to as 'second generation' antipsychotics.

Antipsychotics today have many uses aside from psychoses, such as bipolar disorder and behavioural disorders in autism. Therefore, dental practitioners should be aware of their increasing use across a wider cohort of the population (13, 14, 22). See Table 15.2 for drugs associated with tardive dyskinesia.

Older antipsychotics are also used for off-label indications, such as paralytic ileus, neuropathic pain, intractable hiccups, chronic itch and migraine treatment and prevention.

Levodopa, used in Parkinson's disease, is also associated with a variety of movement disorders, including dystonia and TD. The rate of development of dyskinesias in Parkinson's disease ranges from 3–94% (23). The clinical manifestations of movement tend to correlate with the plasma concentrations of levodopa. Dental appointments should be scheduled to coincide with the patient's medication regimen and the time the patient's symptoms are most settled.

Table 15.2 Drugs associated with tardive dyskinesia. Adapted from (13).

Drug class	Drug
Antipsychotics	Amisulpride Aripiprazole Chloropromazine Clozapine Droperidol Flupenthixol Fluphenazine Haloperidol Lurasidone Olanzapine Paliperidone Pericyazine Quetiapine Risperidone Trifluoperazine Ziprasidone Zuclopenthixol
Dopamine antagonists	Metoclopramide Prochlorperazine
Drugs for Parkinson's disease	Levodopa

15.4 Drug-associated hairy tongue

15.4.1 Definition

Hairy tongue is defined as acquired, benign staining of the elongated filiform papillae on the dorsal surface of the tongue. It is caused by defective desquamation of epithelial cells and subsequent accumulation of exogenous debris, including chromogenic organisms (24, 25).

15.4.2 Clinical effects

Asymptomatic staining of the tongue can manifest in various colours including brown, yellow, green or blue (24).

15.4.3 Drugs associated and mechanism

Several antimicrobials are associated with causing hairy tongue, thought to be due to their capability to alter the composition of oral flora. These drugs include penicillins, doxycycline, erythromycin, griseofulvin, linezolid and metronidazole (24, 26–29). Case reports have been published where chlorpromazine and olanzapine have been associated with causing hairy tongue, the mechanism of which is unknown (24, 30). Drugs that can cause xerostomia may also contribute to hairy tongue, making desquamation on the tongue more difficult to clear (25). See Table 15.3 for drugs associated with hairy tongue.

Table 15.3 Drugs associated with hairy tongue. Adapted from (13).

Drug class	Drug
Antimicrobials	Amoxicillin Amoxicillin/clavulanic acid Ampicillin Doxycycline Erythromycin Griseofulvin Linezolid Metronidazole Phenoxymethylpenicillin
Antipsychotics	Olanzapine Chlorpromazine

15.5 Drug-induced gingival overgrowth

15.5.1 Definition

Drug-induced gingival overgrowth (DIGO) is defined as hypertrophy or enlargement of the gingiva, which can be due to interactions between the host and the environment, or induced by medication (31, 32).

15.5.2 Clinical effects

DIGO tends to affect the buccal and labial surfaces of the anterior gingiva causing swelling. The affected gingivae usually have a granular-like appearance; the interdental papillae can enlarge and eventually can partially obscure the crowns of the teeth (31). DIGO is not only disfiguring but can be functionally compromising and can lead to problems with speech and eating.

15.5.3 Drugs associated and mechanism

While much research has been undertaken to understand the mechanism of DIGO, including effects on gingival fibroblasts and molecular mechanisms involving cytokines and genetic predisposition, there is currently no definitive explanation for the pathogenesis (31, 33). In addition, it is unclear whether the association with medication is related to the dosage or pharmacology of the offending drug (33).

The anticonvulsant phenytoin is a well-established causative agent, with DIGO appearing between 1–3 months after drug commencement, and a prevalence of 13–50% of patients taking phenytoin (13, 34, 35). DIGO has also been reported with other anticonvulsants including valproic acid in children, vigabatrin and phenobarbitone, but the frequency is rare (13, 36–39).

DIGO is a well-documented adverse effect of the immunosuppressant drug cyclosporin, with a prevalence of 25–30% in adults and > 70% in children; gingival overgrowth tends to appear between 1–4 months after starting therapy (34, 35). It is probable that a threshold plasma level of cyclosporin is required for overgrowth to develop, with the likelihood of gingival enlargement corresponding to plasma concentrations of cyclosporin (31).

Calcium channel blockers of the dihydropyridine type (e.g. amlodipine, nifedipine) and non-dihydropyridine type (e.g. verapamil, diltiazem) are also associated with gingival overgrowth. The average time to onset of DIGO with these drugs is 2–14 months, so it is recommended that patients be monitored during this time as gingival enlargement can develop later than with cyclosporin or phenytoin. Current literature suggests the prevalence of gingival overgrowth is greatest with nifedipine (5–80%), diltiazem (5–20%) and verapamil (<5 %) and is rare with amlodipine and felodipine (32, 34).

Table 15.4 Drugs associated with gingival enlargement (13).

Drug class		Drug
Anticonvulsants		Phenytoin
Calcium channel blockers	Dihydropyridines	Amlodipine Felodipine Nifedipine
	Non-dihydropyridines	Diltiazem Verapamil
Immunosuppressants		Cyclosporin

15.6 Drug-associated taste disturbance

15.6.1 Definition

Drug-induced taste disturbance is defined as the modification of a person's sense of taste, due to the chemosensory adverse effects of drugs. Taste disturbances can reduce food, fluid and nutrient intake and, ultimately, quality of life, especially when the causative drug is used long-term (40).

15.6.2 Clinical effects

Taste disorders are classified as:

- **dysgeusia:** taste distortion or altered perception of taste
- **ageusia:** loss of one or more of the basic taste sensations, including sweet, sour, salty and bitter
- **hypergeusia:** heightened perception of taste
- **hypogeusia:** reduced perception of taste
- **parageusia:** perception of a spoiled taste
- **phantogeusia:** experience of taste without any stimulus (40, 41)

The most common taste disorder induced by medication is dysgeusia, often causing a bitter or metallic taste, altered taste perception, or hypogeusia (42). Drug-induced taste disturbance can start immediately from commencement of the drug and may persist for several weeks after the medication is ceased (13).

15.6.3 Incidence

The reported incidence of drug-induced taste disturbances is 3–11% (41). Incidence increases with age as older people report this adverse effect more frequently (41–43).

15.6.4 Drugs associated and mechanism

Up to 350 drugs from all major drug classes have been associated with taste disturbances. Causality is difficult to determine due to the subjective nature of this adverse effect, as well as the lack of standardised measurements of chemosensory processes (42). Individual susceptibility to drug-induced taste disturbance may contribute; however, other risk factors include advanced age, polypharmacy, genetic polymorphisms relating to taste sensation, medical conditions and concurrent dry mouth (42). Various mechanisms have been proposed, including altered relaying of neurotransmitters involved in taste bud signalling.

Antibiotics such as azithromycin, clarithromycin, doxycycline, levofloxacin and moxifloxacin are well known for causing taste disturbances, which are thought to be due to inhibition of zinc absorption and alteration of other cations, such as calcium and magnesium, and their role in taste bud function (40).

Metronidazole, commonly prescribed by dentists, is frequently associated with causing a metallic taste (14).

Mineral supplements, particularly zinc and copper, have also been associated with causing a rapid onset, metallic taste disturbance that may persist long after the drug is stopped.

When administered systemically, the antifungal drug terbinafine is well known for being associated with reversible ablation of taste sensation, which usually takes weeks to return after drug cessation (14). See Table 15.5 for drugs associated with taste disturbance.

Table 15.5 Some drugs associated with taste disturbance. Adapted from (13).

Drug class	Drug
Anticonvulsants	Topiramate
Antifungals	Griseofulvin Terbinafine
Antibacterials	Metronidazole
Antihypertensives and other cardiac medications	Amiodarone Candesartan Diltiazem Losartan Nifedipine
Immuno-modifying agents	Auranofin Interferon alfa Penicillamine
Antineoplastics	Carboplatin Cyclophosphamide
Antipsychotics	Lithium
Carbonic anhydrase inhibitor	Acetazolamide
Hypnotics	Zolpidem Zopiclone

15.7 Drug-associated tooth, gum and alveolar bone discolouration

15.7.1 Definition

Tooth discolouration can be extrinsic or intrinsic. Extrinsic staining occurs on the external surface of the tooth after the tooth has erupted and can be removed with mechanical cleaning. Intrinsic staining occurs during the process of odontogenesis and is permanent. Gum and alveolar bone discolouration can also occur due to medication use (44).

15.7.2 Extrinsic staining

15.7.2.1 Clinical effects and associated drugs

Chlorhexidine is frequently associated with causing brown extrinsic staining of the teeth, restorations and tongue. To avoid staining, it is recommended to use chlorhexidine for less than two weeks continuously (44, 45).

Iron supplements in oral liquid formulations can temporarily stain teeth black, which can occur within days of commencing treatment. In order to avoid staining, it is recommended to dilute the liquid iron with water, drink it using a straw, then rinse out the mouth after the dose with plain water (14).

The antibiotic linezolid has been associated with causing a yellow extrinsic discolouration of the teeth and tongue in several paediatric case reports (13, 26).

15.7.3 Intrinsic staining

15.7.3.1 Tetracyclines

If tetracycline antibiotics are ingested by the patient during tooth development (>18 weeks gestation, <8 years of age), they form a tetracycline–calcium orthophosphate complex by chelating with the calcium inside developing teeth (46, 47). On exposure to visible light, this complex oxidises and, over time, produces a yellow/brown stain and enamel hypoplasia in the cervical one-third of the crown.

Clinical effects

The yellow-stained complex has fluorescent properties on exposure to UV light, but as time progresses the oxidation products of tetracycline turn the stain to a non-fluorescent permanent brown discolouration (46). The degree of staining is influenced by the dose and duration of the tetracycline antibiotic, the stage of calcification of the teeth and the mineralisation rate, and does not go away with drug cessation (46).

15.7.3.2 Minocycline

Minocycline can cause permanent intrinsic staining in teeth after they have fully erupted that may fade over time. Pigmentation of other tissues, including gingiva and alveolar bone, can also occur. The mechanism is unknown.

The incidence of minocycline-induced intrinsic staining is both dose and time dependent. For tooth staining, the incidence has been estimated at 3–6% with exposure of a daily dose greater than 100mg (48). For staining of alveolar bone, the incidence is estimated to be 10% after one year, and 20% for those taking 100–200mg daily for four years (48).

Clinical effects

Minocycline staining appears as a grey-blue discolouration in the incisal-middle thirds of the crown (which contrasts with that of tetracycline). Minocycline can cause pigmentation and discolouration of other tissues, including the skin, nails and sclera of the eye, but also a green/black stain on tooth roots, staining of the gingiva and a black staining of the alveolar bone (47–49). It should also be noted that while the mucosa clinically appears dark due to 'black' pigmented bone showing through the translucence of the gingiva, the overlying mucosa itself is normal. This should therefore be differentiated from a pigmented lesion of the oral mucosa which would have a different aetiology (49).

15.7.3.3 Other drugs

Doxycycline and ciprofloxacin have also been associated with discolouration of fully erupted teeth and causing an intrinsic green stain in infants (48, 50). However, it should be noted that doxycycline is unlikely to cause dental staining when used for up to 3 weeks in children younger than 8 years old (14).

Table 15.6 Drugs associated with tooth and alveolar bone discolouration (13). Adapted from (44).

Tooth discolouration	Drug class	Drug
Extrinsic	Miscellaneous	Chlorhexidine Linezolid Oral liquid iron
Intrinsic	Fluoroquinolones	Ciprofloxacin
	Tetracyclines	Doxycycline Minocycline Tetracycline

15.8 Drug-associated salivary secretory disorders

Salivary secretory disorders are common and drugs are a common cause (51). Both hyper- and hyposalivation can negatively affect a patient's quality of life as well as reduce the health of their teeth and gums.

Saliva is a hypotonic solution, around 90% of which is secreted by the major salivary glands including the parotid, submandibular and sublingual glands, and the remaining 10% by the minor salivary glands (52). Neural control of salivation is mostly exerted via parasympathetic efferent pathways from the facial and glossopharyngeal nerves that act via releasing the neurotransmitter acetylcholine acting on the muscarinic M3 receptors to increase saliva secretion (51). There is also some minor innervation by the sympathetic nervous system where noradrenaline acts on β-adrenoreceptors to increase protein levels in the saliva (52).

While there is a variation in salivary flow rates and the amount produced by individuals, it is accepted that normal unstimulated salivary flow ranges from 0.3–0.5mL/min (51). Flow rates in the range of 0.01–0.1mL/min are diagnosed as hyposalivation.

Stimulated salivary flow of 1–2mL/min is accepted as normal, with <0.7mL/min acknowledged as reduced salivation (51). Normal daily production of saliva ranges from 500–1500mL (52).

15.8.1 Hypersalivation

15.8.1.1 Definition

Hypersalivation (or sialorrhea) is defined as increased secretion of saliva diagnosed by quantitative sialometry (51). Drooling can accompany hypersalivation but may not always be a consequence; drooling occurs where there is inadequate manipulation of the saliva, where the flow and quantity may be normal (51).

15.8.1.2 Clinical effects

Chronic hypersalivation can cause salivary gland swelling, parotitis, skin irritation and infection and, potentially, aspiration pneumonia (52). In addition, sialorrhea can be socially stigmatising which can lead to medication non-adherence and sleep disturbance from anxiety (52).

15.8.1.3 Drugs associated and mechanism

The mechanism of sialorrhea is thought to arise either from increased parasympathetic innervation of the salivary glands, or inhibition of the enzyme acetylcholinesterase, thereby reducing the breakdown of acetylcholine and leading to increased agonist activity on salivary muscarinic receptors. Clozapine is currently the drug most frequently associated with hypersalivation, with an incidence of 31%, and hypersalivation develops early in the treatment course and more frequently at night (52, 53).

In addition to increased cholinergic stimulation, hypersalivation is thought to be attributed to a decrease in sympathetic stimulation of the salivary glands by inhibition of α-2 adrenergic receptors, coupled with inhibition of dopamine receptors that are associated with movement disorders. All three mechanisms are thought to contribute to both hypersalivation and increased drooling (51, 54). Other antipsychotics associated with hypersalivation include chlorpromazine, amisulpride, olanzapine, haloperidol, fluphenazine, quetiapine, risperidone and zuclopenthixol.

Acetylcholinesterase inhibitors for myasthenia gravis, neostigmine and pyridostigmine are also associated with hypersalivation (14, 51). The antidementia drugs donepezil, galantamine and rivastigmine have a weak association with hypersalivation (55–57). See Table 15.7 for drugs associated with hypersalivation.

Table 15.7 Drugs associated with hypersalivation (13).

Drug class	Drug
Acetylcholinesterase inhibitors	Donepezil Galantamine Pyridostigmine Rivastigmine

Table 15.7 (cont.)

Drug class	Drug
Antipsychotics	Amisulpride Chlorpromazine Clozapine Fluphenazine Haloperidol Olanzapine Quetiapine Risperidone Zuclopenthixol
Other	Betel nut

15.8.2 Xerostomia/hyposalivation

15.8.2.1 Definition

Xerostomia is defined as a subjective sensation of dry mouth. Hyposalivation is defined as an objective reduction in salivary quality and quantity, the latter being measured by sialometry (45).

15.8.2.2 Clinical effects

Xerostomia is associated with an increased risk of dental decay, non-carious wear (e.g. erosion), periodontitis, oral mucosal disease, increased infection risk (e.g. oral candidosis) and difficulties with denture retention, chewing, swallowing and speech (45). Xerostomia is also negatively associated with oral health quality of life scores, due to causing pain in the salivary glands, a burning sensation and difficulties with speech and eating (58).

15.8.2.3 Incidence

Xerostomia is common, with a prevalence ranging between 17–29% (51). A cross-sectional study conducted in Australia showed that 20% of patients had self-reported dry mouth (59). There is also the increased association of xerostomia with older age and polypharmacy (59, 60).

15.8.2.4 Drugs associated and mechanism

Xerostomia is the most common oral ADR, being cited in the product information of 43 of the top 100 drugs subsidised on the PBS in Australia (2). A wide variety of drugs are associated with xerostomia, with varying degrees of evidence. The majority are drugs that either reduce salivary gland function by inhibiting cholinergic innervation of the salivary glands, such as anticholinergic or antimuscarinic drugs, or drugs that enhance sympathetic stimulation by acting as agonists on adrenoceptors, such as dexamphetamine (51).

Nevertheless, many other drugs have been associated with dry mouth symptoms, and their mechanisms are unknown. Table 15.8 shows the varied list of drugs associated with xerostomia as determined from a systematic review by Wolff et al., where medications were classified according to the strength of the substantiating evidence (61).

Table 15.8 Drugs associated with xerostomia or salivary gland hypofunction (13). Adapted from (61). Classifications of drugs are from the *Australian Medicines Handbook* (14).

Drug class	Medications with a higher level of evidence	Medications with a moderate level of evidence	Medications with a weaker level of evidence
Anticholinergic/ antimuscarinic medicines	Atropine Oxybutynin Propantheline Scopolamine Solifenacin Tolterodine	Darifenacin Hyoscine	Ipratropium
Anticonvulsants	Gabapentin	Pregabalin Sodium valproate	
Antidepressants	Amitriptyline Citalopram Duloxetine Escitalopram Fluoxetine Imipramine Nortriptyline Paroxetine Reboxetine Sertraline Venlafaxine Vortioxetine	Desvenlafaxine Dothiepin Doxepin	Clomipramine Mirtazapine Moclobemide Phenelzine
Antihistamines	Doxylamine	Azelastine Cetirizine Desloratadine	Chlorpheniramine Dimenhydrinate Diphenhydramine Pheniramine
Antihypertensives	Clonidine Verapamil	Atenolol Enalapril Lisinopril Methyldopa Metoprolol Terazosin	Diltiazem Perindopril
Antipsychotics	Aripiprazole Chlorpromazine Olanzapine Paliperidone Quetiapine Risperidone Ziprasidone	Amisulpride Asenapine Haloperidol Lurasidone	

Table 15.8 (cont.)

Drug class	Medications with a higher level of evidence	Medications with a moderate level of evidence	Medications with a weaker level of evidence
Antivirals		Didanosine Etravirine Lamivudine Maraviroc Nevirapine Raltegravir Saquinavir	
Diuretics	Frusemide	Tolvaptan	Amiloride
Muscle relaxants	Baclofen Orphenadrine		
Opioid analgesics	Buprenorphine	Dihydrocodeine Fentanyl Morphine Tapentadol Tramadol	Pethidine
Sedatives and hypnotics	Zolpidem	Zopiclone	
Other medicines	Alendronate Bevacizumab Brimonidine Bupropion Lisdexamfetamine Lithium Methylphenidate Phentermine Rotigotine Timolol Tiotropium	Dexmedetomidine Naltrexone Nicotine Orlistat	Apraclonidine Atomoxetine Cisplatin Disopyramide Granisetron Levomepromazine Modafinil Moxifloxacin Pseudoephedrine Selegiline

15.9 Medication-related osteonecrosis of the jaw

See Chapter 10.

15.10 Drug-associated oral lichenoid reactions

15.10.1 Definition

Oral lichenoid reactions (OLRs) are defined as oral lesions that are clinically and histo-logically similar to oral lichen planus.

15.10.2 Clinical effects and mechanism

Oral lichen planus is an immunologically mediated reaction driven by lymphocytes, which has a variety of presentations, including white or red plaques, erosions or ulcerations.

15.10.3 Evidence for association

Many drugs have been implicated with causing OLRs but the lack of detail in many case reports, such as confirmation of a diagnosis using an accepted method with biopsy and histopathology, or lack of substantiation using an ADR algorithm, make it difficult to conclusively prove causation (62, 63). Furthermore, OLRs are rare adverse drug effects, and their time association with drug administration is variable due to some OLRs taking months to develop and resolve after drug cessation (64).

15.10.4 Drugs associated with OLRs

A systematic review of drug-induced OLRs identified the immuno-modifying agents imatinib, infliximab, interferon alpha, and the antihypertensive methyldopa as the drugs with the most evidence supporting their association with OLRs (62). Case reports involving imatinib describe the OLR presenting between 3–12 months after commencement of therapy (65, 66), between 3–8 weeks for infliximab (67, 68), and from 10 days to 8 months after starting interferon alpha (69, 70).

Other antihypertensives associated with OLRs include atenolol, captopril and enalapril, as well as the NSAIDs naproxen and indomethacin (13, 71–73).

Table 15.9 lists drugs that have been associated with OLRs. While these drugs are only supported by singular or a few case reports, the diagnosis of OLR has been proven by biopsy or immunofluorescence and some have employed a validation tool to confirm the association of the respective drug with an OLR (13).

Table 15.9 Drugs associated with OLRs (74). Adapted from (62).

Drug class	Drug
Antihypertensives	Atenolol Captopril Enalapril Oxprenolol Methyldopa
Immunosuppressants	Adalimumab Imatinib Infliximab Interferon-alpha
NSAIDs	Indomethacin Naproxen
Other	Carbamazepine Certolizumab Clopidogrel Duloxetine Glimepiride Hepatitis B vaccine Lithium carbonate Ribavirin Risperidone Secukinumab

15.11 Drug-associated aphthous ulceration

15.11.1 Definition

Recurrent aphthous ulceration is defined as an 'inflammatory condition of unknown aetiology characterized by painful recurrent, single or multiple ulcerations of the oral mucosa' (75). These lesions can be drug-induced, although they are less likely to be drug-induced than other types of ulceration, such as mucositis (see Section 15.12).

15.11.2 Clinical effects

Presenting similarly to recurrent aphthous ulceration, drug-induced aphthous ulcers are round or oval, with a well-defined periphery, are relatively shallow, and clusters of ulcers can join to form larger ulcers (75, 76). Pain and dysphagia are also present, and their presence coincides with medication intake.

15.11.3 Drugs associated and mechanism

Nicorandil, a drug used for treatment of angina, has a well-documented link with ulceration in the oral and perianal area. Ophthalmic and cutaneous ulcers have also been reported (14). Drug discontinuation is required for healing of these lesions (14).

Aphthous-like ulceration is also a frequent complication of using mTOR inhibitors everolimus, ridaforolimus, sirolimus and temsirolimus (77, 78). While these medicines are used for cancer treatment and immunosuppression, the mouth ulcers they cause are aphthous-like, not to be confused with the mucositis as commonly associated with antineoplastic drugs (74, 77). A review of oncology-related clinical trials of mTOR inhibitors showed that ulceration was their most frequently reported adverse effect, and the third most frequent severe side effect, responsible for dose limitations and in some cases discontinuation of therapy (77, 79). The ulceration predominately occurs during the first cycle of mTOR inhibitor treatment, develops within the first 5 days, and takes around 1 week to resolve (78).

Orally administered bisphosphonates have been associated with oral aphthous-like ulceration in published case reports. Drugs cited include alendronate, risedronate and etidronate. This is different from the well-known adverse effects of oseophageal and gastrointestinal irritation and ulceration associated with these agents, and is possibly due to the cytotoxic effect of nitrogen-containing bisphosphonates on epithelial cells (80). Most case reports involve alendronate, and resolution of the oral ulcers can take several months after drug cessation (74, 80). Captopril and the NSAID piroxicam have also been implicated in case reports with causing oral aphthous-like ulceration (74–76). See Table 15.10 for drugs associated with oral aphthous ulceration.

Table 15.10 Drugs associated with oral aphthous ulceration. Adapted from (74).

Drug class	Drug
Vasodilators	Nicorandil
Antihypertensives	Captopril
NSAIDs	Piroxicam

Table 15.10 (cont.)

Drug class	Drug
Bisphosphonates	Alendronate Etidronate Risedronate
mTOR inhibitors	Everolimus Ridaforolimus Sirolimus Temsirolimus

15.12 Drug-associated oral mucositis

15.12.1 Definition

Mucositis refers to inflammation and ulceration of the mucous membranes, which can occur anywhere along the digestive tract from the mouth to the anus. Oral mucositis is sometimes referred to as 'stomatitis' when it describes general oral tissue inflammation, whereas 'mucositis' describes mucosal inflammation specifically arising from anticancer drugs and/or head/neck radiation therapy. Stomatitis is therefore a type of mucositis (81, 82).

15.12.2 Incidence

Oral mucositis occurs in approximately 40% of patients exposed to cytotoxic chemotherapy, some targeted cancer therapies (e.g. VEGF inhibitors) and up to 90% of patients treated with head/neck radiation (81, 83).

15.12.3 Clinical effects

Oral mucositis presents clinically as ulcerative lesions of the moveable oral mucosa and pharynx. Painful, irregular, ulcerative lesions without a defined border are present on the moveable mucosa that tends to appear 4–5 days after commencing the antineoplastic drug and peaks in severity between days 7–10 (84). Other symptoms experienced by patients with oral mucositis include dry mouth, generalised pain and burning, difficulty eating and swallowing, and shiny red swollen gums.

Treatment of oral mucositis includes cold food and ice chips, saline and sodium bicarbonate mouthwashes, oral lubricants, NSAIDs, topical local anaesthetics, corticosteroids and occasionally opioid analgesics. Mucositis can severely affect the oral ingestion of food and the ulcerative lesions are a source of entry for oral microorganisms and may cause systemic infections in these already immunocompromised patients (74, 83, 84).

15.12.4 Drugs associated and mechanism

While the exact pathophysiology of mucositis is unknown, it is thought to be influenced by factors including the up-regulation of pro-inflammatory cytokines, the composition of the oral flora, immune compromise of the patient and the effect of the specific drug on the oral epithelium (83, 85). See Table 15.11 for some of the many drugs associated with mucositis.

Table 15.11 Drugs associated with mucositis (74).

Drug class	Drug
Alkylating agents	Bendamustine Busalfan Chlorambucil Lomustine Melphalan Procarbazine
Anthracyclines	Daunorubicin Doxorubicin Epirubicin Idarubicin Mitozantrone
Antimetabolites	Azacitidine Capecitabine Clofarabine Cytarabine Fludarabine Fluorouracil Gemcitabine Hydroxyurea Mercaptopurine Methotrexate Pemetrexed Raltitrexed Thioguanine
Platinum compounds	Carboplatin Oxaliplatin
Podophyllotoxins	Etopoxide Teniposide
Taxanes	Carbazitaxel Docetaxel Paclitaxel
Topoisomerase I inhibitors	Topotecan
Vinca alkaloids	Vinblastine Vincristine Vinflunine Vinorelbine
Other cytotoxic antineoplastics	Bleomycin Dactinomycin Eribulin Mitomycin Romidepsin Trastuzumab
Antineoplastic antibodies	Bevacizumab Cetuximab Panitumumab Pertuzumab

Table 15.11 (cont.)

Drug class	Drug
mTOR inhibitors	Everolimus Sirolimus Temsirolimus
Tyrosine kinase inhibitors	Afatinib Axitinib Dasatinib Erlotinib Gefitinib Lapatinib Sorafenib Sunitinib
Other non-cytotoxic antibodies	Cobimetinib Trametinib Tretinoin
Calcineurin inhibitors	Tacrolimus
Other immunosuppressants	Mycophenolate

15.13 Drug-associated lupus

15.13.1 Definition

Systemic lupus erythematosus is an inflammatory autoimmune condition which can affect almost any organ of the body, but mostly affects the skin and joints (86). Drug-induced lupus is defined as a lupus-like syndrome due to medication use, which resolves after drug cessation (87).

15.13.2 Clinical effects

Drug-induced lupus presents similarly to systemic lupus erythematous, with arthralgias, myalgias, malaise, fever and symmetric polyarthritis, and serological examination demonstrating specific autoantibodies present (88). However, some signs including malar rash, photosensitivity and oral ulceration are not usually present in drug-induced lupus (89).

A retrospective diagnosis is based on exposure to a potential lupus-inducing drug for a minimum of one month, clinical signs and symptoms, appropriate serology, no history of systemic lupus erythematous, and resolution of signs and symptoms on drug discontinuation (89).

15.13.3 Drugs associated and mechanism

The onset of drug-associated lupus is variable, ranging from 1 month to up to 10 years of continuous use of the medication prior to development of signs and symptoms, making drug-associated lupus difficult to diagnose (87, 88). The likely mechanism of drug-associated lupus is due to reactive drug metabolites causing activation and disruption of specific immune cells as well as the cytotoxic-mediated release of autoantigens (90). While many drugs are associated with causing drug-associated lupus, evidence is substantial for only a handful of drugs.

Of the drugs available in Australia, hydralazine has the highest risk, with a yearly incidence of 5–8%, despite around 50% of patients taking hydralazine developing autoantibodies (89). As shown in Table 15.12, the other drugs listed are considered to be of low risk. There are other drugs that are associated with inducing lupus, but many have singular case reports and a weak association.

Table 15.12 Drugs associated with lupus (74). Adapted from (90).

Drug class	Drug
High risk	Hydralazine
Low risk	Captopril Carbamazepine Chlorpromazine Isoniazid Methyldopa Minocycline Penicillamine Propylthiouracil Sulfasalazine TNF-α inhibitors

15.14 Drug-associated pemphigoid

15.14.1 Definition

Pemphigoid refers to a group of rare, mucocutaneous, autoimmune, vesiculobullous diseases of which bullous pemphigoid is the most common. Sub-epithelial blistering is present, and drug-induced pemphigoid is a variant of bullous pemphigoid (91, 92).

15.14.2 Clinical effects

Drug-associated pemphigoid presents as sub-epidermal blistering and ulceration in the oral cavity and other mucosa, external skin of the limbs, and trunk (91). On histopathology, intraepidermal vesicles, necrotic keratinocytes and separation of the epithelium from the connective tissue layer is observed (91). Bullous pemphigoid is characterised by autoantibodies directed towards antigens in the cutaneous basement membrane zone in bullous pemphigoid, and it is thought that the antigens are the mostly the same targets in drug-induced pemphigoid (91, 92).

15.14.3 Drugs associated and mechanism

It is likely that drugs trigger pemphigoid mainly in patients who have a genetic predisposition, due to formation of autoantibodies or modification of the structural components of the basement membrane that are targeted antigens in the pathogenesis of pemphigoid (74, 92).

There can be a latency of up to three months between commencement of the offending drug and the development of clinical signs of pemphigoid such as bullous eruption (91).

Many drugs have been associated with drug-induced pemphigoid, but case reports are few and ADR algorithms are not appropriate to apply.

Table 15.13 shows the list of varied drugs associated with bullous pemphigoid (74).

Table 15.13 Drugs associated with bullous pemphigoid (74).

Association	Drug
Likely[1]	Enalapril Frusemide Ibuprofen Influenza vaccine
Probable[2]	Ampicillin Bumetanide Cephalexin Fluoxetine Penicillamine Penicillin Spironolactone
Questionable[3]	Amiodarone Captopril Chloroquine Interleukin-2 Omeprazole Risperidone Sulfonamides Tetanus toxoid Topical fluorouracil

Notes:
[1] Rechallenge evidence supports association.
[2] Young age group with bullous pemphigoid and temporarily administered medication, or spontaneous resolution of bullous pemphigoid after drug withdrawal alone.
[3] Elderly age group and temporarily associated medication.

15.15 Drug-associated pemphigus

15.15.1 Definition

Pemphigus refers to a group of rare, autoimmune, mucocutaneous diseases characterised histologically by intraepithelial lesions; pemphigus vulgaris is the most common; and drugs are the predominant cause (93).

15.15.2 Clinical effects

The oral lesions of pemphigus are characterised by intraepithelial bullous formation and subsequent blistering, erosions and ulcerations, and are generally present on the buccal mucosa, palate and ventrum of the tongue and lips (93). Desquamative or erosive gingivitis can also be present but often at later stages in the disease process. Cutaneous lesions, as well as lesions on other epithelial mucosa—for example, the oesophagus—often follows the oral lesions (93). Histopathological examination demonstrates intraepithelial splits, and subsequent separation of the stratified squamous cells in the epithelial layer (acantholysis) is present. Lastly, IgG autoantibodies are present and are directed against molecules involved in cohesion of the keratinocytes (desmoglein 1 and 3) (93).

15.15.3 Drugs associated and mechanism

Drugs associated with causing pemphigus are divided into three groups based on specific chemical structures that trigger pemphigus (74, 94). These are:

1. drugs that contain a sulfhydryl group
2. drugs that contain a phenol group
3. drugs that do not contain either a phenol or a sulfhydryl group

15.15.3.1 Drugs that contain a sulfhydryl group

- This group includes penicillamine, captopril, penicillin and piroxicam (95) (see Table 15.14).
- Penicillamine is the most common, with 7% of patients on penicillamine for at least 6 months developing pemphigus (96).
- It is thought that the sulfhydryl group in these drugs is integrated into the keratinocyte and changes the antigenicity of the desmogleins, causing the subsequent production of autoantibodies against the membrane desmogleins and leading to the intraepithelial lesions (95).
- Captopril is thought to directly cause acantholysis as well as trigger apoptosis (95).

15.15.3.2 Drugs that contain a phenol group

- This group includes aspirin, cephalosporins, heroin, levodopa, phenobarbitone and rifampicin (95) (see Table 15.14).
- The phenolic group in these drugs is thought to cause pemphigus by triggering the release of cytokines such as tumour necrosis factor and interleukin-1α from keratinocytes. These cytokines are involved in acantholysis in patients who have a genetic susceptibility (95).

15.15.3.3 Drugs that do not contain a sulfhydryl or a phenol group

- This group includes angiotensin-converting enzyme inhibitors, NSAIDs, interferons and others (see Table 15.14).
- Several proposed mechanisms exist for these drugs to trigger pemphigus, including the release of cykokines from keratinocytes that stimulate the acantholytic process, the augmentation and overactivation of the immune response, and an increase in the antigenicity of the keratinocytes (95).

Table 15.14 Drugs associated with pemphigus (74). Based on (93, 95, 125).

Drug groups	Individual drugs
Drugs containing a sulfhydryl group	Captopril Cephalosporins* Penicillamine Penicillin Piroxicam
Drugs containing a phenol ring	Aspirin Cephalosporins* Heroin Levodopa Phenobarbitone Rifampicin
Non-thiol non-phenol drugs	Diclofenac Enalapril Fosinopril Interferon-α Interferon-β Isotretinoin Nifedipine Norfloxacin Progesterone Propranolol Ramipril

Note:
* Some cephalosporins contain a sulfhydryl group or phenol ring.

15.16 Drug-associated erythema multiforme

15.16.1 Definition

Erythema multiforme (EM) is defined as the presence of typical and atypical inflamed 'target' lesions on the skin or mucosa, or both, with less than 10% of the body surface area involved (97). EM can affect the oral cavity alone (98).

15.16.2 Clinical effects

EM is an acute, self-limiting vesiculobullous disorder. Mucosal involvement affects between 25–60% of cases, which includes the oral cavity, eyes, genital tracts, pharyngeal and respiratory involvement (99). Oral lesions initially appear as erythematous, oedematous vesicles, that within hours rupture and progress into irregular, but well-demarcated erosions with a yellow-grey pseudomembrane, and self-heal in around 6 weeks (99, 100). Ulcerations of the gingival mucosa and ulceration and crusting of the lips can also be present (98).

15.16.3 Drug associated and mechanism

Drugs are the second most common cause of EM, the first being viruses (e.g. herpes simplex) (97). The incidence and determination of specific drugs implicated in EM is difficult due to the rarity of the disease and likelihood of unreported cases. An international, prospective, case-control study from 1989 to 1995 from approximately 1800 hospital departments in Europe determined that the highly suspected drugs in EM were oxicam-NSAIDs (piroxicam), phenobarbitone, phenytoin, antibiotic sulphonamides and allopurinol (97, 101, 102).

Allopurinol, diphenhydramine, amoxicillin, ampicillin, erythromycin, diphtheria-tetanus-pertussis vaccination, nitrofurantoin, tetracycline and valproic acid were all implicated in a large population-based study spanning 14 years (from 1972 to 1986) (97, 103). Several other drugs have either been identified in the pathogenesis of EM through case reports, including trimethoprim/sulfamethoxazole, TNF-α inhibitors, alectinib, and some anticancer drugs as shown in Table 15.15 (74, 97, 99, 104, 105).

Table 15.15 Drugs associated with erythema multiforme (74). Adapted from (97).

Drug class	Drug
Antibacterials	Amoxicillin Ampicillin Erythromycin Nitrofurantoin Sulfonamides Tetracycline Trimethoprim/ sulfamethoxazole
Anticonvulsants	Carbemazepine Phenobarbitone Phenytoin Valproic acid
Antineoplastics	Alectinib Nivolumab Vemurafenib
Oxicam-NSAIDs	Piroxicam
TNF-α inhibitors	Adalimumab Etanercept Infliximab
Other	Allopurinol Diptheria-tetanus-pertussis vaccination

15.17 Drug-associated Stevens-Johnson syndrome and toxic epidermal necrolysis

15.17.1 Definition

Stevens-Johnson syndrome (SJS) and toxic epidermal necrolysis (TEN) are both rare, but potentially life-threatening, severe, T-cell mediated cutaneous reactions caused by drug hypersensitivity (106).

15.17.2 Clinical effects

SJS and TEN commence with a prodromal phase of malaise and fever, followed by cutaneous lesions that affect the skin and mucous membranes (106). Lesions present as flat and atypical with detachment of the epidermis and erosions and blister formation. Purpuric macules can also be present, with epithelial sloughing and necrosis as well as dysphagia and haemorrhagic crusting of the lips and oral cavity (101, 106–108).

The main difference between SJS and TEN is the amount of skin involvement: SJS: <10% skin detachment; SJS-TEN overlap: 10–30% skin detachment; TEN: >30% skin detachment (74, 101, 106).

15.17.3 Incidence

The incidence of SJS and TEN is 2 cases/million population/year but has high morbidity. The mortality is reported to be 5% for SJS and 30% for TEN (102, 106).

15.17.4 Drugs associated and mechanism

Association of drugs with SJS and TEN is independent of dose and not predictable (109). The onset of signs and symptoms usually occur within 4–28 days of commencement of the culprit drug, but some drugs cause this reaction up to 30 weeks later (106, 110). While there is a long list of drugs associated with SJS and TEN, there are a relatively small number that account for the majority of cases; difficulties determining causative drugs arise due to the rarity of the condition and confounding medication.

The large, prospective, international case-control study called SCAR (from 1989 to 1995) and the follow up EuroSCAR study (from 1997 to 2001) conducted through hospital departments across Europe identified a variety of medicines that had association with SJS/TEN, including trimethoprim/sulfamethoxazole, piroxicam, allopurinol, phenobarbitone, carbamazepine, nevirapine, lamotrigine and meloxicam (74, 102, 106, 110). The EuroSCAR study showed that allopurinol was the most common cause of SJS and TEN, with doses >200mg/day associated with greater risk, independent of concurrent medication use (111).

A retrospective analysis of the registration databases across multiple Asian countries from 1998 to 2017 showed carbamazepine, allopurinol, phenytoin, lamotrigine, phenobarbital, oxcarbazepine, esomeprazole and strontium ranelate accounted for the most cases. Various antibiotics, NSAIDS and COX-2 inhibitors were also implicated (112). Other case studies, pooled analyses, retrospective analyses of hospitalisations and a systematic review have shown similar medications (or other new ones) in association with SJS and TEN, including aciclovir, antibiotic sulphonamides, fluoroquinolone antibiotics, antivirals and anticonvulsants (106, 108, 113–115).

Pharmacogenomic variability can increase the risk of SJS/TEN for certain populations. In certain Asian populations, patients who have variants of the human leukocyte antigen (HLA)-B*1502 are more at risk of developing SJS/TEN to carbamazepine; variants to the HLA-B*5801 allele has an associated increased risk to allopurinol; variants to the HLA-B*4403 allele in Korean populations to lamotrigine; and variants to the HLA-A*3101 in European populations to carbamazepine (109, 112). Genetic testing may be considered prior to commencing these medications for patients who are at increased risk.

Table 15.16 shows the most commonly implicated drugs with SJS/TEN, adapted from Teoh et al. (74) and Wang et al. (112) (only drugs with at least five case reports have been shown from Wang et al.).

Table 15.16 Drugs associated with SJS and TEN. Adapted from (74, 112).

Drug class	Drugs
Anti-inflammatories	Diclofenac Etoricoxib Indomethacin Ketorolac Meloxicam Piroxicam Sulindac
Anticonvulsants	Carbamazepine Lamotrigine Oxcarbazepine Phenobarbital Phenytoin
Antimicrobials	Amoxicillin Ampicillin Azithromycin Ceftriaxone Cefuroxime Cephalexin Ciprofloxacin Clarithromycin Doxycycline Erythromycin Levofloxacin Minocycline Norfloxacin Ofloxacin Roxithromycin Sulfadiazine Sulfadoxine/pyrimethamine Trimethoprim/sulfamethoxazole

Table 15.16 (cont.)

Drug class	Drugs
Proton pump inhibitors	Esomeprazole
Drugs for osteoporosis	Strontium ranelate
Drugs for gout	Allopurinol
Other	Nevirapine Sulfasalazine

15.18 Pharmacovigilance and reporting ADRs

Pharmacovigilance is the study of drug safety monitoring. It occurs at many levels—from government agencies to the daily activities of health professionals and consumers. Dentists have an important role to play in pharmacovigilance to accurately identify, manage, report and prevent ADRs occurring in and related to dentistry. Unfortunately, voluntary ADR reporting is in general very low and dentistry is no exception. In 2018, the Therapeutic Goods Administration (TGA) advised that reporting of ADRs by dental professionals only accounted for 0.1% of all reports ever received from commencement of reporting in 1971 (116).

In Australia, voluntary ADR reporting is managed by the TGA. ADR reports are also shared with the WHO Program for International Drug Monitoring which is responsible for statistical analysis of ADR reports and 'signal detection', and trends of causality are then identified from accumulated data from global ADR reports (117). Indeed, adverse effects, such as medication-related osteonecrosis of the jaw, were not detected during clinical trials and were only detected by voluntary reporting, the outcome of which has changed the management of susceptible patients in dentistry today.

15.18.1 ADE versus ADRs

The umbrella term for 'things going wrong with medicines' is adverse drug event (ADE). An ADE is 'an injury resulting from the use of a drug' (118). ADEs can be divided into two types: ADRs and medication errors.

An ADR is 'a response to a medicine that is noxious and unintended, and occurs at doses normally used or tested in humans' (1). The key to this definition is that the ADR is due to the action of the drug.

A medication error, however, is 'a failure in the medication process that leads to or has the potential to lead to patient harm' (119). Errors occur when actions do not proceed as planned, either because the plan was faulty or the operator made mistakes, slips or lapses (120). These are human process issues not caused by the drug itself (see Section 2.3).

Figure 15.1 shows the relationship between ADRs and medication errors. Differentiation between errors and ADRs is important, so practitioners understand that reporting ADRs refers to reporting the unintended actions of a drug, not errors made by a practitioner.

Figure 15.1 Relationship between ADEs, ADRs and medication errors. Adapted from (29).

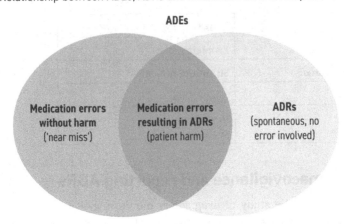

15.18.2 How are drug side effects discovered?

In the past, before the advent of drug safety regulation, side effects of drugs were discovered on a slow and ad hoc basis. Eventually a connection would be made between drug use and unwanted effects, but this process often took decades and, more often than not, the drug was ignored, with adverse effects mistakenly attributed to the patient or their disease instead. Even the catastrophic birth defects caused by thalidomide in the 1960s took 10 years to be identified as drug-induced.

Today, the side effects of drugs are largely determined during pre-marketing clinical trials. Although modern research methods encourage a more timely and structured approach to reporting and identification of potential ADRs, there are still many weaknesses in this system that allow ADRs to remain undetected. These weaknesses include the following reasons:

- Most clinical trials run for short periods (weeks to months) so long-term or delayed adverse effects remain undetected.
- On average, by the time a drug is marketed, it has only been taken by 1000–2000 subjects (121). This may sound like a lot of people, but for rare adverse effects that occur in 1 in 5000, the effect may not have emerged in the trial yet. It has been shown that 3000 at-risk patients are needed to detect an ADR with frequency of 1 in 1000 with 95% certainty (121).
- Vulnerable populations such infants, children, the elderly, pregnant and breast-feeding women are typically excluded from clinical trials. Thus, clinical trial data will not reflect safety issues in these patients.
- People with multiple diseases and/or on multiple medicines are also excluded from clinical trials. As a result, the clinical trial population may not resemble the real-life population the drug is intended to treat. In addition, ADRs due to drug–drug or drug–disease interactions are unlikely to be identified.
- People are more confident to report expected (Type A) ADRs in pre-marketing trials. Therefore, it is not until a drug is approved and used in the wider population that rare and unusual reactions are identified. This is why post-marketing surveillance is so important.

15.18.3 Who reports ADRs?

Unfortunately, ADR reporting is poorly done by most health professionals. In hospitals, less than 10% of serious/severe ADRs are reported, and in general practice <5% of serious/severe ADRs are reported (122).

Despite being plagued by poor participation, ADR reporting remains the most effective, common and inexpensive method of collecting post-marketing drug safety data from the general community. Drug companies contribute most reports, but they are only legally obligated to report serious ADRs which are defined as those causing death, danger to life, admission to hospital, prolongation of hospitalisation, increased investigational or treatment costs, and birth defects (123). Consumers are strongly encouraged to report their own ADRs, as they give a more accurate, first-hand account of the ADR.

15.18.4 Where to report an ADR

ADRs can be reported to a patient's doctor or the drug's manufacturer. However, as useful that might be, it is unlikely the doctor or manufacturer would share the information with anyone else. Therefore, it is recommended that ADRs be reported to the TGA as the report will not only be recorded on the central ADR repository for Australia, but also shared worldwide via the WHO Program for International Drug Monitoring based in Sweden. Worldwide data is collected on their Vigibase® and analysed constantly for drug safety signals.

15.18.5 How to report an ADR

At present, ADR reports can be submitted online via the TGA website, via email or by phone. There is also an online 'blue card' or ADR reporting form which can be downloaded from the TGA website, completed by hand, and emailed, faxed or posted to the TGA.

It is not necessary to be certain the drug is the cause of the ADR, being suspicious will suffice. Every report contributes to knowledge of the product's safety and aids ongoing pharmacovigilance (124).

The following five aspects will give sufficient detail to convey the nature and outcome of the ADR to the TGA. These are:

1. the patient's gender and age
2. a brief medical history
3. a description of the adverse event, including time of onset and outcome
4. all the medicines the patient was on when the adverse event occurred. Give name, dose and duration of each, highlighting timing of use and which drug is the suspected agent/s
5. name of the reporter, so they can contact you if necessary

FURTHER READING

Fortuna G, Aria M, Schiavo JH. Drug-induced oral lichenoid reactions: a real clinical entity? A systematic review. *Eur J Clin Pharmacol.* 2017;73(12):1523–1537.

Lerch M, Mainetti C, Terziroli Beretta-Piccoli B, Harr T. Current Perspectives on Erythema Multiforme. *Clin Rev Allergy Immunol.* 2018;54(1):177–184.

Lerch M, Mainetti C, Terziroli Beretta-Piccoli B, Harr T. Current Perspectives on Stevens-Johnson Syndrome and Toxic Epidermal Necrolysis. *Clin Rev Allergy Immunol.* 2018;54(1):147–176.

Naik BS, Shetty N, Maben EV. Drug-induced taste disorders. *Eur J Intern Med.* 2010;21(3):240–243.

Stavropoulos PG, Soura E, Antoniou C. Drug-induced pemphigoid: a review of the literature. *J Eur Acad Dermatol Venereol.* 2014;28(9):1133–1140.

REFERENCES

1. Australian Commission on Safety and Quality in Healthcare. *Glossary.* 2002. https://www.safetyandquality.gov.au/standards/primary-and-community-healthcare/guide-primary-and-community-healthcare-standards/glossary

2. Teoh L, Stewart K, Moses G. Where are oral and dental adverse drug effects in product information? *Int J Pharm Pract.* 2020;28(6):591–598.

3. Morgan TK, Williamson M Pirotta M et al. A national census of medicines use: a 24-hour snapshot of Australians aged 50 years and older. *Med J Aust.* 2012;196(1):50–53.

4. Roughead E. *Medicine Safety: Take Care.* Pharmaceutical Society of Australia; 2019.

5. Bates DW, Spell N, Cullen DJ et al. The costs of adverse drug events in hospitalized patients. Adverse Drug Events Prevention Study Group. *Jama.* 1997;277(4):307–311.

6. Lobbezoo F, Ahlberg J, Glaros AG et al. Bruxism defined and graded: an international consensus. *J Oral Rehabil.* 2013;40(1):2–4.

7. Lobbezoo F, Ahlberg J, Manfredini D, Winocur E. Are bruxism and the bite causally related? *J Oral Rehabil.* 2012;39(7):489–501.

8. Feu D, Catharino F, Quintao CC, Almeida MA. A systematic review of etiological and risk factors associated with bruxism. *J Orthod.* 2013;40(2):163–171.

9. Lavigne GJ, Montplaisir JY. Restless legs syndrome and sleep bruxism: prevalence and association among Canadians. *Sleep.* 1994;17(8):739–743.

10. Falisi G, Rastelli C, Panti F et al. Psychotropic drugs and bruxism. *Expert Opin Drug Saf.* 2014;13(10):1319–1326.

11. Clark GT, Ram S. Four oral motor disorders: bruxism, dystonia, dyskinesia and drug-induced dystonic extrapyramidal reactions. *Dent Clin North Am.* 2007;51(1):225–243, viii–ix.

12. Garrett AR, Hawley JS. SSRI-associated bruxism: A systematic review of published case reports. *Neurol Clin Pract.* 2018;8(2):135–141.

13. Teoh L, Moses G, McCullough MJ. A review and guide to drug-associated oral adverse effects—Dental, salivary and neurosensory reactions. Part 1. *J Oral Pathol Med.* 2019;48(7):626–636.

14. Editorial Advisory Committee. *Australian Medicines Handbook.* AMH Pty Ltd; 2020.

15. Cornett EM, Novitch M, Kaye AD et al. Medication-Induced Tardive Dyskinesia: A Review and Update. *Ochsner J.* 2017;17(2):162–174.

16. Martino D, Karnik V, Osland S et al. Movement Disorders Associated With Antipsychotic Medication in People With Schizophrenia: An Overview of Cochrane Reviews and Meta-Analysis. *Can J Psychiatry.* 2018;63(11):706743718777392.

17. Abdollahi M, Radfar M. A review of drug-induced oral reactions. *J Contemp Dent Pract.* 2003;4(1):10–31.

18. Jimenez-Jimenez FJ, Garcia-Ruiz PJ, Molina JA. Drug-induced movement disorders. *Drug Saf.* 1997;16(3):180–204.

19. Duma SR, Fung VS. Drug-induced movement disorders. *Aust Prescr.* 2019;42(2):56–61.

20. Bateman DN, Darling WM, Boys R, Rawlins MD. Extrapyramidal reactions to metoclopramide and prochlorperazine. *Q J Med.* 1989;71(264):307–311.

21. Miller LG, Jankovic J. Metoclopramide-induced movement disorders. Clinical findings with a review of the literature. *Arch Intern Med.* 1989;149(11):2486–2492.

22. Pringsheim T, Barnes TRE. Antipsychotic Drug-Induced Movement Disorders: A Forgotten Problem? *Can J Psychiatry.* 2018;63(11):717–718.

23. Tran TN, Vo TNN, Frei K, Truong DD. Levodopa-induced dyskinesia: clinical features, incidence, and risk factors. *J Neural Transm (Vienna).* 2018;125(8):1109–1117.

24. Gurvits GE, Tan A. Black hairy tongue syndrome. *World J Gastroenterol.* 2014;20(31):10845–10850.

25. Thompson DF, Kessler TL. Drug-induced black hairy tongue. *Pharmacotherapy.* 2010;30(6):585–593.

26. Petropoulou T, Lagona E, Syriopoulou V, Michos A. Teeth and tongue discoloration after linezolid treatment in children. *Pediatr Infect Dis J.* 2013;32(11):1284–1285.

27. Pigatto PD, Spadari F, Meroni L, Guzzi G. Black hairy tongue associated with long-term oral erythromycin use. *J Eur Acad Dermatol Venereol.* 2008;22(10):1269–1270.

28. Electronic Medicines Compendium. *Full Product Information: Amoxil/Augmentin Duo Forte/ Cilicaine VK/Ampicillin.* 2021. https://www.medicines.org.uk/emc

29. Aronson JK. *Meyler's Side Effects of Drugs.* Elsevier Science; 2016.

30. Tamam L, Annagur BB. Black hairy tongue associated with olanzapine treatment: a case report. *Mt Sinai J Med.* 2006;73(6):891–894.

31. Hallmon WW, Rossmann JA. The role of drugs in the pathogenesis of gingival overgrowth. A collective review of current concepts. *Periodontol 2000.* 1999;21:176–196.

32. Heasman PA, Hughes FJ. Drugs, medications and periodontal disease. *Br Dent J.* 2014;217(8):411–419.

33. Marshall RI, Bartold PM. A clinical review of drug-induced gingival overgrowths. *Aust Dent J.* 1999;44(4):219–232.

34. Informational Paper: Drug-Associated Gingival Enlargement. *J Periodontol.* 2004;75(10):1424–1431 doi:10.1902/jop.2004.75.10.1424

35. Hatahira H, Abe J, Hane Y et al. Drug-induced gingival hyperplasia: a retrospective study using spontaneous reporting system databases. *J Pharm Health Care Sci.* 2017;3:19.

36. Behari M. Gingival hyperplasia due to sodium valproate. *J Neurol Neurosurg Psychiatry.* 1991;54(3):279–280.

37. Gregoriou AP, Schneider PE, Shaw PR. Phenobarbital-induced gingival overgrowth? Report of two cases and complications in management. *ASDC J Dent Child.* 1996;63(6):408–413.

38. Mesa FL, Lopez C, Gonzalez MA et al. Clinical and histopathological description of a new case of vigabatrin-induced gingival overgrowth. *Med Oral.* 2000;5(2):133–137.

39. Syrjanen SM, Syrjanen KJ. Hyperplastic gingivitis in a child receiving sodium valproate treatment. *Proc Finn Dent Soc.* 1979;75(5–6):95–98.

40. Kan Y, Nagai J, Uesawa Y. Evaluation of antibiotic-induced taste and smell disorders using the FDA adverse event reporting system database. *Sci Rep.* 2021;11(1):9625.

41. Naik BS, Shetty N, Maben EV. Drug-induced taste disorders. *Eur J Intern Med.* 2010;21(3):240–243.

42. Schiffman SS. Influence of medications on taste and smell. *World J Otorhinolaryngol Head Neck Surg.* 2018;4(1):84–91.

43. Hamada N, Endo S, Tomita H. Characteristics of 2278 patients visiting the Nihon University Hospital Taste Clinic over a 10-year period with special reference to age and sex distributions. *Acta Otolaryngol Suppl.* 2002;(546):7–15.

44. Tredwin CJ, Scully C, Bagan-Sebastian JV. Drug-induced disorders of teeth. *J Dent Res.* 2005;84(7):596–602.

45. Oral and Dental Expert Group. *Therapeutic Guidelines Oral and Dental (Version 3).* Therapeutic Guidelines Pty Ltd; 2019.

46. Sanchez AR, Rogers RS, Sheridan PJ. Tetracycline and other tetracycline-derivative staining of the teeth and oral cavity. *Int J Dermatol.* 2004;43(10):709–715.

47. Poliak SC, DiGiovanna JJ, Gross EG, Gantt G, Peck GL. Minocycline-associated tooth discoloration in young adults. *JAMA.* 1985;254(20):2930–2932.

48. Johnston S. Feeling blue? Minocycline-induced staining of the teeth, oral mucosa, sclerae and ears—a case report. *Br Dent J.* 2013;215(2):71–73.

49. Westbury LW, Najera A. Minocycline-induced intraoral pharmacogenic pigmentation: case reports and review of the literature. *J Periodontol.* 1997;68(1):84–91.

50. Ayaslioglu E, Erkek E, Oba AA, Cebecioglu E. Doxycycline-induced staining of permanent adult dentition. *Aust Dent J.* 2005;50(4):273–275.

51. Miranda-Rius J, Brunet-Llobet L, Lahor-Soler E, Farre M. Salivary Secretory Disorders, Inducing Drugs, and Clinical Management. *Int J Med Sci.* 2015;12(10):811–824.

52. Sockalingam S, Shammi C, Remington G. Clozapine-induced hypersalivation: a review of treatment strategies. *Can J Psychiatry.* 2007;52(6):377–384.

53. Safferman A, Lieberman JA, Kane JM et al. Update on the clinical efficacy and side effects of clozapine. *Schizophr Bull.* 1991;17(2):247–261.

54. Ozbilen M, Adams CE. Systematic overview of Cochrane reviews for anticholinergic effects of antipsychotic drugs. *J Clin Psychopharmacol.* 2009;29(2):141–146.

55. Finkel SI. Effects of rivastigmine on behavioral and psychological symptoms of dementia in Alzheimer's disease. *Clin Ther.* 2004;26(7):980–990.

56. Steele LS, Glazier RH. Is donepezil effective for treating Alzheimer's disease? *Can Fam Physician.* 1999;45:917–919.

57. Scott LJ, Goa KL. Galantamine: a review of its use in Alzheimer's disease. *Drugs.* 2000;60(5):1095–1122.

58. van de Rijt LJM, Stoop CC, Weijenberg RAF et al. The Influence of Oral Health Factors on the Quality of Life in Older People: A Systematic Review. *Gerontologist.* 2020;60(5):e378–e394.

59. Villa A, Abati S. Risk factors and symptoms associated with xerostomia: a cross-sectional study. *Aust Dent J.* 2011;56(3):290–295.

60. Guggenheimer J, Moore PA. Xerostomia: etiology, recognition and treatment. *J Am Dent Assoc.* 2003;134(1):61–69;quiz 118–119.

61. Wolff A, Joshi RK, Ekstrom J et al. A Guide to Medications Inducing Salivary Gland Dysfunction, Xerostomia, and Subjective Sialorrhea: A Systematic Review Sponsored by the World Workshop on Oral Medicine VI. *Drugs R D.* 2017;17(1):1–28.

62. Fortuna G, Aria M, Schiavo JH. Drug-induced oral lichenoid reactions: a real clinical entity? A systematic review. *Eur J Clin Pharmacol.* 2017;73(12):1523–1537.

63. Myers SL, Rhodus NL, Parsons HM et al. A retrospective survey of oral lichenoid lesions: revisiting the diagnostic process for oral lichen planus. *Oral Surg Oral Med Oral Pathol Oral Radiol Endod.* 2002;93(6):676–681.

64. P Serrano-Sánchez JB, Jiménez-Soriano, G Sarrión. Drug-induced oral lichenoid reactions. A literature review. *J Clin Exp Dent.* 2010;2:71–75.

65. Ena P, Chiarolini F, Siddi GM, Cossu A. Oral lichenoid eruption secondary to imatinib (Glivec). *J Dermatolog Treat.* 2004;15(4):253–255.

66. Basso FG, Boer CC, Correa ME et al. Skin and oral lesions associated to imatinib mesylate therapy. *Support Care Cancer* 2009;17(4):465–468.

67. Moss AC, Treister NS, Marsee DK, Cheifetz AS. Clinical challenges and images in GI. Oral lichenoid reaction in a patient with Crohn's disease receiving infliximab. *Gastroenterology.* 2007;132(2):488-489, 829.

68. Asarch A, Gottlieb AB, Lee J et al. Lichen planus-like eruptions: an emerging side effect of tumor necrosis factor-alpha antagonists. *J Am Acad Dermatol.* 2009;61(1):104–111.

69. Papini M, Bruni PL, Bettacchi A, Liberati F. Sudden onset of oral ulcerative lichen in a patient with chronic hepatitis C on treatment with alfa-interferon. *Int J Dermatol.* 1994;33(3):221–222.

70. Kutting B, Bohm M, Luger TA, Bonsmann G. Oropharyngeal lichen planus associated with interferon-alpha treatment for mycosis fungoides: a rare side-effect in the therapy of cutaneous lymphomas. *Br J Dermatol.* 1997;137(5):836–837.

71. Wiesenfeld D, Scully C, MacFadyen EE. Multiple lichenoid drug reactions in a patient with Ferguson-Smith disease. *Oral Surg Oral Med Oral Pathol.* 1982;54(5):527–529.

72. Kaomongkolgit R. Oral lichenoid drug reaction associated with antihypertensive and hypoglycemic drugs. *J Drugs Dermatol.* 2010;9(1):73–75.

73. Firth NA, Reade PC. Angiotensin-converting enzyme inhibitors implicated in oral mucosal lichenoid reactions. *Oral Surg Oral Med Oral Pathol.* 1989;67(1):41–44.

74. Teoh L, Moses G, McCullough MJ. A review and guide to drug-associated oral adverse effects—Oral mucosal and lichenoid reactions. Part 2. *J Oral Pathol Med.* 2019;48(7):637–646.

75. Natah SS, Konttinen YT, Enattah NS et al. Recurrent aphthous ulcers today: a review of the growing knowledge. *Int J Oral Maxillofac Surg.* 2004;33(3):221–234.

76. Lisi P, Hansel K, Assalve D. Aphthous stomatitis induced by piroxicam. *J Am Acad Dermatol.* 2004;50(4):648–649.

77. Martins F, de Oliveira MA, Wang Q et al. A review of oral toxicity associated with mTOR inhibitor therapy in cancer patients. *Oral Oncol.* 2013;49(4):293–298.

78. Lo Muzio L, Arena C, Troiano G, Villa A. Oral stomatitis and mTOR inhibitors: A review of current evidence in 20,915 patients. *Oral Dis.* 2018;24(1–2):144–171.

79. de Oliveira MA, Martins EMF, Wang Q et al. Clinical presentation and management of mTOR inhibitor-associated stomatitis. *Oral Oncol.* 2011;47(10):998–1003.

80. Kharazmi M, Persson U, Warfvinge G. Pharmacovigilance of oral bisphosphonates: adverse effects manifesting in the soft tissue of the oral cavity. *J Oral Maxillofac Surg.* 2012;70(12):2793-2797.

81. Sonis ST. Oral mucositis. *Anticancer Drugs.* 2011;22(7):607–612.

82. Soliman Y. What to know about mucositis. *Medical News Today;* 2022. https://www.medicalnewstoday.com/articles/mucositis

83. Sonis ST. Mucositis as a biological process: a new hypothesis for the development of chemotherapy-induced stomatotoxicity. *Oral Oncol.* 1998;34(1):39–43.

84. Sonis S, Treister N, Chawla S, Demetri G, Haluska F. Preliminary characterization of oral lesions associated with inhibitors of mammalian target of rapamycin in cancer patients. *Cancer.* 2010;116(1):210–215.

85. Logan RM, Stringer AM, Bowen JM et al. The role of pro-inflammatory cytokines in cancer treatment-induced alimentary tract mucositis: pathobiology, animal models and cytotoxic drugs. *Cancer Treat Rev.* 2007;33(5):448–460.

86. Australasian Society of Clinical Immunology and Allergy. *Systemic Lupus Erythematosis (SLE).* 2019. https://www.allergy.org.au/patients/autoimmunity/systemic-lupus-erythematosus-sle

87. Vedove CD, Del Giglio M, Schena D, Girolomoni G. Drug-induced lupus erythematosus. *Arch Dermatol Res.* 2009;301(1):99–105.

88. Rubin RL, Haluptzok RF, Davila LM. Severe hydralazine-induced lupus presenting as systemic lupus erythematosus. *Lupus.* 2020;29(5):509–513.

89. Araujo-Fernandez S, Ahijon-Lana M, Isenberg DA. Drug-induced lupus: Including anti-tumour necrosis factor and interferon induced. *Lupus.* 2014;23(6):545–553.

90. Rubin RL. Drug-induced lupus. *Expert Opin Drug Saf.* 2015;14(3):361–378.

91. Stavropoulos PG, Soura E, Antoniou C. Drug-induced pemphigoid: a review of the literature. *J Eur Acad Dermatol Venereol.* 2014;28(9):1133–1140.

92. Lo Schiavo A, Ruocco E, Brancaccio G et al. Bullous pemphigoid: etiology, pathogenesis, and inducing factors: facts and controversies. *Clin Dermatol.* 2013;31(4):391–399.

93. Scully C, Mignogna M. Oral mucosal disease: pemphigus. *Br J Oral Maxillofac Surg.* 2008;46(4):272–277.

94. Brenner S, Goldberg I. Drug-induced pemphigus. *Clin Dermatol.* 2011;29(4):455–457.

95. Ruocco V, Ruocco E, Lo Schiavo A et al. Pemphigus: etiology, pathogenesis, and inducing or triggering factors: facts and controversies. *Clin Dermatol.* 2013;31(4):374–381.

96. Pisani M, Ruocco V. Drug-induced pemphigus. *Clin Dermatol.* 1986;4(1):118–132.

97. Lerch M, Mainetti C, Terziroli Beretta-Piccoli B, Harr T. Current Perspectives on Erythema Multiforme. *Clin Rev Allergy Immunol.* 2018;54(1):177–184.

98. Lozada-Nur F, Gorsky M, Silverman Jnr S. Oral erythema multiforme: clinical observations and treatment of 95 patients. *Oral Surg Oral Med Oral Pathol.* 1989;67(1):36–40.

99. Huff JC, Weston WL, Tonnesen MG. Erythema multiforme: a critical review of characteristics, diagnostic criteria, and causes. *J Am Acad Dermatol.* 1983;8(6):763–775.

100. Du Y, Wang F, Liu T et al. Recurrent oral erythema multiforme: a case series report and review of the literature. *Oral Surg Oral Med Oral Pathol Oral Radiol.* 2020;129(4):e224–e229.

101. Auquier-Dunant A, Mockenhaupt M, Naldi L et al. Correlations between clinical patterns and causes of erythema multiforme majus, Stevens-Johnson syndrome, and toxic epidermal necrolysis: results of an international prospective study. *Arch Dermatol.* 2002;138(8):1019–1024.

102. Roujeau JC, Kelly JP, Naldi L et al. Medication use and the risk of Stevens-Johnson syndrome or toxic epidermal necrolysis. *N Engl J Med.* 1995;333(24):1600–1607.

103. Chan HL, Stern RS, Arndt KA et al. The incidence of erythema multiforme, Stevens-Johnson syndrome, and toxic epidermal necrolysis. A population-based study with particular reference to reactions caused by drugs among outpatients. *Arch Dermatol.* 1990;126(1):43–47.

104. Ahdout J, Haley JC, Chiu MW. Erythema multiforme during anti-tumor necrosis factor treatment for plaque psoriasis. *J Am Acad Dermatol.* 2010;62(5):874–879.

105. Edwards D, Boritz E, Cowen EW, Brown RS. Erythema multiforme major following treatment with infliximab. *Oral Surg Oral Med Oral Pathol Oral Radiol.* 2013;115(2):e36–e40.

106. Lerch M, Mainetti C, Terziroli Beretta-Piccoli B, Harr T. Current Perspectives on Stevens-Johnson Syndrome and Toxic Epidermal Necrolysis. *Clin Rev Allergy Immunol.* 2018;54(1):147–176.

107. Adams L, Creamer D. Controlling oral hemorrhages in Steven-Johnson syndrome/toxic epidermal necrolysis. *J Am Acad Dermatol.* 2020;82(1):e3–e4.

108. Sen SS, Sil A, Chakraborty U, Chandra A. Stevens-Johnson syndrome–toxic epidermal necrolysis: a fatal cutaneous adverse reaction to oral acyclovir. *BMJ Case Rep.* 2020;13(8):e238555. doi:10.1136/bcr-2020-238555

109. Park HJ, Kim SR, Leem DW et al. Clinical features of and genetic predisposition to drug-induced Stevens-Johnson syndrome and toxic epidermal necrolysis in a single Korean tertiary institution patients—investigating the relation between the *HLA-B*4403* allele and lamotrigine. *Eur J Clin Pharmacol.* 2015;71(1):35–41.

110. Mockenhaupt M, Viboud C, Dunant A et al. Stevens-Johnson syndrome and toxic epidermal necrolysis: assessment of medication risks with emphasis on recently marketed drugs. The EuroSCAR-study. *J Invest Dermatol.* 2008;128(1):35–44.

111. Halevy S, Ghislain PD, Mockenhaupt M et al. Allopurinol is the most common cause of Stevens-Johnson syndrome and toxic epidermal necrolysis in Europe and Israel. *J Am Acad Dermatol.* 2008;58(1):25–32.

112. Wang YH, Chen CB, Tassaneeyakul W et al. The Medication Risk of Stevens-Johnson Syndrome and Toxic Epidermal Necrolysis in Asians: The Major Drug Causality and Comparison With the US FDA Label. *Clin Pharmacol Ther.* 2019;105(1):112–120.

113. Levi N, Bastuji-Garin S, Mockenhaupt M et al. Medications as risk factors of Stevens-Johnson syndrome and toxic epidermal necrolysis in children: a pooled analysis. *Pediatrics.* 2009;123(2):e297–e304.

114. Sousa-Pinto B, Araujo L, Freitas A et al. Stevens-Johnson syndrome/toxic epidermal necrolysis and erythema multiforme drug-related hospitalisations in a national administrative database. *Clin Transl Allergy.* 2018;8:2. doi:10.1186/s13601-017-0188-1

115. Patel TK, Barvaliya MJ, Sharma D, Tripathi C. A systematic review of the drug-induced Stevens-Johnson syndrome and toxic epidermal necrolysis in Indian population. *Indian J Dermatol Venereol Leprol.* 2013;79(3):389–398.

116. Personal Communication. *Dental Practitioner ADR Reports 1971–2018.* Drug Safety Monitoring Unit. Therapeutic Goods Administration; 2018.

117. Uppsala Monitoring Centre. *Global pharmacovigilance. What is a signal?* https://www.who-umc.org/research-scientific-development/signal-detection/what-is-a-signal/

118. Nebeker JR, Barach P, Samore MH. Clarifying adverse drug events: a clinician's guide to terminology, documentation, and reporting. *Ann Intern Med.* 2004;140(10):795–801.

119. Aronson JK. Medication errors: definitions and classification. *Br J Clin Pharmacol.* 2009;67(6):599–604.

120. Teoh L, McCullough MJ, Moses G. Preventing medication errors in dental practice: an Australian perspective. *J Dent.* 2022;119:104086. doi:10.1016/j.jdent.2022.104086

121. Lee A. *Adverse Drug Reactions.* 3rd edition. Pharmaceutical Press Ltd; 2022.

122. Hazell L, Shakir SA. Under-reporting of adverse drug reactions: a systematic review. *Drug Saf.* 2006;29(5):385–396.

123. Martin JH, Lucas C. Reporting adverse drug events to the Therapeutic Goods Administration. *Aust Prescr.* 2021;44(1):2–3.

124. Australian Government Therapeutic Goods Administration. *Reporting Adverse Events.* 2023. https://www.tga.gov.au/resources/resource/guidance/reporting-adverse-events

125. Ruocco E, Aurilia A, Ruocco V. Precautions and suggestions for pemphigus patients. *Dermatology.* 2001;203(3):201–207.

16 EMERGENCY MEDICINES

KEY POINTS

- Medical emergencies in dental practice are rare, but knowledge about the medications used in these situations is essential.
- The medicines used in dental emergencies are presented on the practical aspects of their use.
- These medicines include adrenaline, glyceryl trinitrate, aspirin, glucose, glucagon, salbutamol and oxygen.

16.1 Introduction

Medical emergencies rarely occur in dental practice (1). When they do occur, they can be both dangerous for the patient and unnerving for the clinician. If the practice has planned for these events occurring, then staff will be adequately trained, the correct medications will be on hand and their method of use easily recalled, so these rare and disturbing events can be managed with good outcomes.

Staff training in cardiopulmonary resuscitation (CPR) with regular updates is essential. Previous studies have reported very high uptake of CPR training, yet about 20% of dentists felt inadequately prepared and were less likely to have the necessary drugs and equipment in their practice (2). Despite this, dentists should be competent at providing basic life support as outlined in the algorithm in Figure 16.1 from the Australian and New Zealand Resuscitation Councils, supported by various emergency medications and equipment.

Years ago, a long list of drugs and devices were recommended for dental practices to keep as stock for management of medical emergencies.

The current list of medications required for the management of a medical emergency in a general dental practice provided in the *Therapeutic Guidelines Oral and Dental (Version 3)* includes only five drugs:

1. adrenaline (epinephrine) for the management of anaphylaxis, preferably in preloaded autoinjectors in adult and paediatric strengths

Figure 16.1 Australian and New Zealand Committee on Resuscitation basic life support flowchart (4).

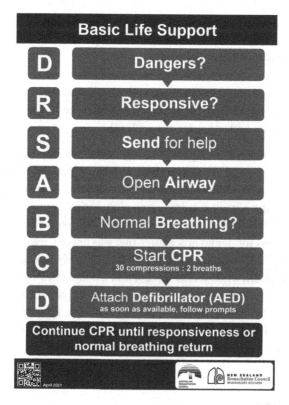

2. glyceryl trinitrate spray for the management of angina or an acute coronary syndrome
3. glucose for management of hypoglycaemia, either as food-containing readily available glucose such as fruit juice or honey, or as pure glucose in the form of glucose gel or tablet
4. a short-acting bronchodilator inhaler such as salbutamol for the management of an acute asthma attack, and
5. aspirin for the management of a suspected acute myocardial infarction (3, 15).

The single most important factor for prevention of medical emergencies in dental practice is the taking of a thorough medical history for each patient. Key elements include previous allergies and adverse drug reactions (ADRs) because, when these are well documented, emergencies can be more readily prevented. It is recommended that patients with asthma or angina bring their emergency medication to their dental appointment so it is readily available if required.

With regard to emergency medical equipment in a dental setting, the *Therapeutic Guidelines Oral and Dental (Version 3)* states that the most important item is an easily transportable source of oxygen for patients who are still breathing (see Section 16.6) (3). For a patient who is not breathing, a bag-valve mask for mouth-to-mask resuscitation is undoubtedly the second most important item (see Figure 16.1) (4).

The devices required for managing a medical emergency in a dental practice include (3):

- a pulse oximeter for measuring arterial oxygen saturation
- a blood pressure monitor for the assessment of patients with cardiovascular symptoms and patients who have collapsed
- a blood glucose monitor for the assessment of patients with diabetes
- a spacer device for emergency salbutamol administration
- an automated external defibrillator for the management of cardiac arrest
- a source of oxygen and bag-valve mask (3, 15)

Rubber dams are another deivce required in every dental practice, with one function being to protect patients' airways from foreign body inhalation. In the 20th century, the incidence of foreign body inhalation in dentistry was as high as 15–18% (5). However, it is now well recognised that the airway requires protection during dental procedures, so dental practitioners employ various measures to reduce the likelihood of foreign body inhalation. The use of rubber dams for dental procedures that was encouraged worldwide during the COVID-19 pandemic further reduces the risk of foreign body inhalation. Nevertheless, it is of considerable concern when it is suspected that a patient has swallowed or inhaled an object during a procedure. While most swallowed objects pass through the gastrointestinal tract without harm, they occasionally require removal. Foreign objects entering the patient's airway require urgent removal to avoid airway obstruction (3).

Medications used for medical emergencies in dentistry are outlined below (see Sections 16.2 to 16.6).

16.2 Adrenaline

16.2.1 Anaphylaxis

Anaphylaxis is a rapid-onset life-threatening hypersensitivity reaction that has a range of systemic manifestations and clinical presentations (6) (see Section 3.4.1). Stinging insects and medications are the leading triggers for anaphylaxis in adults, and medications prescribed by dentists can also be a cause (7).

Adrenaline is the first-line treatment for anaphylaxis. Its immediate administration is required as delay can lead to increased risk of morbidity and mortality (8). Adrenaline is a non-selective adrenergic agonist that rapidly increases peripheral vascular resistance through vasoconstriction, increases cardiac output, and reverses bronchoconstriction and mucosal oedema. Diagnoses of anaphylaxis requires one of the following signs or symptoms, minutes to several hours after the exposure to a likely allergen or trigger:

- sudden respiratory distress
- decreased blood pressure
- sudden skin or mucosal changes with hives or swelling of the lips of tongue
- sudden-onset gastrointestinal symptoms of cramping or vomiting (8)

After the episode resolves, all anaphylaxis patients require subsequent monitoring as there are two types of anaphylaxis—uniphasic and biphasic—with the latter recurring up to 72 hours after the initial phase (8). Follow-up education is required for all patients who have experienced anaphylaxis regarding avoidance of identified triggers, awareness of presenting signs and symptoms, and future use of adrenaline autoinjectors (8).

16.2.2 Angioedema

Acute onset angioedema is caused by mast cell degranulation releasing histamine and other vasoactive peptides causing rapid swelling of deep layers of the skin. This can be life threatening if oral swelling compromises the patient's airway. Precipitants include latex and medications such as penicillin; however, angioedema can also be idiopathic. Skin swelling around the eyes and lips occurs, and oedema of the larynx and bronchus can lead to a clinical picture identical to anaphylaxis and should be treated as such with the administration of adrenaline (7).

For both anaphylaxis and angioedema, adrenaline is ideally administered intramuscularly into the anterolateral thigh using a preloaded autoinjector. For adults and children over 20kg, 300mg should be administered; for children between 10–20kg, half this dose (i.e. 150mg) should be administered (3).

16.3 Glyceryl trinitrate

16.3.1 Angina

The definition of angina is a 'retrosternal chest discomfort, pain or tightness, that lasts 10 minutes or less and subsides promptly with rest' (9). Angina is caused by constriction or obstruction of the blood vessels supplying the coronary muscle. The principal symptom of angina is diffuse, crushing central chest pain that is often described as feeling like a band tightening around the chest. Glyceryl trinitrate administered sublingually can usually relieve the pain of angina very quickly, within seconds or a few minutes, so patients suffering from frequent angina often carry this medicine with them. As management of acute myocardial infarction (AMI) involves more than just relieving angina pain, drugs in addition to glyceryl trinitrate must be administered. AMI symptoms include sweating, nausea, palpitations, breathlessness, vomiting and potentially a loss of consciousness.

Glyceryl trinitrate works by vasodilation, reducing cardiac preload and venous pressure, thus reducing cardiac oxygen requirements and redistributing coronary flow towards ischemic areas and relieving coronary spasm (10). Glyceryl trinitrate is available in either a spray or a tablet that is given sublingually. The spray delivers a single dose of 400mg, while tablets are 600mg. Half to one tablet can be given every 3–4 minutes until pain resolution to a maximum of 2–3 tablets. The spray can be given as 1–2 sprays every 5 minutes until pain resolves to a maximum of 3 sprays (3, 7).

Patients experiencing angina in the dental practice should use their own glyceryl trinitrate product, if they have it with them, according to their doctor's instructions. Nevertheless, glyceryl trinitrate should also be included in dental practice emergency supplies (3, 7).

If a myocardial infarction is suspected, or the angina pain does not resolve quickly from the use of glyceryl trinitrate within 10 minutes, then emergency assistance should be immediately summoned and CPR undertaken if required. Patients should be given 300mg of aspirin as soon as possible, either chewed or dissolved prior to swallowing, unless the patient is allergic to aspirin (3, 7).

16.4 Glucose

16.4.1 Diabetic emergencies: hypo- and hyperglycaemia

Each individual's diabetic control, history of hypoglycaemic episodes, and recent blood glucose and HbA1c levels give an indication of the patient's risk of developing hypoglycaemia during dental treatment. Some simple rules for these patients are to:

- treat earlier in the day
- ensure they have taken their scheduled antidiabetic medication
- ensure they have eaten prior to their dental appointment
- assess the impact if any food or medicines have been skipped

Hypoglycaemia is low glucose levels in the patient's blood, usually less than 4mmol/L (11). This can be caused by using too much medication, such as insulin, delaying or skipping meals, unplanned or excessive strenuous activity, or stressful events. Thus, attending a dentist can be a cause of hypoglycaemia as the pain of toothache, for example, is not only stressful, but it may be compounded by practical aspects of travelling to the dental practice, such as the patient not eating sufficiently on the way to their appointment or due to their dental pain.

Patients experiencing hypoglycaemia usually display weakness, shaking, dizziness and light-headedness. They are likely to look pale, sweaty and can feel hungry. If not treated, these symptoms can worsen to developing confusion with slurred speech, difficulty swallowing or difficulty following instructions. These patients may eventually lose consciousness and experience seizures. A thorough medical history taken prior to the appointment can avoid these acute hypoglycaemic episodes. Should an episode occur, prompt treatment is necessary (11).

The ideal immediate treatment for hypoglycaemia is glucose in any form. If the patient can cooperate and swallow, administration can be by mouth as a tablet, syrup or sugary drink (3, 7). A simple protocol can be to administer to the patient:

- about 6 regular glucose jelly beans
- 3 teaspoons of sugar or honey, or
- a glass or small box of fruit juice or about a third of a can of soft drink (not the 'diet' version) (3)

If this has not been effective after 15 minutes, this step should be repeated. Once the patient has improved, complex carbohydrates such as bread should be given orally (3, 12). If the patient remains unresponsive, unconscious, drowsy, uncooperative or not able to take the above glucose, then seek emergency assistance and commence basic life support (see Figure 16.1) (4).

If the patient is unconscious or unable to swallow oral glucose, intramuscular glucagon can be administered (11) from which clinical improvement should be seen in about 10 minutes (12). Glucagon mobilises hepatic glucose production and increases blood glucose levels (12). The Glucagen Hypokit® delivers 1mg, which is appropriate for children >25kg; for children less than 25kg, the dose is 0.5mg (12).

Hyperglycaemia is very rare in a dental setting, but common in the community. Patient symptoms from hyperglycaemia tend to develop slowly with a feeling of 'unwellness' and can experience fatigue, nausea, abdominal pain and vomiting. As this develops over a long time—at least hours, most likely days—a diabetic patient who is unwell should be strongly advised to seek medical assistance. A diabetic patient who attends the dental practice feeling very unwell should be considered to be developing hyperglycaemia and potential diabetic ketoacidosis for which treatment is intravenous rehydration and further management. These are beyond the clinical scope for a dentist; however, recognition of its occurrence and timely referral is critical (7).

For management of diabetic ketoacidosis occurring in association with sodium glucose co-transporter 2 inhibitors, see Section 11.4.4.

16.5 Salbutamol

16.5.1 Asthma

Asthma is a potentially life-threatening condition with factors such as infection having the potential to precipitate a profound asthma attack. Careful questioning and listening by the dental practitioner should elicit the patient's asthma history to judge how well the patient is involved in their own management. The patient should bring their asthma inhalers to their dental appointment to be used according to their asthma action plan, which advises how to manage their asthma both for maintenance and acute exacerbations.

Despite this planning and preparation, acute asthmatic attacks can occur in the dental setting with very serious outcomes. Asthma attacks result from inflammation and constriction of the bronchioles, causing difficulty in breathing, coughing and wheezing. Asthmatic attacks can be divided into mild/moderate, severe and life threatening. These categories will have different symptoms, ranging from a continued ability to walk and speak (even though with difficulty); to labouring in breathing with the use of neck and chest muscles, difficulty in speaking, and respiratory distress; to finally loss of consciousness, collapse and cyanosis (13).

Salbutamol is the most commonly used treatment for acute asthma in adults and children. Salbutamol is a short-acting β-2 receptor agonist that works by causing relaxation of bronchial smooth muscle (12). Salbutamol is delivered by a metered dose inhaler, which consists of a device containing a pressurised canister full of propellant that sprays out the drug. When pressing down on the canister, it rapidly propels the drug into the air and, if placed in the mouth and inhaled at the right time, into the lungs (12). Good technique relies on excellent hand–breath coordination for adequate drug delivery. Use of a spacer attached to the inhaler allows the patient to pump several doses into the balloon and take their time to inhale, eliminating the need for precise coordination and promoting increased drug delivery to the lungs (12, 13). Spacers should be used on all metered-dose inhalers in emergency management of asthma.

For management of an acute asthma attack, refer to current national asthma guidelines, such as the National Asthma Council or *Therapeutic Guidelines Respiratory* (13, 14).

16.6 Aspirin

16.6.1 Severe chest pain

Soluble aspirin tablets are required for potential use in emergency management of severe chest pain suspected to be due to acute coronary syndrome or acute myocardial infarction. One 300mg tablet should be administered to the patient, which can be chewed or dissolved in water before swallowing (3, 4). Patients with a documented allergy to aspirin or bleeding disorder should not be given aspirin (4).

16.7 Oxygen

16.7.1 Potential causes of loss of consciousness

Patients experiencing loss of consciousness is common in the dental setting. Common causes for lost consciousness include fainting, vasovagal syncope and venous pooling. Recovery from these is invariably rapid, but if not, other more sinister diagnoses must be rapidly considered. Adverse events such as a stroke, a heart attack, hypoglycaemia and epileptic seizure must be considered.

Arguably the most important intervention needed for emergency treatment in dental practice is oxygen. Apart from the above-mentioned medications, such as adrenaline, glyceryl nitrate, salbutamol, and glucose, and often as a conjunct to their administration, provision of oxygen via a simple safe method can be critical in a medical emergency.

If the patient is still breathing, they should inhale oxygen through a mask that supplies around 6–8L/min of oxygen (3). It is possible to supply the same level of oxygen via the nose with use of 'nasal prongs' at a reduced rate, about 2L/min.

If a patient is unable to breathe, CPR should be commenced, the airway needs to be secured, and the use of oxygen or ventilation with oxygen is ideal. As an adjunct, if the dentist is familiar with the use of a pulse oximeter to measure arterial oxygen saturation, then this is a mechanism for continually monitoring the patient's blood oxygenation. If the patient's oxygen saturation is below 90% then they should be placed on supplemental oxygen until such time that this level reaches 90–96% (3, 7).

FURTHER READING

Australian Resuscitation Council. *Australian and New Zealand Committee on Resuscitation Guidelines.* 2023. https://resus.org.au/the-arc-guidelines/

National Asthma Council. *Managing acute asthma in adults.* Australian Asthma Handbook. https://d30b7srod7pe7m.cloudfront.net/uploads/Managing-Acute-Asthma-in-Adults_final160123.pdf

Shaker MS, Wallace DV, Golden DBK et al. Anaphylaxis—a 2020 practice parameter update, systematic review, and Grading of Recommendations, Assessment, Development and Evaluation (GRADE) analysis. *J Allergy Clin Immunol.* 2020;145(4):1082–1123.

REFERENCES

1. Atherton GJ, McCaul JA, Williams SA. Medical emergencies in general dental practice in Great Britain. Part 2: Drugs and equipment possessed by GDPs and used in the management of emergencies. *Br Dent J.* 1999;186(3):125–130.

2. Atherton GJ, McCaul JA, Williams SA. Medical emergencies in general dental practice in Great Britain. Part 3: Perceptions of training and competence of GDPs in their management. *Br Dent J.* 1999;186(5):234–237.

3. Oral and Dental Expert Group. *Therapeutic Guidelines Oral and Dental (Version 3).* Therapeutic Guidelines Pty Ltd; 2019.

4. Australian Resuscitation Council. *Australian and New Zealand Committee on Resuscitation Guidelines.* 2023. https://resus.org.au/

5. Atherton GJ, McCaul JA, Williams SA. Medical emergencies in general dental practice in Great Britain. Part 1: Their prevalence over a 10-year period. *Br Dent J.* 1999;186(2):72–79.

6. Shaker MS, Wallace DV, Golden DBK et al. Anaphylaxis—a 2020 practice parameter update, systematic review, and Grading of Recommendations, Assessment, Development and Evaluation (GRADE) analysis. *J Allergy Clin Immunol.* 2020 Apr;145(4):1082–1123.

7. Greenwood M. Medical emergencies in the dental practice. *Periodontol 2000.* 2008;46:27–41.

8. Shaker MS, Wallace DV, Golden DBK et al. Anaphylaxis—a 2020 practice parameter update, systematic review, and Grading of Recommendations, Assessment, Development and Evaluation (GRADE) analysis. *J Allergy Clin Immunol.* 2020;145(4):1082–1123.

9. Expert Group for Cardiovascular Guidelines. *Therapeutic Guidelines Cardiovascular (Version 7).* Therapeutic Guidelines Pty Ltd; 2018.

10. Ritter JFR, Henderson G, Loke YK et al. *Rang and Dale's Pharmacology.* 9th edition. Elsevier; 2020.

11. Diabetes Australia. *About diabetes: Diabetes Australia.* 2022. https://www.diabetesaustralia.com.au

12. Editorial Advisory Committee. *Australian Medicines Handbook.* AMH Pty Ltd; 2020.

13. National Asthma Council Australia. *Australian Asthma Handbook Version 2.0.* National Asthma Council Australia; 2022. https://www.asthmahandbook.org.au/

14. Expert Group for Respiratory Guidelines. *Therapeutic Guidelines Respiratory.* Therapeutic Guidelines Pty Ltd; 2020.

15. Weston A. Staying up-to-date saves lives. *TeamWise.* 2020;22:8–9.

INDEX

Printed in the United States
by Baker & Taylor Publisher Services